Nursing Issues and Nursing Strategies for the Eighties

SOUTHERN MISSIONARY COLLEGE
Division of Nursing Library
711 Lake Estelle Drive
Orlando, Florida 32803

Bonnie Bullough, R.N., Ph.D., F.A.A.N., is Dean of the School of Nursing at the State University of New York at Buffalo. She is the senior editor of the Springer sequence on Issues in Nursing, of which this is the fourth volume. A certified family and pediatric nurse practitioner, she has done research in that field as well as in the history of nursing, nursing law, human sexuality, and the delivery of health care.

Vern Bullough, R.N., Ph.D., is Dean of the Faculty of Natural and Social Sciences at the State University of New York at Buffalo. Trained as a historian of medicine and science at the University of Chicago, he became interested in the history of nursing, and later earned a bachelor's degree in nursing at California State University, Long Beach. He is the author, coauthor, or editor of over 20 books, 200 journal articles, and numerous reviews and encyclopedia articles. His research interests in recent years have concentrated on nursing, women in the professions, human sexuality, achievement, and historical sociology.

Mary Claire Soukup, R.N., M.S., received her master's degree from The Catholic University of America and her bachelor's degree in nursing from Canisius College. She has been an Associate Professor in Nursing at the State University of New York at Buffalo since 1968. She has edited the book, *Reading in Professional Nursing Seminar,* that serves as a basis for a course currently in the curriculum of the undergraduate program at the State University of New York at Buffalo.

Nursing Issues and Nursing Strategies for the Eighties

Bonnie Bullough, R.N., Ph.D., F.A.A.N.
Vern Bullough, R.N., Ph.D.
Mary Claire Soukup, R.N., M.S.
Editors

WY
16
N974
1983

11071

SPRINGER PUBLISHING COMPANY New York

SOUTHERN MISSIONARY COLLEGE
Division of Nursing Library
711 Lake Estelle Drive
Orlando, Florida 32803

Copyright © 1983 by Springer Publishing Company, Inc.
All rights reserved
No part of this publication may be reproduced, stored in a
retrieval system, or transmitted in any form or by any means,
electronic, mechanical, photocopying, recording, or otherwise,
without the prior permission of Springer Publishing Company, Inc.

Springer Publishing Company, Inc.
200 Park Avenue South
New York, New York 10003

83 84 85 86 87 / 10 9 8 7 6 5 4 3 2 1

Library of Congress Cataloging in Publication Data

Main entry under title:
Nursing issues and nursing strategies for the eighties.
    Includes bibliographies and index.
    1. Nursing. I. Bullough, Bonnie. II. Bullough, Vern L. III. Soukup,
Mary Claire. [DNLM: 1. Nursing—Trends. 2. Education, Nursing—Trends—
United States. WY 16 N9746]
RT42.N86 1983   610.73   83-499
ISBN   0-8261-4441-1 (soft)

Printed in the United States of America

Contents

II. The Ethical Dimension in Patient Care

III. Nurse Practitioners and Other Specialists

IV. Educational Issues

V. Nursing Law and Politics

Preface

This is the fourth in a sequence of volumes on Issues in Nursing. The sequence grew out of a discussion between Bonnie and Vern Bullough and Bernhard Springer in 1964. The first volume was published in 1966, and was one of the first, if not the first, book of its kind in nursing. Since then, we have periodically reexamined the issues, and this book represents our latest effort in this direction. As we put it together, it became evident that some of the problems we discuss have been with us throughout the entire sequence while others represent new or emerging issues. The economic problems of nurses and issues related to the nursing educational system have been covered in all four volumes. Concerns related to the developing nursing specialties emerged as an issue in the second volume (1971). Although nursing law was the subject of an occasional article in the first three volumes, law and politics now merit an entire section. Ethical dilemmas related to patient care have also grown in complexity as nurses gain in decision-making power, and so we have a new section devoted to this issue.

Several other changes have occurred over the years, to the editors personally, and to the content of the volumes. Bonnie Bullough acquired her Ph.D. soon after the appearance of the first volume while Vern Bullough, who already had his Ph.D., became an R.N. in 1980. This volume also indicates that we have a third associate, Mary Claire Soukup, on our editorial team. The original issues book consisted entirely of reprints of articles, and our own introductions were, at the request of the publisher, kept to a minimum. Over the years, we have reprinted fewer articles, since many of them are available to the interested reader through photocopies or offprints. The amount of original material has increased, and the longer introductory sections furnish background knowledge to elucidate the issues. The aim, however, has remained the same: to inform the reader of the many sides and dimensions of the problems nurses face.

The production of this volume involves the work of many persons. We feel it is important to acknowledge the advice and support of the publisher, Dr. Ursula Springer, and of Carole Saltz and Linda Eisenberg, editors at Springer Publishing Company. Mary Boldt deserves special thanks for her patient and careful preparation of the manuscript. We would also like to thank our contributors for their willingness to modify and change their chapters in order to meet the page constraints demanded in a book of this type. Lastly, we would like to thank our many readers of past editions. It is our fervent hope that they will find this book as useful as its predecessors.

Bonnie Bullough
Vern Bullough
Mary Claire Soukup

Contributors

Linda H. Aiken, Ph.D., F.A.A.N., Vice President for Research, The Robert Wood Johnson Foundation, Princeton, New Jersey

Mila Ann Aroskar, R.N., Ed.D., Department of Public Health Nursing, School of Public Health, Minneapolis, Minnesota

Nancy Baker, R.N., M.S., Instructor, School of Nursing, University of Rochester, Rochester, New York

Steve Barr, R.N., Community Hospital, Indianapolis, Indiana

Michael Beebe, R.N., D.N.S., Chairman, Division of Nursing, Point Loma College, San Diego, California

Robert J. Blendon, Sc.D., Senior Vice President, The Robert Wood Johnson Foundation, Princeton, New Jersey

Buckeye State Nurses Association, State of Ohio

Patricia T. Castiglia, R.N., Ph.D., Assistant Professor, School of Nursing, State University of New York at Buffalo

Ruth E. Colavecchio, R.N., M.S., Director of Nursing, American River Hospital, Carmichael, California

Sister Rosemary Donley, Ph.D., F.A.A.N., Dean, School of Nursing, The Catholic University of America, Washington, D.C.

Ruth Elder, R.N., Ph.D., F.A.A.N., Associate Professor and Associate Dean, School of Nursing, State University of New York at Buffalo

Claire M. Fagin, Ph.D., F.A.A.N., Dean, School of Nursing, University of Pennsylvania, Philadelphia, Pennsylvania

Jane Garvey, R.N., Ed.D., Evaluation Coordinator, School of Nursing, State University of New York at Buffalo

Jane Greenlaw, R.N., M.S., J.D., Associate Faculty, School of Nursing, University of Rochester, New York

Ira Gunn, C.R.N.A., F.A.A.N., Visiting Professor and Director of the Nurse Anesthesia Program, School of Nursing, State University of New York at Buffalo

Mary Hamilton, R.N., D.N.S., Chairperson, Department of Nursing, Marian College, Indianapolis, Indiana

Juanita Hunter, R.N., M.S., Assistant Professor, School of Nursing, State University of New York at Buffalo

Beatrice J. Kalisch, Ed.D., F.A.A.N., Professor of Nursing and Chairperson, Parent-Child Nursing, University of Michigan, Ann Arbor, Michigan

Philip A. Kalisch, Ph.D., Professor of History and Politics of Nursing, University of Michigan, Ann Arbor, Michigan

Marlene Kramer, Ph.D., F.A.A.N., Dean and Professor, School of Nursing, University of Connecticut, Storrs, Connecticut

Carrie B. Lenburg, Ed.D., F.A.A.N., Coordinator, Regents External Degrees, Nursing, University of the State of New York, Albany, New York

Linda McCausland, R.N., M.S., Assistant Professor, School of Nursing, State University of New York at Buffalo

Anna C. Mullins, R.N., D.N.S., Administrator of Nursing Service, Children's Hospital, San Francisco, California

The National Advisory Council on Vocational Education, Washington, D.C.

David E. Rogers, M.D., The Robert Wood Johnson Foundation, Princeton, New Jersey

Margaret Scobey, M.A., Resource Associate, Nursing in the Mass Media Research Project (with Beatrice and Philip Kalisch), University of Michigan, Ann Arbor, Michigan

Mark B. Silber, Ph.D., Mark Silber Associates, Ltd., San Diego, California

Corinne T. Stuart, R.N., M.S., Associate Professor, School of Nursing, State University of New York at Buffalo

Russell C. Swansburg, R.N., M.A., Professor of Nursing and Assistant Dean for Nursing Services, University of South Alabama, Mobile, Alabama

Barbara E. Tescher, R.N., D.N.S., Langley Porter Psychiatric Institute, San Francisco, California

Fay Whitney, R.N., Ph.D., Associate Professor and Director of Nurse Practitioner Programs, Health-Related Professions, State University of New York Upstate Medical Center, Syracuse, New York

I

The Crisis
in Nursing Practice

1. Introduction—
Needed: Better Salaries and
More Autonomy for Nurses

Bonnie Bullough and Vern Bullough

A major emerging issue of the 1980s is the shortage of nurses, a problem compounded by a more fundamental issue, the discontent of a significant portion of the nursing work force. The papers in this section analyze this problem from a variety of vantage points and propose several solutions, including more autonomy and better salaries for nurses. This introduction will furnish the historical background to put the current situation in context.

In 1978 there was an unsuccessful law suit by the nurses employed by the City and County of Denver. They sued for salaries commensurate with their levels of education and responsibility. Craig Barnes, the attorney for the nurses, argued that the problem had started at least 600 years ago when nursing emerged as a poorly paid, sex-segregated occupation (Barnes, 1980). In the early medieval period nursing monastic orders had been organized for both men and women, but in the late medieval period nursing orders for men dwindled and the field was left primarily to the sisterhoods, all of whom required vows of poverty.

With the advent of Protestantism more lay nurses were used, but these too tended to be women who were of low status and poorly paid. Thus, by the middle of the nineteenth century when Florence Nightingale entered the picture, nursing was already somewhat sex-segregated and there was a long-standing tradition of minimal monetary reward.

The Nightingale Influence

The Nightingale reforms did little to correct either the sex segregation or the economic plight of nurses. Rather, Nightingale's focus was on improving patient care and establishing secular nursing as a respectable occupation for women. She in fact reinforced the norms related to sex segregation because she saw nursing as an extension of the traditional female virtues. She not only argued in *Notes on Nursing* that every woman is a nurse (Nightingale, 1860), but she herself emphasized some of the manipulative aspects of the stereotypic female role. She proved to be a master manipulator who was able to get other people, usually men, to speak for her while she pretended helplessness. In Scutari, although she came with significant power delegated to her by the secretary of war, she refused to allow the nurses under her command to give any care to the suffering men until the surgeons "ordered" them to do so. This mechanism temporarily gained her the support of the army doctors, who were very suspicious of her as well as the 38 nurses who came with her, but it also helped maintain the concept that the surgeon was superior to the nurse (Woodham-Smith, 1951, pp. 98–110), even on matters about which he knew little.

After the war, Florence Nightingale started her monumental work of reforming the army to secure better pay and more humane treatment for the common soldier. She accomplished this reform in a proper, ladylike fashion by getting men to act for her. She herself retired from public view, gradually withdrawing into seclusion until she finally simply took to her bed, where she stayed for the last 50 years of her life. Sitting in her bed she wrote letters, collected data, and drafted lengthy, well-documented position papers. She never, however, appeared in public to defend these positions. Instead, she convinced her various male friends and admirers (including Sidney Herbert, the former secretary of war) that they should present her arguments to Parliament and wage the public fight for reform. She claimed that she was a weak, feeble woman, and the work of public struggles should be handled by great, strong men (Woodham-Smith, 1951, pp. 162–366; Bullough and Bullough, 1978, pp. 95–100).

In 1860, Nightingale used funds which had been raised to honor her to set up the famous nursing school at St. Thomas' Hospital. As the news of the school spread, people from around the world traveled to her bedside to seek advice on how to set up similar "Nightingale schools" in their hospitals, as well as to get hints on how to better run their hospitals or district nursing services. Her mark on nursing was indelible. She insisted that nurses should be clean, chaste, quiet, and religious. She agreed with hospital authorities that nurses should work long hours, never complain, and be obedient to their superiors and physicians. She was against any self-determination on the part of nurses and fought against the organization of the British Nurses Association. She argued that good character was more important than knowledge in producing a good nurse, so the Nightingale model in nursing education stressed apprenticeship training in the simple procedures, with long hours and stringent rules to help the students avoid temptation (Bullough and Bullough, 1978, pp. 94–100).

It is, of course, an oversimplification to lay all of the blame for the subordination of nurses on Florence Nightingale, just as it is an oversimplification to accuse Sigmund Freud of subordinating twentieth century housewives. Both of these people were great innovators in their own specialty who adhered to traditional beliefs about the proper role and status of women. This is particularly true of Florence Nightingale, even though she helped create a work role for women which took them outside of the home. Under her direction the nursing role was shaped in a completely traditional female manner and the accepted interaction patterns of the sexes were not disturbed.

Hospital Training Schools

The major social structure which institutionalized and perpetuated the nineteenth century sex segregation and subordination of nurses was the hospital training school. The two primary functions of the modern hospital are to assist physicians in their practice of medicine and to serve patients who are ill (Rosen, 1963). Thus, when American hospital nursing schools were established, their goal was clearly one of service rather than education. Nurse training schools were opened to improve patient care and to save money; educating students was seen as a method for achieving these objectives but certainly not as a goal in and of itself. Student nurses in this period were expected to work long hours and were allowed to hear lectures only when it would not interfere with their ward duties.

Because the educational process was primarily by apprenticeship, nurses learned by doing, although eventually more class work was added to the curriculum as graduate nurses pressed for reform. The student was considered the lowest person in the status hierarchy and was responsible for much of the work now done by aides and cleaning women, as well as for patient care. Students were answerable to members of the hospital administrative hierarchy, physicians, and teachers (if separate teachers were hired). The physician was considered the most significant of these three and was such an awesome authority figure that, until about 30 years ago , student nurses were taught to stand up when a doctor entered the room. A distinctly harmful aspect of the extreme subordination which students were taught was the intellectual subordination. A cornerstone of the hospital nursing school education was a belief that the physician was always right, and even when he was wrong he should be made to appear right.

This system tended to exclude the rebels and the serious scholars who had other alternatives for an education, including most of the men. According to census figures, 7 percent of the working nurses in 1910 were men, and that figure probably represents a decline from earlier decades (Strauss et al., 1963, p. 205). The men who did not exclude themselves were often excluded by the hospital schools on the grounds of a housing problem. In the tradition of live-in servants and to protect their morals, student nurses were required to live in a dormitory called a nurses' home. The norms of the day and the high moral stance of the schools precluded men from living in the nurses' home, and the lower status of student nurses precluded their being housed in the interns' quarters. Thus, to avoid the problem, men were often simply not admitted to the schools. The few men who did graduate in the first half of the twentieth century came primarily from a few all-male Catholic or mental hospital schools which were gradually closing in the first half of the twentieth century. The number of men in the nursing work force reached its lowest ebb in 1960, when less than 1 percent of the employed registered nurses were men (ANA, 1967). The figure has now climbed to 2.7 percent, while 5 percent of the student population is male (ANA, 1981; USDHHS, 1982). This suggests that the desegregation process has started but that it has a long way to go. This problem is discussed in more detail by Beebe in this section.

The Doctor-Nurse Game

The sex segregation, the norms of poverty, and the extreme subordination of nurses have left their mark on present day nurses and institutions. The legacy is evident in the communication patterns between nurses and physicians, the lack of autonomy over nursing care, and in the difficulties nurses face in accepting collective bargaining and achieving equitable salaries.

The lack of autonomy in the work place is tied to the communication patterns. Based on the past and supported by the norms of male-female interaction, a pattern, called the doctor-nurse game, has evolved. It is characterized by an avoidance of decisions or, more accurately, avoidance of the appearance of decision making. When nurses make decisions, they handle the situation by invoking the name of the doctor to the patient and pretending to the doctor that their idea was his idea. They do this by means of hints, flattery, and feminine wiles rather than by making open statements. Such an approach is not unusual among groups of people who have little formal power because they have learned to negotiate power by devious means. For example, oriental wives and grandmothers are renowned for the power they are able to accrue through manipulation. Similar patterns are fairly common among minority groups, so that the ghetto walls are often as well policed from the inside as the outside (Bullough, 1967, 1969). Unfortunately, feelings of powerlessness and fear of punishment can prevent people from challenging the status quo with honest assertiveness, and the fact that the fear is based on former traditions and past punishments rather than present realities is often overlooked.

The classic description of the doctor-nurse game was written by the psychiatrist Leonard Stein in 1967 (Stein, 1967). Though his article was originally prepared for a psychiatric journal, it has been reprinted several times in nursing publications because it points out the games so clearly. Stein was fascinated by the strange way in which nurses make recommendations to physicians and the reciprocal pretense on the part of physicians that nurses never make recommendations; yet, he noted, successful physicians are careful to follow nurses' recommendations. Stein called the pattern a transactional neurosis. No matter what name is attached to it, this tortuous communication pattern is a serious deterrent to good patient care. It prevents nurses from being accountable for their own decisions and from the sense of personal and professional worth which comes from honest accountability.

Economic Problems of the Profession

The training school movement which used students as the major hospital staff produced a surplus of graduate nurses during the first part of the twentieth century. This surplus was partly a paper one since many nurses followed the standard convention of the day and left the job market for marriage. Some of these women were available for an occasional case or for emergencies, such as the influenza epidemic of 1918, but usually not for full-time work. Yet their potential availability was an additional factor keeping salaries low. During World War II the nursing surplus changed to a shortage. In spite of this shortage, a survey done by the U.S. Department of Labor in 1946–1947 indicated that nurses worked longer hours, did more night and shift work, carried more responsibility, received less overtime pay, had fewer fringe benefits, and were paid less than most workers in industry and/or comparable occupations (U.S. Dept. of Labor, 1947).

In spite of this disparity, the House of Delegates of the American Nurses' Association in 1946 adopted its first economic security package with a no-strike pledge as a prominent feature. On the positive side the program endorsed collective bargaining, a 40-hour week, minimum salaries, increased participation in planning for nursing care, and plans to eliminate racial barriers to nursing (Zimmerman, 1971; "The Biennial," 1946). When the statement was voted on, hospitals were under the provisions of the 1936 Wagner Labor Relations Act, which obliged them to bargain with their employees. The next year, 1947, the Taft-Hartley Labor Management Relations Act was passed. It specifically exempted nonprofit hospitals from the necessity of bargaining and hospitals quickly took advantage of this exemption to refuse to bargain. Yet once again, at the 1950 biennium, the ANA reiterated its no-strike pledge; it was argued that moral persuasion was the better tool (Scott et al., 1966; Kleingartner, 1967).

Perhaps it was inevitable that some nurses would find the moral persuasion insufficient. In 1952, when negotiations broke down between nurses and management at a hospital in Eureka, California, all but one of the nurses resigned (Belote, 1967). In 1961, nurses in Kewanee, Illinois petitioned the hospital administration and board of directors to meet with them to talk about salaries and substandard care for patients. When their request was denied, 24 of the staff of 26 resigned and were supported by the state nurses association (Peters, 1961). That same year, at an institution in Brandenton, Florida, five nurses were fired when they informed the administration of their concerns about personnel policies; the Florida Nurses Association supported them and took their case to court ("The Brandenton Story," 1962).

In 1966 nurses in New York City employed in the 19 New York City municipal hospitals decided that their situation had become intolerable and about half of them (nearly 1,500) submitted their resignations. Five days before the resignations were to take effect, starting salaries were increased from $5,100 to $6,400 with differential pay for evening and night shifts, academic preparation, and experience (Lewis, 1966). Thus, gradually dissident nurses took action in spite of their organization and sometimes even gained the support of the state nurses associations.

Finally, the California Nurses Association took the logical next step of voting to revoke the no-strike pledge. Such action was only taken when nurses in the San Francisco area considered leaving the association to join a union (Mittman and Bumgarner, 1967; Schutt, 1968). In 1968 the ANA voted to rescind its no-strike pledge, and in 1969 the National Federation of Licensed Practical Nurses repealed a no-strike pledge they had taken in 1958 ("LPN . . . , " 1969; Bullough, 1971). This change in policy opened up the way for lobbying at the national level for a change in the 1947 Taft-Hartley Law, and in 1974 the Labor Relations Act was extended to include employees of nonprofit health care institutions.

State nurses associations are now moving to expand the collective bargaining activities. For some this is difficult because staff do not know how to bargain, but they are learning. Nurses themselves are more favorable toward collective bargaining than they were in 1946 but they remain divided. An example of this is the 1978 survey of 373 readers of the magazine *RN;* only 58 percent indicated they felt nurses would be justified in going out on strike (Donovan, 1978).

The Current Crisis

From this historical summary it is clear that neither the salary problems nor lack of autonomy for both registered and practical nurses is new. Why, then, is there now a crisis in nursing? There are several reasons. First, there has been a rapid escalation in the need for nurses as the technology of health care and the acuity level of the illnesses of hospitalized patients have increased. Second, nursing has also increased its scope to include more social and psychological patient support. These changes have increased the need for knowledge on the part of the average nurse. Both the educational system and the individual nurse have responded to these needs with increased education preparation. Third, the occupational choices for women have changed. There were few options for women in the nineteenth century, but now a variety of work roles are possible and most of those roles do not include the heavy load of responsibility and the shift work. Fourth, women as a group, and nurses are still mostly women, have become conscious of the discriminatory practices to which they have been subjected. All of these variables have left nurses with a sense of frustrated entitlement.

Some nurses have voted with their feet and left the field, but most have stayed, albeit with a growing sense of dissatisfaction.

Several prestigious bodies have investigated this problem recently: the National Commission on Nursing, the Robert Wood Johnson Foundation, and the Institute of Medicine. The National Commission on Nursing started gathering data in 1980. A series of open hearings were held around the country and the final report is now available from the commission. Preliminary findings highlighted the observation of the commission that there was a general lack of recognition of the worth of the nurse in patient care. Articles about the other two reports are included in this section along with papers which look at the crisis in nursing practice from a variety of other vantage points.

References

American Nurses' Association. *Facts About Nursing*. New York: ANA, 1967, p. 12.

American Nurses' Association. *Facts About Nursing 80–81*. New York: American Journal of Nursing Company, 1981, pp. 3, 144.

Barnes, C. "Denver: A Case Study." In *The Law and the Expanding Nursing Role*, pp. 125–137. Edited by Bonnie Bullough. New York: Appleton-Century-Crofts, 1980.

Belote, M. "Nurses are Making it Happen," *American Journal of Nursing* 67 (1967):285–289.

"The Biennial," *American Journal of Nursing* 46 (1946):728–746.

"The Brandenton Story: A Community Crisis," *American Journal of Nursing* 62 (1962):58–63.

Bullough, B. "Alienation in the Ghetto," *American Journal of Sociology* 72(5) (1967):469–478.

Bullough, B. *Social Psychological Barriers to Housing Desegregation.* Special Report No. 2. Housing, Real Estate and Urban Land Studies Program, Los Angeles, 1969.

Bullough, B. "The New Militancy in Nursing," *Nursing Forum* 10(3) (1971):173–188.

Bullough, V. and Bullough, B. *The Care of the Sick: The Emergence of Modern Nursing.* New York: Prodist, 1978, pp. 85–100, 94–100.

Donovan, L. "Is Nursing Ripe for a Union Explosion?" *RN* (May 1978):63–65.

Kleingartner, A. L. "Nurses, Collective Bargaining and Labor Legislation," *Labor Law Journal* 18 (April 1967):236–245.
Lewis, E. P. "The New York City Hospital Story," *American Journal of Nursing* 66 (1966):1526–1533.
"L.P.N. Group Asks More Pay, Rescinds No Strike Policy," *Hospitals* 43 (November 16, 1969):107.
Mittman, B. and Bumgarner, B. "What Happened in San Francisco," *American Journal of Nursing* 67 (1967):80–84.
Nightingale, F. *Notes on Nursing.* New York: D. Appleton, 1860; reprint ed., Philadelphia: J. B. Lippincott, 1946, preface.
Peters, D. "The Kewanee Story," *American Journal of Nursing* 61 (1961): 74–79.
Rosen, G. "The Hospital: Historical Sociology of a Community Institution." In *The Hospital in Modern Society*, edited by E. Freidson. New York: Free Press of Glencoe, 1963, pp. 1–36.
Schutt, B. G. "The Right to Strike" (editorial), *American Journal of Nursing* 68 (1968):1455.
Scott, W. G., Porter, E. K., and Smith, D. W. "The Long Shadow," *American Journal of Nursing* 66 (1966):538–554.
Stein, L. I. "The Doctor-Nurse Game," *Archives of General Psychiatry* 16(6) (1967):699–703.
Strauss, A., Schatzman, L., Ehrlich, D., Bucher, R., and Sabshin, M. "The Hospital and Its Negotiated Order." In *The Hospital in Modern Society*, edited by E. Freidson. New York: Free Press of Glencoe, 1963, p. 205.
U.S. Department of Labor, Bureau of Labor Statistics. *The Economic Status of Registered Professional Nurses, 1946–47.* Bulletin 931. Washington, D.C.: U.S. Government Printing Office, 1947.
U.S. Department of Health and Human Services, Division of Health Professions Analysis, Bureau of Health Professions. *The Registered Nurse Population: An Overview from National Sample Survey of Registered Nurses*, Report No. 82-5, November, 1980; Revised June, 1982; p. 9.
Woodham-Smith, C. *Florence Nightingale, 1820–1910.* New York: McGraw-Hill, 1951, pp. 98–110, 162–366.
Zimmerman, A. "The ANA Economic Security Program in Retrospect," *Nursing Forum* 10(3) (1971):313–321.

2. What! Another Report on Nursing?

Ruth Elder

In 1979, Congress ordered a 2-year study to find out whether or not there was a need to continue a program of federal financial support for nursing education. The study was to examine the rate at which nurses leave their professions, the reasons they leave, and the reasons they do not practice in medically underserved areas. Information was to be provided about the need for nurses from *each* type of educational program (diploma, associate degree, baccalaureate) as well as the extent to which nurses would be needed if national health insurance legislation were passed or increased use of ambulatory care became a fact. Comparative cost of each type of nursing education was to be assessed also. Recommendations were to spell out what actions could be taken to encourage nurses to remain in nursing, to reenter nursing, or to practice in underserved areas. If a need for continued federal support was found, Congress wanted to know exactly what form it should take and asked that it be supplied with a rationale for the choice made (IOM, 1981).

Why did Congress mandate such a global study of nursing just at this time? Since 1964, nursing education had been receiving relatively large amounts of federal financial support through the Nurse Training Act. Well over 1.5 billion federal dollars during a period of 16 years had been assigned to schools of nursing in order to increase the country's *total* supply of nurses as well as the number of nurses with advanced training. This federal program was successful in that the number of nurses increased dramatically, doubling between 1962 and 1980, and outstripping population growth. Toward the end of the 1970s, the Carter administration, faced with ever increasing governmental spending, inflation, and economic recession, developed a budget which decreased federal financial support for all the health professions. With the exception of small amounts of support for the preparation of selected specialties, nursing was designated to receive severe financial cuts. Nurses, nursing organizations, and their supporters fought vigorously for the rescission of these financial cutbacks and Congress, concerned about the potential impact on the country's supply of nurses, finally did reinstate a considerable portion of the lost funds.

In the process of deliberating over what stand they should take, the members of Congress were given a great deal of conflicting information about the shortage of nurses and the importance of educational institutions in alleviating such a shortage. They were made aware that the administration no longer considered federal support for nursing education beneficial. They finally decided that they needed more objective, impartial information in order to make wise decisions in the future, and thus the mandate for the aforementioned study was written into the 1979 Nurse Training Act Amendments and became public law.

In 1980, the government awarded a preliminary contract to the Institute of Medicine (IOM) of the National Academy of Sciences to plan the study. The IOM planning group decided that a thorough examination of policy issues underlying the functioning of nursing would have to be addressed before the questions set out in legislation could be answered. It also decided that a study committee would review and analyze the research and information already available rather than engage in collecting new data.

A 26-member study committee was selected, made up of IOM members, nationally recognized experts in public policy analysis and formulation, and experts in disciplines related to the study issues; approximately one-third of the members were nurses. A support staff to do literature searches and prepare background materials was organized and plans for the 2-year study were forwarded to the Department of Health and Human Services. The government accepted the Institute of Medicine's plans and awarded a 2-year contract for the study proper, which began January 1981.

In the first 6 months, the committee and their staff conducted an extensive literature search, identified additional subsidiary questions, held an open meeting at which individuals and representatives of organizations concerned with nursing testified, solicited written statements from a wide range of interested groups, and identified gaps in information. In addition, a series of background papers was prepared on topics ranging from a review of state licensure laws to a critical review of the literature on nurses' satisfaction/dissatisfaction with their roles (IOM, 1981).

In July 1981, a 6-month interim report was released, made up of the committee's findings to that point. A summary of the report was sent to the Committee on Labor and Human Resources of the Senate, the Committee on Energy and Commerce of the House of Representatives, and the Secretary of the Department of Health and Human Services. Obviously, both this interim and the final report, which is due in January 1983, could have far-ranging implications for nursing, and both deserve to be watched closely. A summary of the interim report follows.

Findings of the 6-Month IOM Interim Report

Nursing Shortage

The committee became convinced that in many institutions the demand for nurses did outstrip the supply, although they found no evidence for the widely quoted estimate of 100,000 nurse vacancies throughout the country. They found that shortages occurred very unevenly and varied widely in different regions, among different employers, and in different units of the same institution. All types of hospitals, however, reported shortages of staff nurses prepared to provide direct care at the bedside or to work on intensive care units, especially during weekends and night shifts. Municipal, county, and state hospitals experienced both chronic and acute shortages. In view of the fact that employers sought to fill more nursing positions than there were nurses willing to fill them under the salary and working conditions offered, the committee concluded that there was, in this sense, clear evidence of a nursing shortage (IOM, 1981).

The reasons commonly given for the shortage, however, were considered by the committee to be riddled with error. They identified three pervasive myths frequently offered as explanations of the nurse shortage.

Myth 1: The supply of nurses has decreased, at least in relation to population growth.

Reality: The supply of nurses has been increasing steadily both in absolute numbers and in relation to population growth. For example, in the last decade the number of full-time equivalent nurses increased from 313 to 427 per 100,000 population.

Myth 2: A disproportionately large number of nurses choose not to work or have moved to other work outside the profession.

Reality: The labor force participation of nurses is *much* higher than that of women in general. In 1980, approximately one-half of all women 16 years and over were in the labor force whereas the latest figures (1977–1978) indicate that well over two-thirds of female nurses were employed in nursing itself. In 1977, only 4 percent of nurses were employed in a field other than nursing and only 3 percent of those not working were looking for work. Furthermore, a large percentage of nurses not working were either 50 years of age or older or had children 17 years of age or younger. One study found that the primary reason found for nurses not working 5 years after graduation was responsibility for children. So, although nurses are frustrated and complain, they do not leave nursing.

Myth 3: Nurses have been leaving hospitals and nursing homes for other types of nursing because of unsatisfactory working conditions.

Reality: More nurses are working in hospitals now than ever before (in 1978, 70 percent of full-time equivalent licensed nurses did so). Furthermore, the ratio of nurses to hospitalized patients increased dramatically in the 1970s. Nurse staffing ratios in nursing homes have remained about the same over the last decade and there is no evidence that nurses are leaving nursing homes for other types of work (IOM, 1981).

Factors Increasing Demand for Nurses

Because of the evidence that the demand for nurses was outstripping the supply despite dramatic increases in numbers over the past two decades, the committee examined carefully both sides of the demand/supply equation. They first identified a number of factors which have an important impact on demand for nursing care. One of these is the demographic changes taking place in America. More people are living to the age at which they are likely to have chronic, incapacitating, and life-threatening illnesses requiring the attention of nurses. Closely related to this is the change in health care financing which came about with the 1965 Social Security Act Amendment (Medicaid/Medicare). This act made it possible for many of the sick elderly (and also the poor) to obtain hospital and nursing home care. In particular, there was a tremendous increase in the number of nursing homes and nursing home beds following the act, all of which had to be staffed, thus increasing the demand for nurses.

Another factor affecting demand is the constantly changing medical technology. The number and intensity of services provided to sick people has increased dramatically in the last few decades due to the continuing development of complex life-saving and diagnostic equipment. Intensive care units become more complex every year and require very high staff/patient ratios. Furthermore, in efforts to decrease health care costs, policies have been instituted to reduce hospital stay to the minimum. Thus, the overall intensity of care in the hospital has been increased not only because of changing technology but also because of policies which send people home early once they no longer require intensive attention. This, of course, again increases the demand for nurses because personnel are now dealing with a higher proportion of patients requiring a great deal of care (IOM, 1981).

The committee discussed another often overlooked cause of increased demand—the substitution of nurses for other personnel. They referred to the theory that when the labor market provides insufficient distinction between RNs, LPNs, and other technical support staff, hospitals have incentives to employ high proportions of registered nurses because they have broad, flexible competencies and do not cost that much more. Thus, because of their depressed salary situation, nurses tend to be used for many tasks which do not require their full professional skills. Conversely, hospitals are also assigning tasks traditionally performed by physicians to nurses because physicians command much higher pay and nurses are therefore cost-effective. Both of these practices may create an unusually high demand for nurses (IOM, 1981).

Factors Affecting Supply

The committee first noted a number of factors which had actually increased the supply of nurses over the last few decades, such as the extra financial support for nursing education from public and private sources. They also commented on the many special "reentry" programs which had been established (orientation, inservice, continuing education) which had made it easier for nurses to return to nursing after having dropped out for awhile. They thought that innovations such as the new temporary agencies, flexible time schedules, and childcare facilities might also be attracting inactive nurses back to work (IOM, 1981).

The committee next turned their attention to the factors *decreasing* nurse supply: low salary and fringe benefits, poor working conditions, and the lack of professional autonomy and authority relative to nurses' knowledge, skill, and responsibility. They pointed out that the nursing occupation does not fit labor market theory because despite the cries of "nursing shortage" there has been no dramatic increase in salaries beyond cost-of-living gains. There has also been failure to reward experience and proficiency; failure to pay adequately for nights, weekends, and holidays; and little differential for RNs with varying education preparation. The committee observed that those patterns are typical of female-dominated professions in which one can expect to find depressed wage rates and flat age-earning profiles. Male-dominated occupations are more likely to have salaries and other benefits increase with age, experience, competence, and education. An additional factor which may decrease the nurse supply in the future is the increasing costs of education. These are steadily growing and act as a disincentive to entering this low-paying occupation. Furthermore, there are more attractive opportunities available to women in many other fields than there were several decades ago (IOM, 1981).

Areas of Uncertainty and Contention

The committee listed a number of issues that the IOM study group was planning to grapple with. They considered "resource allocation" to be an overarching theme linking together concerns about utilization of nurses and policies for nursing education. They stated that these two areas cannot be considered by themselves but must be studied in relation to the intense competition in the country for resources—especially health and education resources. Thus, they decided to study areas of uncertainty and contention in terms of the allocation decisions that will probably be required and the likely authority over such decisions.

They pointed out that the extent of the future demand for nurses depends on the needs of future patients and on the ability of employers to pay for services to meet these needs. If present trends continue, more nurses will be needed to look after the high-technology units in hospitals and the increasing number of elderly people receiving long-term care both at home and in institutions. Whether the needs for nursing service will be translated into demand, however, will depend on the resources society provides for health/illness care. Changes in the way nurses are paid, the number of physicians, and the insurance benefits patients receive could all affect demand for nurses (IOM, 1981).

The substitutability of one level of nurse for another, and

substituting nurses for other health personnel, was a hotly debated issue. The committee noted that the role of the nurse will have to be considered in relation to the role and contribution of the physician and other health professionals whose work may complement or overlap. They wondered if there was an artificially high demand for nurses because of current economic incentives for the substitution of nurses for both LPNs and physicians (IOM, 1981).

A serious problem in making recommendations about the most efficient use of the nurse was foreseen because of the role ambiguities and overlapping responsibilities, not only between RNs and LPNs, but also between RNs with different levels of education. In addition, they noted considerable conflict or at least uncertainty about the boundaries between the responsibilities and decision-making powers of nurses, physicians, and managers (IOM, 1981).

A particularly contentious issue outlined by the committee concerned the mismatches between the kinds of nursing knowledge and skill nurse employers and nurse educators thought important for new graduates. Educators tend to believe that hospitals have unrealistic job expectations whereas hospitals are more likely to believe that excessive investment is necessary to orient and train new graduates. It was the committee's view that this area of disagreement as well as the criticism that hospitals fail to use nurses' knowledge and skills appropriately are going to require "dispassionate assessment" (IOM, 1981).

The committee plans to deal with controversies over which types of basic nursing education should be supported by examining the effects of the programs on supply/demand problems. They hope to evaluate each type of program as to its effectiveness in meeting patients' needs, its costs, and the availability of other sources of support. The expense of orienting new graduates and providing continuing education will be counted as part of the overall costs when comparing one type of program with another.

The committee recognized that a major policy issue was embedded in the controversy over which basic educational programs should receive support. The fact that health care delivery is increasingly complex suggested to them that "highly trained, flexible nursing professionals" should be developed. However, their discussion of costs constraints along with increased differentiation of technical tasks indicates that they might recommend other solutions (IOM, 1981).

A question was raised as to whether graduate programs in nursing have placed enough emphasis on producing skilled nurse administrators. The production of so many nurse practitioners for primary care rather than for clinical specialties, such as geriatrics, was also questioned. In addition, the committee began to grapple with factors which inhibited nurses from serving inner city and rural populations. Among the most important of these was the existence and attractiveness of the institutions located in these areas. Interestingly, no mention was made of the legal and third party payment barriers which curb nurses from moving to areas such as these, which are noted for physician shortages (IOM, 1981).

Response of Hospitals and Nurses
to Shortage Issues

The committee observed that employers have already begun to respond to the nursing shortage by intensive recruiting. A number of "temporary nurse" agencies have sprung up and are being utilized, and some institutions have begun to develop their own on-call systems. New staffing patterns are being tried out, and attempts are being made to improve management practices in some localities. There has also been some substitution of nonnursing personnel for nurses. The effect of these developments on the availability and cost of care has not been determined (IOM, 1981).

Although nurses are not leaving nursing, they have reacted by expressing strong dissatisfaction and discontent with their working conditions, high-pressure responsibilities, schedules, salary, fringe benefits, and pay increments relative to clinical experience. They are becoming increasingly involved in collective bargaining, not just to obtain salary increases but also to gain more control over the organizations in which they work. Furthermore, nurses are becoming more politically involved in that they are seeking changes in nurse practice acts and supporting candidates for state legislatures and Congress (IOM, 1981).

The committee noted that the American Nurses' Association (ANA) had responded by attempting to increase control over standards of nursing practice through modifying the nation's system of accrediting educational programs and service agencies; they also were attempting to modify the system of licensing and certifying nurses. Another response of the ANA was to propose the baccalaureate degree as minimal preparation for beginning professional nursing. At the point of writing the committee was unconvinced that such changes would ensure quality, and they expressed concern that such actions might *increase* costs and shortages (IOM, 1981).

Cross-Cutting Factors

Finally, the committee pointed out that a number of cross-cutting factors would be taken into account in their final report, e.g., women's issues, especially women's labor market participation; possible changes in how the health care system is organized and financed; trends in state support; relationship of nurses' roles/responsibilities to those of other health workers; the drive toward further professionalism in nursing; and the movement toward collective bargaining (IOM, 1981).

In concluding, the committee outlined a central dilemma that they were facing. Information from all sources suggests that maintaining the supply of nurses involves serious problems which require policy changes, yet budget constraints indicate that any plan requiring major expenditures would not be acceptable (IOM, 1981).

Discussion

Because this is only the 6-month interim report, there is little one can say about it except that the nursing profession should be aware of the activities of this committee and alert to the publication of the final report, which may have a significant impact on policies dealing with support for nursing education. Nursing itself is divided on a number of the issues discussed in the report. An informal paper circulated at the National League for Nursing's Baccalaureate and Higher Degree Program in late 1981 complained of the report's bias against baccalaureate education for nurses; other nurses at the same meeting disputed the bias and thought the paper was only being realistic and fair to associate degree and diploma nurses. It will no doubt be difficult for the committee to reach their goal of "dispassionate assessment," in light of the conflicts not only between medicine and nursing but also within nursing itself.

More important, there is little in this preliminary report to suggest that the committee is going to move beyond status quo health and illness care to search for answers more fundamental to the problems of the health care system. The larger questions of how to define and provide better health and illness care were not addressed. These questions need to be considered *prior* to thinking through how the nurse should or could be utilized and the implications this might have for funding nursing education.

The health care labor force reflects the sex, class, and race divisions of the economic, political, and social structure of society in general. White, higher socioeconomic status males dominate medicine and medicine dominates the other health occupations. Nursing in particular holds a subordinate position on two counts—both to medicine and to hospital management. The prevailing power relations among the health professions are reflected in the nature of the health care provided. Patient care, the nurse's primary function, is held in low esteem as compared to the more highly rewarded research, teaching of medical students, and high-technology activities of medicine. If the committee first looked at the type of care required to meet the health needs of the population—prevention, primary care, well-managed hospital care responsive to patient concerns, rehabilitation—they might emerge with many suggestions about how nurses could be better utilized and educated. This, in turn, might resolve the dilemma with regard to costly solutions in a tight-budget area.

In conclusion, this observer was amazed at one further point made by the committee. Because they were oriented to the status quo, they did not seem to seriously consider the necessity of removing the barriers to nurses functioning freely in inner city and rural areas—barriers related to absence of third party payment rights and licensure to practice legally the functions they have been prepared to fulfill. Instead, they spoke of nurses going where doctors go as if this were etched in stone. But we do not know where nurses will go nor what their potential role might be until the barriers to their full functioning are removed and rewards are substituted.

Reference

Institute of Medicine. *Six-month Interim Report by the Committee of the Institute of Medicine for a Study of Nursing and Nursing Education: Myths, Realities, and Public Policy Dilemmas in Nursing.* Washington, D.C.: National Academy Press, July 1981.

3.   The Shortage of Hospital Nurses: A New Perspective

*Linda H. Aiken, Robert J. Blendon,
and David E. Rogers*

*There appears to be a critical shortage of hospital nurses in the
United States, despite a 15-year national effort to bring the supply of nurses into balance with increased demand. Careful review
of supply and requirement data does not provide an adequate
explanation for the persistent shortage, and common misconceptions about the nature of the nurse shortage have clouded the
debate. Several popular explanations for the shortage do not appear to be valid. Evidence strongly favors the explanation that the
shortage has been caused by the depression of nurses' incomes
relative to incomes of other workers. The present wage structure
has both short- and long-term effects on the shortage of nurses;
allowing nurses salaries to rise to levels of comparable workers
may be the only solution.*

Much national attention recently has been focused on what appears to be a critical shortage of nurses, particularly hospital-
based nurses in the United States. Almost daily, the media tell of
hospitals that have been forced to close facilities because nurses
are unavailable, and that nursing coverage, especially in intensive
care units, is dangerously low. Opinions on the causes and solutions to this problem have frequently appeared in the health care
literature (1-4).

Over the past 15 years the nation has made great efforts
and invested many dollars in trying to solve this problem. Para-
doxically, it now seems worse than ever. Further, careful review

Aiken, L. H., Blendon, R. J., and Rogers, D. E. "The Shortage of Hospital Nurses:
A New Perspective." Published simultaneously by *Annals of Internal Medicine* 95(3)
(September 1981):365–375 and *American Journal of Nursing* 81(9) (September
1981):1612–1618. Reprinted with permission of *Annals of Internal Medicine* and
the authors.

of supply and requirement data makes it difficult to understand how a "shortage" can still exist. The following facts should be considered:

1. Overall growth in hospitals has been declining for the past 3 decades. Since 1950, the ratio of hospital beds to population has dropped by more than one third (5, 6). One might logically assume that this would reduce the need for hospital-based nurses.
2. Since 1950, general hospital occupancy rates have declined significantly. Now on average only three fourths of the nation's general hospital beds are being used (5). Decreasing occupancy rates should again lead one to predict a reduced need for nurses.
3. The nation's output of nurses has doubled in the past 3 decades. Since 1950, the increase in active nurses has outstripped population growth by 139% (Figure 3–1).

How can one then conclude that the country is facing one of the worst shortages of nurses seen in years? In fact, these data have led our last three presidents to conclude that the shortage could not be acute enough to warrant federal intervention. Nevertheless, all three presidents were overruled by Congress, whose members were acutely aware that hospitals in their districts were closing units for lack of nurses. It follows that some unexplained factors not reflected in traditional indicators must be present to explain this paradox.

Labor economists have noted that nursing is one of the few occupations in the American economy affected by monopsony: the presence of only a few firms that employ the majority of those in a particular occupation (9–12). Sixty-six percent of nurses work in hospitals. In most communities there are fewer than 10 hospitals; many communities have only one or two hospitals. It follows that if nurses want to work in health care, they must for the most part work in those hospitals. Further, the nature of nurses' education is such that it does not seem to allow them to move easily out of nursing or health care into other positions of comparable status. In short, nurses are in a captured labor market.

Because geographic mobility of nurses tends to be limited by family obligations, and because there is little competition for nurses in other settings, hospitals have not generally competed with each other by increasing wages. It has been the conventional wisdom that such competition will not attract additional nurses to

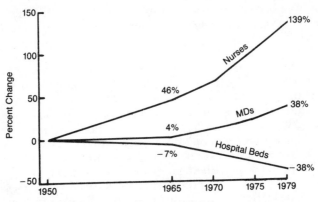

Figure 3–1 Percent change in ratio of RNs, MDs, and hospital beds to population, 1950–1979. Data from *Hospital Statistics* (Chicago: American Hospital Association) and References 7 and 8.

hospitals in the community but will only increase turnover of existing nurses, causing hospital costs to rise even faster without resolving the community's nursing shortage.

This belief has, however, largely been applied only to nurses but has not prevailed when hospitals have sought to fill other positions. Many hospital workers have employment options in other industries. When shortages occur in other sectors of the economy, hospitals must match the wage rates if they want the services. Computer experts, for example, are in high demand across many industries, and workers with these skills are recruited by those willing to offer the largest salaries. The same is true of managers, electricians, accountants and even health professionals such as pharmacists, physical therapists, dieticians, and social workers. All have employment options outside the hospital sector. To attract these workers, hospitals pay the market rate. For nurses, however, hospitals have been and remain the dominant employer and thus are freer of the pressures from other industries that might compete and push nurses' salaries up.

The attitude on the part of those responsible for hospitals is understandable: hospitals have been under enormous pressure to slow the increase of their costs. Beginning in late 1971, federal wage and price controls, state rate controls, the voluntary hospital cost-containment effort, and Medicaid caps have all placed tremendous pressures on hospitals. Moreover, hospitals have been unable to control the costs of energy, supplies, the minimum wage, the growth of unions, or the salaries of personnel whose rates are determined by competition in the economy. Thus, hospitals have sought to contain costs any way they can, and nurses' salaries, which represent at least 25% of hospital costs, have been one area of focus.

We believe that limiting the growth of nurses' salaries relative to salaries of others may be a prime factor in the current shortage of hospital nurses. But before discussing the evidence for this belief, it would be useful to consider the three most popular explanations for the perceived shortage of nurses.

Common Explanations for the Perceived Shortage

Nurses are not working at all, or are working in jobs outside the health field.

Not true. Nurses have one of the highest labor force participation rates of any occupation predominantly engaged in by women. Seventy-five percent of all nurses are actively employed in nursing at any one time (up from 55% in 1960). Further, and contrary to popular opinion, nurses are not leaving nursing in large numbers to work in other fields. Only 3% of nurses are employed in a field outside nursing—strong evidence that nurses are not able to move into positions of comparable status in other areas (13). Thus, inactivity or flight from nursing to other areas does not offer a plausible explanation for the perceived shortage.

All of the increase in the supply of nurses has been absorbed by rapid increases in nonhospital employment.

Again, contrary to belief, the proportion of nurses working in hospitals has remained stable at approximately 65% over the past 15 years. Although the actual numbers of nurses employed in ambulatory care increased after the introduction of Medicare and Medicaid, increases in hospital employment have kept pace. Thus, rising nonhospital employment of nurses does not offer a convincing explanation for the perceived shortage.

Increasing intensity of hospital care and more hospitalizations for an aging population have increased the need for nurses faster than additional nurses can be employed.

The intensity and complexity of hospital care have increased over the past decade, leading to the belief that the need for nurses has increased faster than the number of nurses employed by hospitals.

The most obvious reason for potential demands for more nurses is an increase in inpatient days. As indicated in Figure 3–2, inpatient days increased by 9% in nonfederal, short-term community hospitals between 1972 and 1979. A generous estimate of the effect of this increase on the requirements for nurses would be to assume that a similar increase in the number of nurses would be required—that is, 9%. However, the likely economies of scale when nurses care for additional patients are not considered in such an estimate.

The second source of new demand for nurses is the increasing intensity of nursing services needed because the patients are sicker and length of stay has been shortened, requiring greater intensity of services within a shorter period. Two methods developed by the National Center for Health Statistics have been used to estimate these changes (16). Between 1972 and 1979, the overall severity of the problems of patients treated has increased by approximately 6%. During the same period, length of stay asso-

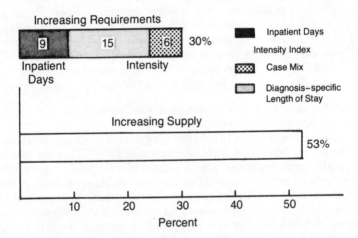

Figure 3–2 Percent change in requirements for and supply of hospital nurses (full-time equivalent nurses employed in nonfederal short-term community hospitals), 1972–1979. Data from *Hospital Statistics* (Chicago: American Hospital Association); the National Center for Health Statistics; and Reference 16.

ciated with specific diagnoses declined by approximately 15%. Both the changing case mix and shorter hospital stays require additional nursing personnel. However, during this 1972-to-1979 period, not only has the number of nurses kept pace with the growing intensity of care, but the increase in the number of nurses in hospitals has exceeded any reasonable estimate of increased patient need. The number of full-time equivalent nurses employed by nonfederal, short-term community hospitals increased from 370,000 to 560,000—a 53% increase (17, 18).

Clearly these changes (increased number of inpatient days, a changed case mix, and reduced length of stay) would require employing additional nurses. These factors are interrelated, and it is difficult to believe their effects are entirely additive. Even if we consider them together, however, to estimate the need for additional nurses, we find that the number of nurses working in hospitals in the 1972-to-1979 period is at least 23% higher than the resulting generous estimate of need for additional nurses. Nurses who actually work in hospitals but are employed by temporary nursing services agencies are not represented in these calculations. Adding this group of nurses would yield an even greater increase in the number of hospital nurses over this period.

Thus, the three commonest explanations for the nursing shortage do not seem to provide a complete answer. There is another explanation, however, that has received comparatively little attention in the recent debates over the nursing shortage.

Relation of Relative Wages to the Shortage of Hospital Nurses

Analysis of trends over the past 2 decades suggests a relation between vacancy rates for hospital nurses and nurses' incomes relative to those of other workers (9). Between 1946 and 1966, nurses' salaries increased by 53% while teachers' salaries increased by 100% and those of other female professional, technical, and kindred workers by 73%. However, after the introduction of Medicare in 1966, nurses' salaries increased at twice the rate of those in these other groups. With the introduction of new insurance programs, hospitals were able to raise nurses' salaries and transfer the costs to third-party insurers. During this period, hospital nursing vacancy rates also dropped rather dramatically from over 23% in 1961 to 9% in 1971, a decline that corresponds to the income increases accompanying improved reimbursement to hospitals by Medicare. In 1960, nurses' incomes were 77% of what teachers received and 93% of the incomes of female professional, technical, and kindred workers. Beginning in 1966, nurses' incomes began to rise relative to the gains experienced by teachers and other female professional workers. By 1969, nurses had gained on teachers, making 87% of teachers' incomes, and had surpassed the average income of other female professionals. During this period, a significant number of inactive nurses came back to active practice. Over one third of the net increase in the number of employed nurses from 1966 to 1972, an increase that profoundly reduced hospital vacancy rates, came from the existing pool of inactive nurses (27).

Wage and price controls introduced in late 1971 were soon followed by states setting rates and by voluntary cost containment efforts. As a result, nurses' incomes again declined relative to those in other jobs predominantly filled by women. Hospital nursing vacancy rates again began to climb, approaching pre-Medicare levels. Thus, there is compelling evidence from the Medicare period that there is a direct relation between the incomes of nurses and their availability for hospital employment.

The improvement in income of other health care providers relative to that of nurses has highlighted the problem. Salaries of other hospital health care personnel have been moving upward more swiftly than those of nurses, narrowing the gap between the two groups. In 1960, licensed practical nurses' incomes were 70% of nurses' incomes; now they are 76%. Incomes of nurses aides rose from 65% of nurses' incomes in 1960 to 71% today (28–31).

In contrast, the gap between incomes of nurses (32, 33) and physicians (34, 35) has widened dramatically. In 1945, nurses' incomes were one third of physicians' incomes; now they are less than one fifth. Thus, during a period when there has been significant transfer of technologies from medicine into standard nursing practice, nurses have not shared in the economic rewards of these advances.

Perhaps of greatest concern, nurses' current incomes do not compare well with those in other occupations predominantly filled by women. Nurses' salaries are on a par with the national average salaries for secretaries (Figure 3–3) even though the educational preparation is considerably greater for nurses. Teachers and female professional, technical, and kindred workers earn more than nurses in the current market. Health professionals, whose work

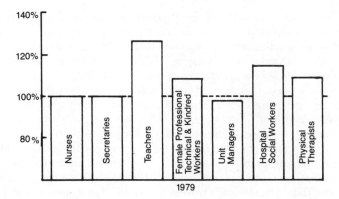

Figure 3–3   Nurses' incomes compared to those of persons in other jobs predominantly filled by women, 1979. Data from References 24–26, 36.

and general responsibilities are roughly similar to those of nurses—social workers, physical therapists, occupational therapists, and pharmacists—all appear to be earning more in the current economic climate than nurses.

Thus, there is considerable evidence to suggest that when nurses' incomes rise relative to those of other workers, more nurses are available for hospital employment and vacancy rates decline. Likewise, as nurses' incomes decline compared to those in other occupations predominantly filled by women, hospital nursing vacancy rates increase.

Despite the fact that the number of nurses has doubled since 1960, estimates indicate a hospital shortage of at least 100,000 nurses (4). Although economists have suggested that depressed wage rates may be important in continuing the shortage, only recently has the overall supply of nurses increased dramatically enough to allow this theory to be more adequately examined. An inadequate wage structure for nurses may have both short-term and long-term effects.

Short-Term Effects of Inadequate Wages

More nurses may choose part-time employment.

Although 75% of nurses are actively employed, less than half work full time, a rate considerably lower than many believe it could be. A unique aspect of nursing, especially hospital-based nursing, is that nurses can work almost any number of hours they choose. Teachers, for example, except for a relatively small proportion of part-time substitutes, must accept a full-time assignment if they want to work. Figure 3–4 shows the variability of part-time employment among nurses. In 1966, for example, as salaries increased, both full-time and part-time employment increased. In recent years, more nurses have been choosing part-time employment.

Contrary to popular opinion, a large proportion of nurses with young children are employed. Women with small children are quite sensitive to the wage rate, however, because their income has to finance child care and homemaker substitute services, costs that are rising faster than nurses' incomes. Thus, many may have reduced the number of hours they work because the additional income from full-time employment does not adequately offset increased expenses.

In lieu of increasing overall salaries, hospitals have begun to offer full-time salaries for part-time work—for example, working

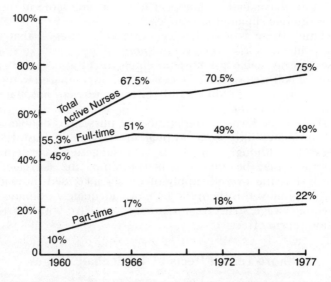

Figure 3–4   Labor force participation of nurses, 1960–1977. Data from References 10, 14, 15, 37, 38. Note: The sum of full- and part-time percentages does not equal total active nurses in some cases due to missing data.

two 12-hour shifts on the weekend may be reimbursed at full-time salary levels. Nurses with responsibilities outside the hospital find these offers increasingly attractive and tend to work as few hours as possible. Greater part-time employment contributes to the hospital shortage of nurses.

An increasing number of nurses are working for temporary nursing services agencies to maximize incomes while minimizing hours worked.
Over the past 5 years, temporary nursing services agencies have proliferated. An ongoing national study has identified 3000 such agencies. The agency hires the nurse and supplies the hospital with nurses. Frequently agency nurses can select the units and shifts they will work and are paid higher wages than full-time hospital staff. Hospital vacancy rates do not reflect the use of agency nurses, which makes it more difficult to assess the extent of the current shortage. For example, if the 3000 agencies employ an average of 20 nurses apiece, a pool of 60,000 nurses could be available for hospital nursing, a resource that is not taken into account in reported hospital vacancy rates.

Temporary services agencies may have proliferated in response to the decline in relative incomes of nurses and the lack of adequate incentives to work unpopular hours. Temporary agencies do offer nurses a way of avoiding caps on hospital nurses' wages but they may have some negative short-term consequences. Agencies may add to the costs of hospital care, encourage nurses to reduce the number of hours they work, increase the fragmentation of care, and add to the frustration of nonagency hospital nurses who are left to work less convenient hours. Nevertheless, in the present climate temporary agencies seem here to stay.

The differential cost of a nurse over that of other personnel is so small that hospitals may be having nurses do jobs that could be done by others.
Nurses are versatile hospital employees; they can do most or all of the tasks of allied nursing personnel and other hospital support staff and can fill many of the roles of other allied health professionals in the hospital. Because of this versatility, when nurses' relative wages fall, hospitals tend to substitute as many nurses as they can recruit for jobs previously done by other personnel. There has been a dramatic increase in the percentage of nurses within the total hospital nursing personnel over the past decade, from 33% in 1968 to 46% in 1979. That there seems to have been a direct substitution of nurses for nurses' aides is sug-

gested by the fact that the percentage of nurses' aides has declined from 51% in 1968 to 35% in 1979 (5, 39, and unpublished data from the Current Population Survey, Bureau of Labor Statistics). During this period, the proportion of licensed practical nurses has remained constant at about 19% of total hospital personnel. Because salaries of nurses versus those of nurses' aides differ by only 29%, which usually amounts to a difference of only $4000 to $5000 a year, substitution of nurses for aides may be viewed as quite reasonable by hospitals. Indeed, some administrators have estimated that aides actually cost hospitals more than twice their salaries because of turnover, continuing education, and, supervision costs.

This substitution effect in hospitals is analagous to the phenomenon of homeowners and industries switching from fuel oil or even coal to natural gas. As a result of the artificially low cost of natural gas resulting from federal price controls, many are converting to a fuel source that is actually in shorter supply. Where we would expect to see hospitals reacting to a critical shortage of nurses by substituting practical nurses, aides, unit managers, and ward clerks for nurses, the opposite seems to be occurring. Current salary rates make it financially advantageous to have nurses do many different jobs rather than just those that require their special training.

Clearly this form of substitution can be beneficial in those hospitals with successful recruitment programs and convenient locations. But substitution accentuates the nursing shortage for hospitals located in unsafe inner city areas or far from middle-class residential areas where nurses live. These institutions have critical shortages, sometimes have to operate with unsafe staffing ratios, or have closed units. Thus, substitution results in stockpiling of nurses by some hospitals while creating a shortage in others.

Long-Term Consequences of Inadequate Wages

Nursing school enrollments may continue to decline, resulting in fewer nurses.

The number of high school graduates applying for nursing school admission appears to have declined gradually since 1962. The only exception was during the 1970-to-1974 period when the admission rate sharply exceeded the increase in high school graduates. This period, as discussed earlier, may have represented the lag time between relative salary gains made by nurses after introduction of Medicare and increased enrollments. Actually, only an increase in the number of older students seems to have saved nursing schools from dramatic decreases in enrollments. Between 1962 and 1975, the percentage of students over 21 years old admitted to nursing schools increased from 10% to 37%, primarily because of community college programs (40). However, growth in all programs has now leveled off. There has been a steady decline in the rate of growth of nursing school graduations since 1974. By 1979, there were fewer graduations than in the preceding year, and a continued, sustained reduction in numbers of new graduates is predicted.

The qualifications of nursing school applicants are likely to fall.

Given the many career options now available to young women, it is not surprising that they are choosing fields with greater economic rewards. Between 1970 and 1980, the number of women enrolled in law school increased from 7000 to 42,000 (42 and unpublished 1980 data from the American Bar Association). The same trend is evident in medicine, with women increasing from 9% of the entering class in 1969 to 28% in 1979, an increase of 13,000 women enrolled in medical school (43). Of special concern is the potential decline in the number of nursing school applicants with high science aptitudes and the background for advanced clinical training at the very time when the technologic complexity of nursing care is rising significantly. With the costs of education rising every year, it will become less attractive for anyone to invest 3 to 4 years of potential earning capacity and up to $25,000 or more to enter a field where the expected income is no greater than that in fields requiring no such investment. To maintain enrollments, greater public subsidies will be required to attract a sufficient number of qualified students.

Dissatisfaction of nurses in hospitals may increase significantly and contribute to costly, high turnover rates.

In hospitals where nurses have been substituted to carry out duties that should be done by others, nurses' frustration may escalate because they will not have challenging jobs that fully utilize their knowledge and expertise. In hospitals left with high vacancy rates, the remaining nurses may find the responsibilities of patient care too overwhelming to handle satisfactorily.

Attempts at collective bargaining may increase.
The rapid growth of temporary nursing services agencies may be a prelude to growth of collective bargaining in various forms. In the short run, at least, collective bargaining may have detrimental effects on the day-to-day operation of hospitals and the quality of patient care.

Potential Solutions to the Shortage

The evidence suggests that adjustments in nurses' incomes to make them more compatible with those of other professionals with comparable responsibilities may be the best way of swiftly overcoming the perceived hospital nursing shortage. Increasing the relative incomes of nurses might bring about a resolution to the crisis by a combination of the following:

1. Raising nurses' incomes would tend to halt the large-scale substitution by hospitals in favorable locations of nurses for health workers with less training.
2. If substitution were reduced in the more favorably located hospitals, nurses might, when offered better financial incentives, seek employment in less desirably located hospitals that often house the sickest patients and are now most desperately in need of nurses.
3. Increasing nurses' incomes might encourage part-time nurses to work more hours and could bring additional inactive nurses into the labor force. Given a labor pool of over 1.4 million nurses, a rather modest increase in the hours each worked might add enough additional nursing services to eliminate the current hospital nursing shortage.
4. Applicants to nursing schools might increase in numbers and quality, ensuring an adequate supply of nurses for the future.

But here is the problem. Obviously, a significant increase in nurses' salaries will lead to an increase in hospital costs—something the nation is now desperately trying to avoid. In a period of severe economic restraint, it is difficult to make such a recommendation. If, however, the way to eliminate the present perceived nursing shortage in hospitals lies in the economic arena, perhaps tradeoff strategies should be examined to see if this can be accomplished without large overall additions to hospital costs. Federal, state, and local subsidies for nursing education over the past 15 years have been enormous. But if our thesis is correct, simply continuing the subsidies and expanding the numbers of nurses will not make hospital nursing a more desirable career. Ever-increasing subsidies will be required to maintain nursing school enrollments, and the quality of applicants may decline at the very time more knowledgeable people are needed in nursing.

Other strategies might be considered to offset the costs of increasing nurses' salaries. First, would it not be wise to proceed carefully to reduce the country's excess hospital bed capacity? In 1976, the Institute of Medicine estimated that the United States had at least 100,000 excess short-term general hospital beds (44). Elimination of these beds might not only bring about significant cost savings, but would also modestly reduce the number of nurses required in hospital settings. Second, many studies have suggested that a substantial number of patients in hospitals would not actually require hospitalization if effective alternatives were available. Would it not be sensible to more aggressively explore ways to significantly reduce hospital use where appropriate? This reduction would lead to considerable savings that could help offset the expense of raising nurses' salaries while reducing the number of nurses required in hospitals.

In closing, we recognize that there are other problems that affect nurses in American hospitals. Dissatisfaction with the conditions of nursing practice in hospitals is causing high turnover rates and a general disillusionment among nurses employed by hospitals (45). During the next decade, resolving these problems could lead to a significant improvement in the quality of patient care in hospitals. We suggest, however, that we are not likely to bring an end to the shortage of hospital nurses without giving similar serious attention to the economic rewards for becoming and remaining a nurse in hospital practice.

Acknowledgment

The authors would like to acknowledge the importance of the published research of Donald E. Yett in this analysis.

References

1. Fagin CM. The shortage of nurses in the United States. *J Public Health Policy.* 1980; **1**(4):293–311.
2. Aiken LH. Nursing priorities for the 1980s: hospitals and nursing homes. *Am J Nurs.* 1981; **81**(2):324–30.

3. Demkovich LE. The nurse shortage—do we need to train more or just put them to work? *Natl J.* 1981 May 9:837–40.
4. The nurse shortage: there's a long road ahead. *Hospitals.* 1980; 54(9):63–4. Editorial.
5. American Hospital Association. *Hospital Statistics.* Chicago: American Hospital Association; 1980:4.
6. U.S. Bureau of the Census. *Statistical Abstract of the United States, 1980.* Washington, D.C.: U.S. Bureau of the Census; 1980.
7. Health Resources Administration. *Supply of Manpower in Selected Health Occupations: 1950–1990.* Bethesda, Maryland: Department of Health and Human Services; 1980:59. (DHHS publication no. [HRA]80-35.)
8. National Center for Health Statistics. *Health Resources Statistics.* Rockville, Maryland: National Center for Health Statistics; 1976–1977:305.
9. Yett DE. *An Economic Analysis of the Nurse Shortage.* Lexington, Massachusetts: Lexington Books; 1975.
10. Altman S. *Present and Future Supply of Registered Nurses.* Bethesda, Maryland: Department of Health Education and Welfare; 1971:9–14. (DHEW publication no. [NIH]72-134.)
11. Sloan FA. *Equalizing Access to Nursing Services: The Geographic Dimension.* Hyattsville, Maryland: Department of Health, Education, and Welfare; 1978:57–66. (DHEW publication no. [HRA]78-51.)
12. Feldstein PJ. *Health Care Economics.* New York: John Wiley & Sons; 1979.
13. McCarty P. Survey shows a million RNs employed. *Am. Nurse.* 1980; 12(9):1, 6, 10.
14. Roth AV, Walden AR. *The Nation's Nurses: 1972 Inventory of Registered Nurses.* Kansas City, Missouri: American Nurses' Association; 1974:44.
15. American Nurses Association. *RNs, 1966: An Inventory of Registered Nurses.* New York: American Nurses' Association; 1969:17–8.
16. National Center for Health Statistics. *Health, United States 1980.* Rockville, Maryland: National Center for Health Statistics; 1980:109–10. (DHHS publication no. [PHS]81-1232.)
17. American Hospital Association. *Hospital Statistics 1972.* Chicago: American Hospital Association; 1973:35.
18. See Reference 5, p. 21.
19. See Reference 9, Tables 3–13, p. 136; and Table 4-2, p. 160.
20. Maryland Hospital Association. *Nursing in Maryland Hospitals—In Critical Condition?* Lutherville, Maryland: Maryland Hospital Association; 1980.
21. New Jersey Department of Higher Education. *An Analysis of the Need for Registered Nurses in New Jersey, 1979–1990.* Trenton, New Jersey: New Jersey Department of Higher Education: 1980.
22. Texas Hospital Association. *Survey of Nursing Staff Requirements.* Austin, Texas: Texas Hospital Association; 1979.

23. California Hospital Association. *A Study of the Recruitment of Registered Nurses by California Hospitals and Nursing Homes.* Sacramento, California; 1978.
24. National Center for Education Statistics. *Digest of Education Statistics, 1979–1980.* Washington, D.C.: U.S. Department of Education; 1980.
25. U.S. Bureau of the Census. *Money, Income, and Poverty Status of Families and Persons in the U.S.: 1979.* Washington, D.C.: U.S. Bureau of the Census; 1980. (Current Population Reports, series P-60, no. 125.)
26. University of Texas Medical Branch at Galveston. *1979 National Survey of Hospital and Medical School Salaries.* Galveston, Texas: University of Texas Medical Branch at Galveston; 1979.
27. See Reference 12, p. 373.
28. Bureau of Labor Statistics. *Occupational Outlook Handbook.* Washington, D.C.: U.S. Department of Labor; 1961.
29. Bureau of Labor Statistics. *Occupational Outlook Handbook.* Washington, D.C.: U.S. Department of Labor; 1970–71.
30. Bureau of Labor Statistics. *Occupational Outlook Handbook.* Washington, D.C.: U.S. Department of Labor; 1980–81.
31. University of Texas Medical Branch at Galveston. *1974 National Survey of Hospital and Medical School Salaries.* Galveston, Texas: University of Texas Medical Branch at Galveston; 1974.
32. American Nurses' Association. *Facts About Nursing.* New York: American Nurses' Association; 1945:74.
33. University of Texas Medical Branch at Galveston. *1980 National Survey of Hospital and Medical School Salaries.* Galveston, Texas: University of Texas Medical Branch at Galveston; 1980.
34. U.S. Bureau of the Census. *Historical Statistics of the U.S.—Colonial Times to 1970.* Washington, D.C.: U.S. Department of Commerce; 1975.
35. Glandon GL, Werner JL. Physicians' practice experience during the decade of the 1970s. *JAMA* 1980; **244**:2514–8.
36. Bureau of Labor Statistics. *National Survey of Professional, Administrative, Technical, and Clerical Pay.* Washington, D.C.: U.S. Department of Labor; 1979.
37. Inventory shows 75 percent of nation's nurses work. *Am J Nurs.* 1980; 80:1948.
38. See Reference 10, p. 102.
39. Health Resources Administration. *Source Book, Nursing Personnel.* Bethesda, Maryland: U.S. Department of Health, Education, and Welfare; 1974. (DHEW publication no. (HRA)75-43.)
40. Johnson WL. Supply and demand for registered nurses: part 2. *Nursing and Health Care.* 1980; **1**:74.
41. National League for Nursing. *NLN Nursing Data Book 1979.* New York: National League for Nursing; 1979:29.
42. American Bar Association. *Review of Legal Education, 1980.* Chicago: American Bar Association; 1980:64.

43. Peterson ES, Crowley AE, Rosenthal J, Boerner R. 80th annual report: medical education in the U.S. 1979–1980. *JAMA* 1980; **244:**2814. Special issue.
44. Institute of Medicine. *Controlling the Supply of Hospital Beds.* Washington, D.C.: National Academy of Sciences; 1976.
45. Wandelt MA, Pierce PM, Widdowson RR. Why nurses leave nursing and what can be done about it. *Am J Nurs.* 1981;**81:**72–7.

4. Anatomy Is Destiny

Michael Beebe, Steve Barr, and Mary Hamilton

Why should we be in such desperate haste to succeed, and in such desperate enterprises? If a man does not keep pace with his companions, perhaps it is because he hears a different drummer. Let him step to the music he hears, however measured or far away.   Thoreau

Most historians agree that Florence Nightingale established the profession of nursing during the Crimean War in the middle nineteenth century. Although Nightingale reportedly possessed qualities of warmth and sympathy, her ability to influence the initiation of a profession must have been affected by the attributes of organizational ability and dynamic leadership (Dolan, 1973).

The popular image of the nurse is based on the attributes of tenderness, caring, and passivity. However, today's nurse must be dynamic, assertive, instrumental, and expressive (Simpson and Green, 1975; Bem, 1974). Contemporary nursing practice requires the maximization of the potentials of all its members. However, the profession is only now learning to draw from the positive qualities of all nurses and to utilize the collective capabilities of its constituents.

Throughout time, instances of men as professional nurses have punctuated the development of the profession to its present state (Beebe, 1978). In recent years the number of men who have selected nursing as their life work has increased, but the total percent of men in the profession remains below 2 percent. Because nursing has been and is a female-dominated profession, questions continue to arise about the need, and indeed the appropriateness, of men in nursing. A discussion of the salient issues associated with the entrance and socialization of men into the profession of nursing is the focus of this chapter.

Although this paper is not intended to be a list of all the problems and prejudices associated with men in nursing, a discussion of the prominent issues will have to include some of them. Research findings about the characteristics of men who choose nursing as a career and the positive attributes and contributions of men to nursing will be discussed.

The role of the man in nursing is changing as rapidly as nursing itself. Stewart Hase in the *Australian Nursing Journal* (1977) suggested an interesting notion, i.e., there are two species of nurses found in every hospital: nurses and male nurses. The implication is that a person with the title "nurse" must possess female attributes, and this is the long-standing image portrayed by the Nightingale schools. What Hase (1977) is also implying is that sex typing is the central issue in the discussion of men in nursing.

Behaviors which are culturally sanctioned and considered characteristic of one sex but which are ridiculed and considered inappropriate when performed by members of the other sex are labeled as sex-typed behaviors. The process by which individuals come to value and acquire the behaviors considered characteristic of and appropriate for their own sex produces this sex typing.

Descriptive research shows that children display definite sex-typed behavior preferences before school age. Boys tend to choose play objects related to sports, aggression, and mechanical aptitudes, while girls select objects associated with home and maternal activities. There is less crossing of sex lines by boys than girls, i.e., girls frequently select objects or activities that are generally associated with boys, while boys seldom choose objects associated with girls. There are plenty of tomboys, but few examples of the male equivalent of that behavior pattern, and the male counterpart is ultimately categorized as a "sissy" by his peers. Boys generally scorn girls' tasks, games, and future life roles; while girls not infrequently express desires that they were boys. Wishes to change sex are virtually unheard of in prepubescent boys (Henderson and Bergan, 1976).

Sex stereotyping represents a psychological phenomenon

which evolves during normal development and may increase the stress experienced when one considers a future profession that traverses usual sex roles. Along with the related peer pressure, sex stereotyping can be a deterrent to school age children considering professions ordinarily associated with the other sex. One study indicated that high-school-aged males overwhelmingly ranked nursing lowest of any profession on a masculinity scale (Vaz, 1968).

Altering the traditional occupational roles so that members of both sexes can achieve their fullest potential may necessitate change at all levels of society. There needs to be a widespread use of children's books which are rewritten to include men in traditionally female roles and a shift in educational curricula which will open the door to men in female-dominated occupations.

Career counseling is said to be a deterrent to men choosing nursing as a profession. Beginning in grammar school and continuing through high school, men have rarely been encouraged toward nursing (Auster and Auster, 1981). What seems necessary is a continuing change in the national climate of opinion concerning sex roles so that more individuals can pursue goals of their own choosing. It is interesting to note that the number of men in nursing dropped steadily from the turn of the century, and only since active recruitment for men students began in the 1970s have there been indications of this trend being reversed ("Men in Nursing," 1973).

In the past men who entered nursing were usually in their late 20s or early 30s (Mannino, 1963; Auster and Auster, 1970). This pattern may have indicated that older men had transcended the sex-typed bridge on the basis of maturity and individual goals. More recent statistics show an increasing number of men entering nursing in their early 20s ("Men in Nursing," 1973). This suggests that contemporary society is relaxing its classical role typing and is beginning to accept individuals in cross-typed roles. Increasing numbers of men entering nursing may also indicate their own realization that nursing is a very secure profession. Nursing offers steady if not lucrative employment. The modern nurse also has the option of high mobility. A recent report from the American Hospital Association indicates that between 90,000 and 100,000 RN vacancies exist throughout the United States ("AHA Commission," 1981).

The role men assume in nursing should be viewed in the same light as women in politics, government, business, or the sciences. The addition of women to the political arena has been welcomed by many as a remedy for the long-standing sexist attitudes generated by male-dominated politics. Not all people accept women as politicians, nor do most of us expect them to.

Rejection by others that takes the form of harassment or discrimination does generate a legitimate concern. It is important to note that individuals who risk peer rejection and criticism are applauded in most instances. However, it is equally important to note that this applause is usually not immediate, but rather is an outgrowth of the populace's experience with the individuals involved. Gradually, the positive contributions of the opposite sex come to be viewed as a real necessity to the rounding out of a profession. Yet, to feign that simply increasing the numbers of members of one sex or the other alone will improve the status of a profession is a risky statement. As always it is not merely quantity but the kind and quality of services which are the key to a profession's status.

In a report for the Indiana Commission for Higher Education, Johnson (1980) projects that the number of high school graduates will decrease by at least 26 percent over the next 20 years. And nursing can expect a concomitant drop in enrollment. Dr. Johnson concludes that nursing must discover a way to attract more minorities, including men, into its ranks (1980). If nursing continues to be a profession of low status and nurses are seen only as maternalistic servants of the sick, one can see why minorities, especially men, reject nursing as a viable career option. The status and image of nursing must change. However, just wanting or even demanding these changes will not bring them about.

One of the tasks incumbent on men already in nursing is to bring the positive career aspects to the high-school-aged males. The role of men in nursing must be portrayed in the same light as that of women in politics, government, business, science, or any of the previously sex-typed professions.

Equilibrium, stability, and steadiness are synonyms for balance, and balancing the profession can bring these attributes to nursing. It is not that men are the only source of balance; it is rather that their presence provides another viewpoint, a sometimes different way of thinking and dealing with problems that face nurses clinically and professionally. Men do not represent a panacea to nurses' problems. Men bring a sense of balance and a different viewpoint to nursing (Christman, 1970b). In our modern society it has become clear that any profession or institution which lacks heterogeneity does not possess the ability to adequately provide services to a heterogeneous society. If the population of health care consumers is mixed, why should there not be a similar mix of health care providers.

Men in nursing interrupt the classic pattern of "sexual politics" which has existed for years between male doctors and female nurses. Contemporary female nurses are often heard encouraging each other to be more assertive. However, in terms of earlier personality development, psychological testing generally portrays males as self-confident and self-assured during the preschool years. During the midchildhood years (ages 5–10) play activities are aggressive and team- or club-oriented. Male adolescents show increased bravado and expansiveness (Vaughn and McKay, 1969). Therefore, it should be natural that men would bring these attributes to the profession of nursing.

Current sexual politics cast the male physician as master and the (female) nurse as unquestioning servant to both physician and patient. This is one example of the traditional male-female role expression as well as the model of health care in which the physician is the pinnacle of the field and all other professionals are subordinate. It is logical to assume that the independent, objective, active, and competitive nature which men would bring to nursing could help to accelerate the liberation of these qualities in their female counterparts. Who would argue that help in changing traditional ways of relating among health care professionals is not needed or wanted?

Nursing needs the very best of both genders and to deny itself the abilities of anyone qualified is to be the poorer for it (Jenny, 1975). We believe that contemporary nurses are becoming more assertive for several reasons, one of which is the increased numbers of men in nursing and sexual liberation in general.

There is a growing body of research literature related to men in nursing. In one study, Segal (1962) interviewed 22 male and 79 female nurses from one large eastern hospital. Two-thirds of Segal's men nurses had wanted to be or be like doctors. None of the women respondents expressed similar interests. The men in Segal's study ranked job security as the dominant reason for entering nursing. Other studies (Mannino, 1963; Beebe, 1981) listed job security as the number two reason for entering nursing. Segal found that although the men in his study tended to be in administrative or management positions, they still expressed anxiety and tension which Segal attributed to their (sexual) "minority status"

(1962, p. 38). The prestige of being a nursing supervisor did not affect the role strain associated with being in a female occupation. How comfortable a man feels in the practice of nursing depends largely on the resolution of conflict between sex role orientation and professional role. We believe this conflict is commonly resolved by finding a specialty which is more likely to be compatible with the perceived sex role.

The study done by Sandy Mannino (1963) can now be considered a classic. Mannino gathered his data from 480 male graduate and 36 male nursing students. Most of his graduates and all the students were from the Pennsylvania School of Nursing for Men. At the time Mannino did his study (1962), many U.S. schools of nursing did not accept male students. However, the Alexian Brothers Schools in Chicago and St. Louis and the Pennsylvania School of Nursing were for men only.

Mannino asked his subjects why they entered nursing. In rank order they answered (1) "because I like people and enjoy helping them," (2) "I wanted to go into medicine but was financially unable to do so," (3) "because of a desire to improve my status in life," (4) "to enter a service occupation and make a contribution to my community," and (5) "for security for myself and my family." Of particular interest, among Mannino's respondents 75 percent were married to nurses, 61 percent said they subscribed to a professional journal, and 57 percent held membership in a professional organization. Mannino interpreted these data to mean men nurses support the profession "to a greater extent than do nurses in general" (1963, p. 187). Mannino also found that men nurses earned approximately $350 a year more than their female colleagues, a trend that has continued to the present day (Goluck, 1981).

Donald and Carol Auster used questionnaires and interviews to gather data from 335 male and 508 female nursing students at 32 degree-granting institutions (Auster and Auster, 1970). They found that men students come from lower socioeconomic groups and that more men were from rural areas and small towns than their female counterparts. The Austers found that men students became interested in and made the decision to nurse later in life than women. Men nursing students tend to be older, married, and to have had previous employment experience. These findings are consistent with those of Mannino (1963) and with data gathered by Beebe (1981). The Austers' men students stated that "personal contacts" helped them make the decision to choose nursing as a career. The men students did not like the institutional atmosphere and the regimen of nursing school. They were more critical of the school of nursing and its curriculm. Men students were more technically and administratively oriented and had more psychomotor skills than the female students (Auster and Auster, 1970).

Of special interest is the fact that the men students said they would "act independently to benefit the patient" (Auster and Auster, p. 505). Many of the men students reported that, though they thought men made better nurses, they might use nursing as a steppingstone to other roles, but most said they planned to stay in health care. The findings of the Austers' study are mentioned in detail because (1) the Austers were very thorough in their data collection from each subject, (2) they maintained a rigorous research methodology, and (3) though Mannino had a larger sample of men nurses (516), the Austers' sample (n=335) was more representative of men nurses throughout the United States.

As previously stated, the studies about the characteristics of men nurses (Mannino, 1963; Auster and Auster, 1970; Beebe, 1981) are fairly consistent in their findings. Though it is clear that the number of men entering the profession is increasing ("Men in Nursing," 1973), the characteristics of male students remain essentially unchanged.

A few studies have been done to assess personality characteristics of men nurses. Van Hoang (1979) had a small sample of 9 ASN, 17 BSN, and 4 MSN male students. Van Hoang administered the Tennessee Self Concept Scale and asked the students about their perceptions of discrimination they may have experienced in nursing school. Discrimination was defined as unequal treatment of individuals of basically equal status. Van Hoang (1979) found that early in their programs, all levels of students reported lower self-concept, but few students perceived discrimination. As students progressed in their programs, their self-concepts improved and their reports of discrimination increased. Van Hoang's results must come under some question because of his convenience sampling in only one school of nursing and small sample size. However, Van Hoang's findings coincide with results of other similar research (Aldag and Christensen, 1967; Aldag, 1970; Williams, 1973; and Auster, 1979).

Aldag and Christensen (1967) used the MMPI to look at personality traits of four groups of students (29 in each group): male and female nursing students and male and female junior college students. These researchers found that the personality profiles of male students of nursing, as measured by the MMPI, were more similar to female students of nursing than the profiles of male junior college students to female junior college students (1967). The male-female scale of the MMPI indicated that "male and female nursing students are more 'feminine' than male junior college students" (p. 376). In addition, "nursing students regardless of sex are more likely to appear as responsible-generous individuals than are junior college students" (p. 376).

Along similar lines, Rutledge and Gass (1968) interviewed 19 black male students and found problems of "masculine identity" because the men felt they were being dealt with as women. Lewis (1980) states that the "scarcity of black males in the nursing field seems to have roots deeply embedded in the black experience" (p. 6). For the black male who is trying to recover his masculinity post-slavery, the choice of nursing as a career may be too paradoxical (Lewis, 1980). Viewing Lewis's comments and the study by Rutledge and Gass, it may be quite a few years before we see a proportionate number of black men in the nursing profession.

In another study, Aldag (1970) administered the Strong Vocational Interest Blank to four equal size groups ($N = 45$) of male and female nursing students and male and female college students. Aldag (1970) found that "interests appear to be vocationally related regardless of sex and that men nurses have interests characterized as more feminine than college males" (p. 533).

Holtzclaw (1981) studied factors which influence the male nurse's ability to negotiate the role strain and possible status contradictions exerted by a feminine sex-typed profession. Holtzclaw was looking for androgyny among men nurses, i.e., the ability to perform both masculine and feminine tasks without discomfort. Holtzclaw hypothesized that androgynous male nurses would have perceptions of greater control of their own destiny. Control may be defined as from whence a person perceives the forces which mold or mandate his or her behavior. Internally controlled individuals are controlled by self. Externally controlled individuals are controlled by forces outside of self (Rotter, 1966).

In comparison of data gathered from a random sample of 26 graduate men students and a normative male sample, there was no difference in sex role identity. In comparison with a group of female nurses, the men nurses were less sex typed but no more androgynous than their female counterparts. Finally, there was no difference in locus of control perceptions, regardless of sex role perceptions of men or women (Holtzclaw, 1981).

R. G. Brown and R. W. Stones are British sociologists who have conducted considerable research on men nurses and men students in Britain (1970–1976). A longitudinal study of over 500 men nursing students in British hospitals was begun in 1968. Brown and Stones (1972) administered intelligence and personality inventories to the students and gathered data from nurse instructors on their assessment of the men students' chances of passing final exams. It was found that men were more extroverted and less neurotic than a normative male sample. However, personality traits did not correlate with the instructors' previous assessment of the students' grades. For a complete description of the Brown and Stones findings the reader is referred to the supplemental articles called "Occasional Papers" found in *Nursing Times* magazine (1970–1976).

Williams (1973) studied 273 men students in 32 schools of nursing, all in the western United States. The male students came from a middle-class environment and were likely to be older and married when they entered school (p. 520). The men students ranked "helping people" as the primary reason for choosing nursing (p. 523). Williams (1973) fashioned his questionnaire after the work of Auster and Auster (1970) and his findings were consistent with theirs.

The research about men in nursing depicts individuals who want to help people, are older, probably married, and make their career choice later in life. Men nurses may have more female-oriented interests than other nonnursing males, but otherwise they have no striking personality differences from any normative sample.

At this point, we will delve further into the social issues of men in nursing. As the total number of men in the nursing profession increases, the patriarchal-authoritarian structure which they bring with them may balance the purely matriarchal structure which has classically characterized nursing. The matriarchal principle is that of unconditional love, institutionalism, natural equality, compassion, and mercy. The patriarchal structure principle is that of conditional love, hierarchical structure, abstract thought, manmade laws, and justice. A purely matriarchal orientation may hinder the true development of an individual, and the purely patriarchal orientation may stifle love and equality and look only at manmade laws and obedience. However, when the matriarchal and patriarchal principles form a union, each principle is enhanced by the other: motherly love by justice and rationality, and fatherly love by mercy and equality (Fromm, 1971).

The applicability of Fromm's comments (1971) lies in what we believe is a need for the liberation of the "feminine" aspects of the male personality along with the "masculine" part of the female. This androgynous person might be both masculine and feminine, both assertive and yielding, and both instrumental and expressive (Lawrence, 1978). There has been and still is a reluctance on the part of many nurses to acknowledge these qualities in themselves. But it is vital that all nurses explore their self-concepts in order to achieve the balance for which our society is searching.

There is no clinical area where men nurses cannot function effectively. Yet recently an Arkansas judge ruled that "due to the intimate touching required in labor and delivery the services of all male nurses are inappropriate [for that area]" ("Arkansas Judge," 1981). Male nurses are not inadequate due to some trait equated with their gender; rather, it is their very sex which makes all male nurses unacceptable—or so said Judge Roy (p. 1253). Judge Roy also contended that "the majority of women patients will object to intimate contact with a member of the opposite sex"; therefore, the performance of "intimate functions" by a male nurse would violate the patient's constitutional rights to privacy (p. 1253). Judge Roy viewed as specious the argument that male nurse and male physician situations are analogous, because the physician is "selected" by his patient but the nurse is not. This litigation emphasizes that men in nursing today must remain cognizant of the obstacles they may encounter in school and in their professional endeavors. They must be prepared to enter a professional world which is primarily composed of women and a society which may not be able to accept or accommodate the man nurse in his own career goals.

We believe that there are trends in society and therefore nursing schools which will ultimately help create a more heterogeneous climate in the profession. Many nursing schools are now recruiting from a wider social base. The experience of studying with individuals from varying backgrounds, vis-à-vis sex, race, culture, etc., will inevitably expand the insight of future nursing professionals. Attending school with a mix of students will not only expand graduate nurses' cultural and psychosexual knowledge base, but will make them less resistant to working in an atmosphere considered untraditional by the establishment.

We believe that greater awareness is needed as to how nursing has viewed and does view men nurses, at both the conscious and unconscious levels. It is our hope that the view of men in nursing in its totality will be such that a constructive relationship will evolve, and that nursing may utilize both men and women to their fullest potential for the betterment of the profession and toward that ever present goal of quality patient care.

References

"AHA Commission Sponsors Hearings on Nursing Shortage," *American Journal of Public Health* 81 (May 1981):926–930.

Aldag, J. C. "Occupational and Nonoccupational Interest Characteristics of Men Nurses," *Nursing Research* 19(6) (1970):529–533.

Aldag, J. C. and Christensen, C. "Personality Correlates of Male Nurses," *Nursing Research* 16(4) (1967):375–376.

"Arkansas Judge Rules Male Nurse Out of Labor/Delivery," *American Journal of Nursing* 81(7) (1981):1253, 1274.

Auster, D. "Sex Differences in Attitudes Toward Nursing Education," *Journal Of Nursing Education* 18(6) (1979):19–28.

Auster, D. and Auster, N. R. *Men Who Enter Nursing: A Sociological Analysis.* Washington, D.C.: Division of Nursing, Public Health Service, Department of Health, Education and Welfare, 1970.

Auster, C. J. and Auster, D. "Factors Influencing Women's Choice of Non-traditional Careers: The Role of Family, Peers, and Vocational Counselors," *Vocational Guidance Quarterly* (March 1981).

Beebe, M. E. "Men in Nursing: Yesterday, Today, Tomorrow." Paper presented at Men In Nursing Symposium, A.N.A. Convention, 1978, Honolulu.

Beebe, M. Data collected from participants at Men in Nursing Symposium at ICN meeting, Los Angeles, 1981.

Bem, S. L. "The Measurement of Psychological Androgyny," *Journal of Consulting and Clinical Psychology* 42(2) (1974):155–62.

Brown, R. G. S. and Stones, R. W. H. "Personality and Intelligence Characteristics of Male Nurses," *International Journal of Nursing Study* 9 (1972):167–177.

Christman, L. "What the Future Holds for Nursing," *Nursing Forum* 9(1) (1970b):13–18.

Dolan, J. A. *Nursing in Society: A Historical Perspective,* 13th Ed. Philadelphia: W. B. Saunders, 1973.

Fromm, E. "Mother," *Psychology Today* 4 (1971):74–77.

Goluck, R. (Ed.). "Just Beginning to Catch Up," *RN* 44 (August 1981):40–43.

Hase, S. "The Role of the Man in Nursing," *The Australian Nurses Journal* 7(1) (1977).

Henderson, R. W. and Bergan, J. R. *The Cultural Context of Childhood.* Columbus, OH.: C. E. Merrill, 1976, Chap. 10.
Holtzclaw, B. J. *The Man in Nursing: Relationships Between Sex-typed Perceptions and Locus of Control.* Doctoral Dissertation, University of Oklahoma, 1981.
Jenny, J. "The Masculine Minority," *Canadian Nurse* (December 1975): 21–22.
Johnson, J. *Report on Nursing Education and Practice for the Indiana Commission on Higher Education.* Indianapolis, IND.: Indiana State Commission on Higher Education, July 1980.
Lawrence, J. "Men in Nursing." Paper presented at the Symposium on Men in Nursing, American Nurses' Association, 1978, Honolulu. Unpublished.
Lewis, M. C. "A Black Perspective: Afro-American Men in Nursing." Paper presented at Rush University, Men in Nursing Meeting, December 1980, Chicago.
Mannino, S. F. "The Professional Man Nurse: Why He Chose Nursing and Other Characteristics of Men in Nursing," *Nursing Research* 12 (1963):185–187.
"Men in Nursing," *RN* 36 (August 1973):33–43.
Rotter, J. B. "Generalized Expectancies for Internal versus External Control of Reinforcement," *Psychological Monographs* 80(1, Whole No. 609) (1966).
Rutledge, A. L. and Gass, G. Z. *Nineteen Negro Men.* San Francisco: Jossey-Bass, 1968.
Segal, B. E. "Male Nurses: A Case Study in Status Contradiction and Prestige Loss," *Social Forces* 41 (1962):31–38.
Simpson, O. W. and Green, Y. N. "Androgynous Nurses," *Canadian Nurse* 71 (1975):20–21.
Van Hoang, N. *Self-concept and Perceptions of Discriminations of Male Nursing Students.* Unpublished study, Indiana University, Indianapolis, 1979.
Vaughn, V. and McKay, R. J. (Eds.). *Nelson's Textbook of Pediatrics.* Philadelphia: W. B. Saunders, 1969, pp. 57–65.
Vaz, D. "High School Senior Boys' Attitudes Toward Nursing as a Career," *Nursing Research* 17 (1968):533–538.
Williams, R. A. "Characteristics of Male Baccalaureate Students Who Selected Nursing as a Career," *Nursing Research* 22(6) (1973):520–525.

5. The Motivation Pyramid in Nurse Retention

Mark B. Silber

Recent best sellers have analyzed the foibles and weaknesses of organizations. In his widely read and oft-quoted publication, *The Peter Principle,* Laurence J. Peter sets forth his observation on organizations of noteworthy size: In a hierarchy, individuals tend to rise to the level of their incompetence. Without delving into the validity of Peter's assertion nor accepting the notion that incompetence and inefficiency are inherent in a large organization, it must be admitted that certain motivational and productivity problems are of prime concern to hospitals today.

There is a costly incidence of on-the-job retirement wherein hospital employees stay on the payroll and their cradle-to-grave existence is not constituted of contribution but, rather, performance stagnation. Granted that in some cases the capability is just not there, sadly enough, in terms of human vitality, there probably are more instances in which a person's talents and motivations are used restrictively or not used at all. Rather than finding her job a vehicle for personal fulfillment and occupational excitement, an individual often drifts into a "work station mentality" that becomes no more than a series of coffee breaks punctuated by long lunch hours. Such "motivation waste" is debilitating to the overall effectiveness of hospital management. This expensive problem might be alleviated in part by an understanding of the nature of the motivation that comes from within the staff nurse, not that generated externally. This view of employee motivation and a grasp of the nuances and complexities of this concept could result in more satisfied, committed hospital employees.

To better present the concept of self-released, internal motivation to the patient care coordinator, I have organized a structure referred to as "The Motivation Pyramid." The pyramid is

Silber, Mark. "The Motivation Pyramid in Nurse Retention." *Supervisor Nurse* (April 1981): 45–46. Reprinted with permission of *Nursing Management* and the author.

appropriate because its structure relies on a layering process—each layer forms the foundation for the next. Also, a pyramid is a complex, many-sided shape and its form suggests the convergence of multiple factors toward the climax that is the release of motivated behavior (see Figure 5–1).

Layer One

The bottom or first layer of the pyramid is composed of the unique biographical background of each individual staff nurse. Just as a gourmet cook is familiar with many spices and seasonings and knows when and how to use each one, so an effective hospital administrator is aware (1) that there are unique motivating factors within each hospital employee, (2) that no two persons are ever "seasoned" alike, and (3) that the handling of life events differs with each of them. In addition to such essential ingredients as skills, abilities, job expectations and work values, careful attention must be given to past job experience (including successes and failures). Careful assessment of biographical history, abilities and motives will help the management team avoid creation of a margi-

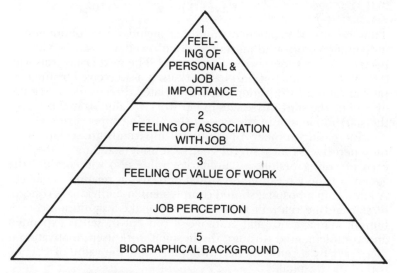

Figure 5–1   The motivation pyramid.

nal job situation and a hospital work climate that promotes low self-initiating behavior and consequently, job dissatisfaction.

Layer Two

The next layer in the Motivation Pyramid takes into account the preconceptions each staff nurse brings to her work. Prior to starting a job, every employee has certain preconceptions about what her hospital work will be like and what she expects for her own growth and job satisfaction. Often these preconceptions do not agree with the reality the individual encounters on the job. Subsequently, situations occur that could be remedied by the practice of Management By Clear Objectives (M-B-C-O). If the nursing administrator defines clearly what the employee's duties include and explains why the first few months on the job may be filled with many unstimulating assignments, a staff nurse will have a far more accurate preconception of the job and hence less frustration. Moreover, the administrator could further enhance the new employee's motivation by showing appreciation through a few honest compliments on her handling of initial assignments.

Layer Three

Thus far the Motivation Pyramid has included the foundation of individual background ingredients reinforced with clarified job expectations and supervisory appreciation. The next layer deals with the utilitarian value of hospital work itself as perceived by the hospital employee. Motivation release is related directly to the amount of "good" the staff nurse sees in her work. "Value" is in the eyes of the staff nurse, not in the eyes of the nursing supervisor.

Increasing numbers of graduates apparently are seeking what they perceive as meaningful goals. An understanding of the concern of young people for utilitarian value also will consider the "good" of the job as the individual perceives it relating to herself. A job within a hospital should complement an individual's concept of self and be relevant to her desire to make a significant contribution. When a hospital employee's concept of self is expanded and complemented through the hospital work itself, motivation is increased by a sense of her own value and the value of her job within the hospital.

Layer Four

It can be said that motivation exists in direct proportion to the degree of association one feels with a job. If high morale depends on the "3 B's" (to belong, to be and to become), a feeling of belonging is important. This "B"—to belong, to be accepted by the group—was mentioned earlier in our discussion of the importance of making each hospital staff nurse aware of her contribution. An employee's sense of belonging to the hospital and to the job is enriched if she feels that others in the group are aware of the importance of her job. Personal recognition by one's manager is vital and meaningful, but group acceptance of one's work also is important for job motivational release. One way to bring this about is to explain at the time a new nurse is introduced to her co-employees what her contribution to the department will be and how her work relates to theirs.

Layer Five

This final supportive layer of the pyramid concerns itself with the need of each individual to feel important. How does a house nursing supervisor generate a feeling of personal and job importance in employees? Contemporary research shows that a person's sense of importance is directly related to the influence she feels that she has through her work. By the establishment of multiple opportunities for a person to exercise influence, a hospital structure can help an individual to feel important.

Due North

If a nursing supervisor is to instill a sense of personal and job importance in a hospital employee, she must be receptive to that employee's influence. An effective head nurse directly solicits hospital employees' advice and establishes a reputation as someone who is always open to suggestions. A nursing care supervisor's actual willingness to spend time intently listening to an employee's ideas is an indication of the importance she gives to this person as a human being.

Due East, Due West

In addition to providing opportunity for upward influence, a hospital supervisor can motivate an employee by letting her influence laterally by allowing her to deal with members of other organizations on a free basis without quizzing her sitting in on their meetings, or "policing" what is done.

Due South

Equally important is a staff nurse's opportunity to exert influence downwards—to manage her subordinates (if she has any) without interference from her hospital executive. Details such as whether a person's subordinates deserve a raise, when her staff should take vacations, etc, should be left up to her.

Due Center

Finally, a staff nurse should be able to influence and give meaning to her own work. True job motivation includes the opportunity not only to initiate new ideas and make decisions, but also occasionally to make some learning errors. The employee who has been given job freedom and managerial support will make mistakes, but she will profit by these occasional mistakes. Because the task is "her baby," she will feel responsibility with regard to an error and will do her best to see that it is not repeated. Recognizing the freedom she has been given and the trust her house nursing supervisor has invested in her, she commits herself to the job as though the boss's job has become her own.

By understanding that a core part of a person's job motivation is pride in one's self-initiated abilities, the house nursing supervisor may discover that her personnel are adept at handling things in her absence, that they can control their projects through self-control and that they enjoy saying, "That was my decision" when a questioned action is confronted. The elements we have explored—the background a staff nurse brings to the job, her job perception, the meaningfulness of her work, the "3 B's" and the opportunity to influence others—interacting together, result in a climate conducive to achievement, a successful hospital and a good place to work.

6. Blowout: An Alternative Conceptual Approach to Nursing Turnover

*Patricia T. Castiglia, Linda McCausland,
and Juanita Hunter*

That a critical shortage of nurses in the United States exists can not be denied. Efforts by the federal government over the past 15 years in terms of traineeships to educate nurses at advanced levels and capitation funds to schools of nursing have not been successful in preventing the existing shortage. This shortage has been most acute in hospital settings (Aiken et al., 1981). Wolf cites the national average turnover rate at 32–40 percent, i.e., 3 or 4 of every 10 nurses quit their jobs each year (Wolf, 1981).

Nursing has traditionally been a women's profession. Therefore, one might speculate that the women's movement was somehow implicated in the nursing shortage, or one might conjecture that factors within the profession itself have caused nursing to decline. Indeed, the decline might well be the combination of these and/or other factors.

Kramer and Baker (1971) studied 220 nurses from the staffs of medical center hospitals to identify if the exodus of nurses from the profession was related to professional-bureaucratic conflict. Individuals with a high bureaucratic role conception exhibited primary loyalty to hospital administration. These nurses tended to acknowledge the legitimacy of rules, external control and supervision, and promotion based on allegiance to organizational policies and requirements. A high professional role conception was indicated if the nurse professed primary allegiance to the profession of nursing and to work principles which would transcend particular work settings. This role conception placed importance on education, individual judgment, continual self-improvement, and support of professional organizations. It was assumed that a nurse who has been socialized into the profession of nursing as a professional and who must

practice in a bureaucratic organization will experience reality or
acculturation shock.

It was found in this nationwide sample that within 2 years of
beginning practice, about half of the 220 nurses exited from hospital nursing and that about one-third left nursing practice alto-
gether. Nurses were rated by employers in terms of success in
nursing. The majority of the nurses with a high bureaucratic role
conception received "highly successful" ratings by their employers. Those with "less successful" ratings tended to congregate
in the low bureaucratic cells. It was further found that success
ratings improved and that the majority of nurses changed their
role value configuration to high loyalty to the bureaucratic system
and low loyalty to the profession.

One interesting question explored in the Kramer-Baker study
was whether or not teachers of nursing are really dropouts from
nursing. The investigators stated that they suspected that more
nurse teachers are actually dropouts from nursing than their operational definition identified. If teachers of nursing were actually
included in the dropout rate for this study, the figure would have
been 33 percent rather than 28.9 percent.

Fagin (1980) cites the number of registered nurses today as
being 1.4 million and identifies that this is probably the most
diverse group licensed in the United States. Variations within the
nursing profession exist in terms of education, type of work, social class, status, and values. These variations, she feels, have led
to both strengths and weaknesses in the profession. In 1980, although 73 percent of registered nurses were in the labor force,
there were "between 90,000 and 100,000 vacant budgeted registered nurse positions in hospitals alone; serious nursing shortages
in nursing homes; and unfilled positions in community health
agencies" (Fagin, 1980, p. 297).

The following factors were identified by Fagin as being responsible for the nursing shortage: (1) increased degree of acute-
ness of condition of hospitalized patients, (2) increased degree of
illness of long-term care patients, (3) increased degree of sophistication of treatment in and out of hospitals, (4) demographic
changes in population with growth in absolute number and percentage of persons over 65, (5) focus on community-based care
and home health care, and (6) emphasis on health and health
maintenance (Fagin, 1980, p. 298). Fagin believes that the first
three factors are the dominant causes of our present and future
problems. In addition, Fagin states that these changes have not

only created an increased demand for nurses but have also changed the nature of the routine day, increased the emotional and physical demands on nurses, and increased the need for nurses to be technologically and interpersonally competent.

The first recommendation Fagin makes to alleviate the shortage, i.e., that working conditions must be improved for nurses, is directed to employers. Salary, benefits, and working conditions, including rotation, double shifts, and "floating," must be addressed. The whole question of whether or not nursing can be considered a competitive profession must also be considered. A resultant question is: What changes need to be made in the power structure of the health care delivery field? The second recommendation is that opportunities should be provided for educational advancement. Support from state and federal sources should be directed at undergraduate, graduate, and continuing education programs for nurses. The third recommendation emphasizes the need to plan and implement the baccalaureate as the entry level of practice. This is important if we are to instill a career orientation rather than a job orientation. Next, Fagin states that the rational planning of nursing education must be done on a state, regional, and national basis. A massive public relations campaign must be developed to improve the image of nursing and, finally, all governmental plans for change in health service should be required to address the implications for nursing resources in such plans.

Wandelt, et al. (1981) studied factors associated with nurse unemployment and sought ways to attract nonworking nurses into the work force. Thirty-five hundred Texas nurses responded via a questionnaire; 30 hospital nurses in 6 small-group interviews supplied reasons for working/not working in nursing and factors that would encourage nurses to return to work; and in a daylong conference consumers, nurses, physicians, and other interested persons produced innovative suggestions for attracting nurses back to work. Each part of the investigation was found to support the findings in each other part.

The questionnaires gave data about how nurses perceived nursing. The interviews gave material for understanding nurses' feelings about patient care and about opportunities for professional practice. The findings indicate that conditions in the job setting that interfere with the practice of nursing cause nurses to leave nursing and to remain outside the work force.

The mean salary increment for a 20-year period in nursing

was found by the Wandelt study to be $100/year. Dissatisfaction factors identified by employed nurses included (in rank order): (1) availability of adequate salaries, (2) the amount of paper work, (3) support given by the administration of the facility, (4) administrators' opportunity for continuing education, (5) adequacy of laws regulating the practice of nursing in Texas, (6) support given by nursing administration, (7) availability of acceptable child care facilities, (8) availability of inservice education, (9) availability of fringe benefits, and (10) competence of nonregistered nursing staff.

The interview methodology elicited some interesting comments. Nurses felt guilty about not having been able to give adequate and complete care. Staffing problems relate to overload and overwork. It was suggested that agencies could use short shifts (with specialized tasks at specific times, i.e., pre-op teaching), that nurses assist in planning staffing, that part-time nurses be offered all inservice opportunities, and that nursing school faculties provide a part-time and substitute pool. Nurses further believe that the tasks they perform constitute a meaningful part of health care delivery. It was suggested that staff nurses serve on all committees making policy about patient care and personnel matters and that a Joint Practice Committee be established to serve as a grievance board to handle disputes between the professions and to offer appropriate counseling.

Nurses also stated that they expect to be able to exercise some discretion and choice over work methods. They suggested establishing primary care with all RN staff on all units, identifying a theory base, allowing RNs to write nursing prescription orders, self-scheduling, and task analysis. Nurses also indicated that they need to have occasional recognition for a job well done. They suggested establishing a quality assurance plan with awards and recognition for outstanding performance and the use of merit awards related to professional growth, e.g., continuing education costs.

The conflict identified in the Wandelt study is the same as that identified by Kramer (1974), Kramer and Baker (1971), and Storlie (1979), which is that nurses perceive themselves as professionals engaged in nursing practice while administration views them as employees carrying out the job of nursing. The data from the Wandelt study indicates that nurses are dissatisfied with employment when job conditions do not allow them to function professionally.

It has seemed apparent to these investigators, as it has to

many concerned nurses, that factors causing the severe nursing shortage must be identified and measures taken to ensure that the nursing profession maintain its identity as a key profession in the health care delivery system. Storlie (1979) has elaborated on the reality shock concept coined by Kramer to describe disillusionment with the actual practice of nursing. Reality shock is, according to Storlie, a "literal collapse of the human spirit" that transforms caring into apathy (Storlie, 1979, p. 2108). A susceptible host, the highly idealistic nurse, is needed for burnout to occur. Burnout is further viewed as a lack of power. Ellis (1980) reiterates that nurses do want control over their practice.

Responsibility has also been cited as a cause of stress and burnout. Responsibility for people is identified as causing more stress than responsibility for things (Calhoun, 1980). Not only patients, but a significant number of other persons, must be satisfied by nurses. It appears that industry has taken more of a lead in recognizing and managing stress than health care delivery systems. Specific ICU/CCU hospital studies have indicated the following techniques to be useful for reducing stress: (1) using an integrated team approach to share responsibility, (2) having regular group meetings for mortality and morbidity discussions and instilling a feeling of team spirit and pride, (3) ensuring immediate physician availability, (4) working staff not more than 8 hours per shift, (5) providing periodic rest and relaxation on other units, (6) providing an area for staff privacy, (7) ensuring that proper instruction has been given on electronic equipment relating to physiology, e.g., monitoring or treatment.

Bullough (1974) studied job satisfaction of nurses in terms of intrinsic satisfiers. Intrinsic factors were concerned with job creativity, job importance, the job's use of their skills, autonomy, and how interesting the job is. It was found that pediatric nurse practitioners rated higher than extended role nurses and other registered nurses in intrinsic and overall job satisfaction.

Price and Mueller (1981) developed a causal model for the turnover in nursing based on a review of the literature. The determinants whose increase resulted in less turnover were intent to stay, job satisfaction, participation in making job-related decisions, the receipt of work-related information, and the chance to get ahead occupationally in hospitals. Increased repetitiveness of work resulted indirectly in greater turnover (Price and Mueller, 1981, p. 109). When the individual nurse was studied, in contrast to the aggregate of nurses, the determinants whose increase resulted in reductions in turnover were intent to stay, job satisfaction, and the existence of local kin.

Utilizing the factors identified in the review of the literature, a study was designed and carried out in the summer of 1980 which indicates that a more appropriate term for the turnover problem occurring in the nursing profession would be that of a "blowout." A blowout in nursing is analogous to the blowout of a tire. A blowout would imply that a variety of causes (not just disillusionment) might contribute to the condition and that the final disablement might be one factor which becomes too much to bear. Blowout also implies the notion of repair and the potential to continue to serve and be useful if conditions are adjusted.

The Western New York Study

The study now being reported was designed and implemented to investigate job satisfaction/dissatisfaction for registered professional nurses. A questionnaire was developed which sought to determine significant factors contributing to job satisfaction or causing job dissatisfaction, if the reasons for changing positions were alleviated in new job settings, if a significant number of nurses are planning on leaving their present position or are considering such a change, and which factors could influence nurses to remain in their current positions.

The Sample

The subjects for the study were randomly selected from the official list of registered professional nurses in western New York State. Four hundred seventy questionnaires were deliverable. A return rate of 57 percent was obtained.

The respondents presented the following picture: 96 percent females, 65 percent married, 99 percent white, 60 percent diploma graduates, and 89 percent received their basic education in New York State. Only 10 males responded to the survey. None of the males were baccalaureate graduates and 8 were graduates of associate degree programs. In terms of employment status, 59 percent of the respondents were employed full time, 31 percent were employed part time, and 10 percent were unemployed. Nearly half of the respondents were staff nurses (47 percent).

Most of the respondents worked in medical-surgical settings. Only diploma graduates were functioning in intensive care and rehabilitation units.

Findings

Factors Perceived as Preventing Turnover

Respondents were asked to rank the five most important items from 16 alternatives in terms of preventing job turnover. A scale of 1–5 with 1 being the highest rank and 5 the lowest was utilized. Respondents could also utilize an "other" category. Table 6–1 illustrates the ranking of the factors. The highest ranking factor was improved salary and fringe benefits. More nursing service backup and sufficient power to function effectively were the next most frequently ranked factors. The item most frequently written in was the need for more nursing staff. The factors selected least often were a distinctive uniform or symbol followed by a 30-hour work week, rotation as a unit coordinator, and periodic rotations to other types of nursing services. These were techniques which Hay and Oken (1972) identified as possible stress reducers. It would appear from these findings that nurses perceive vacations as a means of relieving job related stress (41.1 percent), but that they do not perceive rotation to another setting (22.1 percent) or to another position (19.1 percent) as stress relievers.

Further analysis of the factors showed a discouraging lack of pattern among the conditions. The 16 factors identified through the review of the literature as being potentially in control of employers and as being indicators of job satisfaction failed miserably to account for the nurses' intent to leave their present position. The highest correlation shown by any of the 16 items was .133. Thus, this item, more physician backup, accounts for less than 2 percent of the variance in the plans of nurses in the sample to leave their present positions.

Factoring was carried out automatically as part of the computer program, MODEL (Ackerman and Lohnes, 1981), but factor analysis is largely irrelevant in a situation such as this one which provides so little explained variance with which to work. The conclusion must be that the job arrangements employers are in control of simply did not explain how nurses feel about their jobs or whether they intend to leave their positions.

Table 6–1 Factors perceived as preventing nursing turnover.

Factor	Percent of Nurses Ranking Factors ($n=236$)					Percent of Nurses Ranking the Factor 1–5
	1	2	3	4	5	
A distinctive uniform or symbol	.3	.8	.2	.8	9	12.9
A pay differential	15.7	8.9	5.1	6.3	6.8	42.8
Periodic, brief, extra vacations (R&R)	8.5	8.9	8.9	6.3	8.5	41.1
Periodic rotations to other types of nursing services	3.4	3.4	4.7	3.8	6.8	22.1
Rotation as a unit coordinator (freed from regular nursing duties)	1.3	3.4	5.1	2.5	6.8	19.1
More physician backup	5.9	12.3	9.3	8.1	10.2	45.8
More nursing service backup	19.5	9.3	12.3	9.3	5.9	56.3
Attention to physical setting	4.2	4.7	5.1	5.9	10.2	30.1
More staff orientation	4.7	5.9	10.2	3.8	3.8	28.4
More improved inservice education programs	13.6	9.7	8.9	11.9	6.4	50.5
Four-day work week	4.2	5.1	3.4	7.6	8.9	29.2
Thirty-hour work week	2.1	3.4	3.8	1.3	5.9	16.5
More peer consultation	5.5	3.8	8.5	3	5.5	22.8
Alternate weekends off	5.9	8.5	8.5	4.2	7.6	34.7
Sufficient power to function effectively	19.5	8.5	8.5	4.2	7.6	48.3
Improved salary and fringe benefits	30.1	19.1	10.2	8.9	8.1	76.4
Other	7.2	3.4	1.3	1.7	8.1	21.7

Findings Concerning the Current Position

A most significant finding is that only 23 percent of all the nurses in the study indicated that they were completely satisfied with their present position. While supervisors, clinical nurse specialists and educators appeared to be the most completely satisfied, it must be noted that the sample for these groups is extremely small.

Respondents were asked to consider their positions in relation to 31 factors. These factors were developed as possible indices of power, communication, and assertiveness. The five most satisfying and the five most dissatisfying factors are seen in Table 6-2. Friendliness among co-workers and the opportunity to relate to clients/patients are the most satisfying factors. The factor identified as causing the most dissatisfaction is the reward for education/ experience. Responses to salary and fringe benefits were almost equally divided in terms of satisfaction/dissatisfaction. From Table 6-2 it can be seen that the nurses are most satisfied with communication factors and most dissatisfied with power factors.

In terms of their present positions, only two factors were found to be statistically significant at the .05 level: satisfaction with job security and dissatisfaction with the opportunities available for advancement. Most respondents felt that they were autonomous. However, as in the Wandelt study, a large number of the respondents indicated that salary was a major item of dissatisfaction. Also in support of the Wandelt study, 40 percent of the respon-

Table 6-2   Factors selected most frequently as a source of satisfaction or dissatisfaction.

Satisfaction Factors	% of Nurses	Dissatisfaction Factors	% of Nurses
Friendliness among co-workers	82	Reward for education/ experience	60
Ability to maintain professional standards on the job	77	Opportunities for advancement	58
Opportunity to relate to clients/ patients	71	Promotion possibilities	56
Job security	69	Incentive pay	56
Consultation with peers	67	Opportunities for creativity	50

dents indicated that inservice education was less than adequate. Other factors rated as less than adequate by 25 percent or more of the respondents were expertise of the nursing supervisor, the evaluation process, the opportunity for leadership, the effect the job has on emotional well-being, fringe benefits, grievance procedures, communication with superiors, opportunities to be creative, and opportunities to provide comprehensive patient care. Fifty-five percent of the nurses rated autonomy as better than adequate while half of the respondents felt that the opportunity to be creative is less than adequate.

Findings Concerning the Previous Position

Respondents were asked to identify the most important reason for leaving their previous positions. The three most important reasons were family obligations, dissatisfaction with the organization, and moving to a new location. Dissatisfaction factors common to both the previous and present position are found in Table 6–3. It can be seen that more nurses are identifying salary, fringe benefits, and opportunities for promotion as being dissatisfying in their present position than the number of nurses who named these same factors as dissatisfying in their previous positions. This may be due to the general economic climate today and to the emphasis on higher education for leadership positions in nursing.

Table 6–3   Dissatisfaction factors common to the previous and present nursing position.

Factors	% of Nurses Identifying Factors in Previous Position	% of Nurses Identifying Factors in Present Position
Position is emotionally and physically demanding	41	34
Salary	28	43
Fringe benefits	18	40
Opportunities for promotion	18	56
Shift rotation	14	11

Findings Concerning Nurses Intending to Change Positions

Of the 32 percent of the respondents who indicated that they were currently thinking of leaving their present position, the reasons most frequently given were that the position was emotionally/physically demanding and that they were dissatisfied with the type of nursing in their present situation. This is interesting because, in general, most of the nurses (55 percent) state that they are satisfied with the specialized type of nursing in which they are engaged.

It appears that not receiving support from nursing administration when they are in conflict with doctors or administration is a major reason for intending to leave positions; 47 percent of those nurses intending to leave their present positions feel that they rarely or never receive this support. Stress related to the job also appears to be a major influencing factor; 55 percent of those respondents intending to leave their present positions feel that the job is usually to always stressful. This is interesting because stress did not appear to be alleviated by changing positions. Forty-four percent of the respondents stated that the amount of stress in their present position as compared to their previous position was greater (38 percent indicated that the stress was the same). It would appear, therefore, that stress reduction was not accomplished by changing positions even though stress factors were motivators for the change.

Another factor investigated concerned the collegial relationship with physicians as reflected by discussing and developing patient/client plans of care. One-third of those who would change their positions indicated that they never or rarely discussed the patient/client's plan of care with the physician. Hay and Oken (1972) indicated that predictability in terms of incessant repetitive routine is a negative factor for intensive care nurses. In this study 22 percent of the respondents who indicated that they would change their positions said that their positions were always predictable (40 percent of all nurses indicated that the routine is predictable).

It would seem from these responses that nurses appear to be thinking of changing positions more because of feelings of powerlessness than because of factors associated with satisfaction or dissatisfaction related to patient care or with aspects of a particular setting.

Educational Preparation Similarities and Differences

Will the educational preparation of the respondents influence the respondent's perception of job satisfaction? Cross-tabulations of data revealed the following findings: 84 percent of the AD graduates, 78 percent of the diploma graduates, and 50 percent of the baccalaureate graduates rated the opportunities for advancement in their present position as less than adequate (poor to fair). None of the AD graduates rated the opportunities for advancement as excellent.

The responses rated as very good to excellent concerning the basic educational preparation are found in Table 6–4. There were more associate degree graduates than any other group who felt that their basic preparation in terms of their present position was less than adequate. Most of the nurses (92 percent) felt that their basic nursing preparation was adequate to excellent. In terms of salary, there were no diploma or associate degree graduates who made over $21,000. Approximately three times as many baccalaureate graduates earn over $18,000 as diploma and associate degree graduates.

In addition to assessing their basic nursing education, the nurses were asked to evaluate inservice education and orientation programs. Ninety percent of the nurses stated that inservice education is very important. This finding agrees with Wandelt's 1981 study. However, 49 percent indicated that the inservice education programs at their place of employment were either poor or just fair. The same response was given in terms of the orientation programs.

Table 6–4   Responses concerning the basic education of RN's in western New York.

Response Item	Very Good to Excellent Ratings (%)		
	AD	Diploma	BS
Rating of the quality of basic education preparation	37	74	50
How the basic education prepared for the current position	10	25	50

In terms of their present position, the most dissatisfied group was the baccalaureate graduates. The most completely satisfied graduates were the master's-prepared nurses. The latter were also 67 percent of the total number of respondents who rated their salary as being more than adequate. Two-thirds of the master's graduates also felt that the fringe benefits were either excellent or very good. Except for the master's-prepared nurses, the other nurses indicated that the rewards for education and experience were less than adequate (82 percent diploma graduates, 83 percent AD graduates, and 75 percent baccalaureate graduates). The evaluation process was rated as poor or fair by 40 percent of the diploma, 45 percent of the AD, 50 percent of the baccalaureate, and 44 percent of the master's-prepared nurses. Whether or not the nurses viewed the positions as being emotionally and physically demanding (a dissatisfaction factor for previous and present positions) appears to be directly related to length of educational preparation: 89 percent of the master's-prepared nurses, 71 percent of the baccalaureate-prepared nurses, 54 percent of the diploma nurses, and 52 percent of the associate degree nurses responded positively.

Findings Concerning Collective Bargaining and Grievance Procedures

The study sought to identify how nurses felt about their representation and which collective bargaining units represented them. Thirty percent of respondents stated that they are currently represented by collective bargaining agents and 68 percent felt that nurses needed to be represented by collective bargaining units. Examples of the collective bargaining agents named include the New York State Nurses Association, AFL-AFT, Civil Service Employees Association (CSEA), Professional Employees Federation (PEF), and Buffalo Teachers Federation. Sixty-six percent of all the respondents stated that they felt that a collective bargaining agent could improve job conditions and 59 percent felt that nurses do have more input into working conditions with a collective bargaining agent. More AD (84 percent) than diploma (65 percent) or baccalaureate (59 percent) graduates indicated that they needed to be represented by collective bargaining agents. The most satisfied nurses who had been represented by collective bargaining agents were the diploma graduates.

Being able to bring grievances before an appropriate body is a benefit sought by most workers. It is viewed as a means of having arbitrary matters settled and provides a mechanism for staying in a position despite differences once those differences are negotiated. A majority of the respondents (72 percent) indicated that the grievance procedures in their job settings were less than adequate.

Summary

The study of the nurses in western New York State indicates that there are a variety of factors which influence job satisfaction and subsequent job turnover. Respondents rated job security as high in satisfaction and opportunities for advancement as low in satisfaction. The most important reasons for leaving their previous positions were family obligations, dissatisfaction with the organization, and moving to a new location. While most nurses rated stress as high in their current position, stress was not reduced by changing jobs. More associate than diploma or baccalaureate nurses indicated a need to be represented by collective bargaining agents.

In terms of professionalism and directions for the future of the nursing profession, almost three-fourths of the respondents indicated that membership in professional organizations is not important. A large majority of the respondents indicated that in-service education is important but almost half of the nurses stated that inservice education at their places of employment is less than adequate.

The significant job satisfiers were friendliness among co-workers, the ability to maintain professional standards on the job, the opportunity to relate to clients/patients, job security, and consultation with peers. The factors adding to dissatisfaction include rewards for education/experience, opportunities for advancement, promotion possibilities, incentive pay, and opportunities for creativity. These factors tend to confirm those identified by Wolf (1981). The current study found that nurses are most satisfied with communication factors and most dissatisfied with power factors.

Most of the respondents indicated that they would not change their profession but might change their employment settings. Over half of the respondents indicated that they would want to change who has control over their working conditions. The highest ranking items for impacting on remaining in the

current position were improved salary and fringe benefits, sufficient power to function effectively, and more nursing service
backup. Almost three-fourths of the respondents indicated that
grievance procedures were less than adequate. Most of the respondents were satisfied with the specialty area in which they
worked.

Of the respondents who intend to leave their current positions or who are thinking of leaving, the reasons most frequently
given were that the position was emotionally/physically demanding and that they were dissatisfied with the type of nursing in
which they were presently engaged. However, only 32 percent of
the respondents indicated that they were thinking of leaving their
current positions. In terms of their present position, the baccalaureate graduates were the most dissatisfied group and the most
satisfied were the master's-prepared nurses.

Most of the nurses stated they were adequately prepared for
their profession and their present position by their basic nursing
program. The nurses did reflect feelings of powerlessness and
dissatisfaction with salary and associated benefits. This study
lends support to the premise that current nurses are in stress
situations and that they remain in stress situations despite changing positions. This study further supports the notion that satisfiers relate to what the individual does and dissatisfiers relate to
the context or environment in which he does the job (Herzberg
et al., 1959).

Although the literature reviewed indicates that turnover rates
may be decreased by attending to factors which may be employer-
controlled, this study indicates that none of these factors are sufficiently powerful enough to influence decreased turnover. The
interpretation may be that personal factors tied to the woman's
role in society may continue to significantly influence turnover
and that employers may have little real control. If this is so, however, there may be ways in which nurse employers could capitalize
on the turnover factors. Certainly day care centers in hospitals
and health care settings is one means. Another might be to have
hospitals unite as employers and allow nurses to transfer from
one geographic area to another without the loss of job benefits
accrued. Not only would employees benefit but so would the employers because they would experience more satisfied nursing
personnel. The multiplicity of factors found in this study support
the alternative conceptualization of blowout as a more relevant
description of nursing turnover today.

70   THE CRISIS IN NURSING PRACTICE

References

Ackerman, W. B. and Lohnes, P. R. *Research Methods for Nurses*. New York: McGraw-Hill, 1981.

Aiken, Linda, Blendon, Robert, and Rogers, David. "The Shortage of Hospital Nurses: A New Perspective," *American Journal of Nursing* 81(9) (September 1981):1612–1618.

Bullough, Bonnie. "Is the Nurse Practitioner Role a Source of Increased Work Satisfaction?" *Nursing Research* 23(1) (January/Febrary 1974):14–19.

Calhoun, Gary L. "Hospitals Are High Stress Employers," *Hospitals* (June 16, 1980):171–172.

Ellis, Barbara. "Winds of Change Sweep Nursing Profession," *Hospitals* (January 1, 1980):95–98.

Fagin, C.M. "The Shortage of Nurses in the United States." *Journal of Public Health Policy* (December 1980):293–311.

Hay, D. and Oken, D. "The Psychological Stresses of Intensive Care Unit Nursing," *Psychosomatic Medicine* (2) (March/April 1972):109–118.

Herzberg, F., Mausner, B., and Snyderman, B. *The Motivation to Work*, New York: Wiley, 1959.

Kramer, M. *Reality Shock: Why Nurses Leave Nursing*. St. Louis: Mosby, 1974.

Kramer, Marlene and Baker, Constance. "The Exodus: Can We Prevent It?" *Journal of Nursing Administration* (May/June 1971):15–30.

Price, James L. and Mueller, Charles W. *Professional Turnover: The Case of Nurses*. New York: SP Medical and Scientific Books, 1981.

Storlie, Frances. "Burnout: The Elaboration of a Concept," *American Journal of Nursing* 79(12) (December 1979):2108–2111.

Wandelt, M., Pierce, P., and Widdowson, R. "Why Nurses Leave Nursing and What Can Be Done About It," *American Jounal of Nursing* 81(1) (January 1981):72–77.

Wolf, G. "Nursing Turnover: Some Causes and Solutions," *Nursing Outlook* 29(4) (April 1981):223–226.

7. Reflections on a Television Image

Beatrice J. Kalisch, Philip A. Kalisch, and Margaret Scobey

Editor's Note: Though the authors primarily address the content of The Nurses, *which was televised in 1962–65, CBS-TV has recently launched a six-episode series of* Nurse. *Although the authors provide an in-depth analysis of the television image of nurses in an older dramatic series, the readers are offered tools to use in the assessment of a popular series being televised today.*

In the December 1980 issue, Nursing and Health Care *ran a story on the National League for Nursing's involvement as consultant on the* Nurse *series.*

The CBS television network has recently introduced a dramatic series about nurses. The new show, *Nurse,* stars Michael Learned in the role that she created in a made-for-TV movie of the same name, shown in the spring of 1980. Ultimately, the new series will be judged by its ability to attract a sufficiently large audience to guarantee its survival. Should *Nurse* do well in the ratings war (the pilot was quite successful) and win a solid place in the weekly programming schedule, it will be in a strong position to influence the way in which the American public of the 1980s perceives the nursing profession (1,2). Registered nurses interested in the promotion of positive and realistic portrayals of contemporary nurses on television would do well to turn a critical eye toward *Nurse.*

Criteria for judging the new series do exist. In the entire history of television programming, only one other prime-time, national network series focused primarily on nursing: *The Nurses* (CBS, 1962–1965). The image of nursing found in this series proved to be the strongest and most positive image in any series to

Kalisch, B. J., Kalisch, P. A., and Scobey, M. "Reflections on a Television Image." *Nursing and Health Care* (May 1981):248–255. Reprinted with permission of Technomic Publishing Co., Inc., Westport, CT. Copyright © 1981.

feature nurses as regular characters. A retrospective examination of what elements contributed to the positive image of the nursing profession in *The Nurses* and an explanation of the series' unfortunate fate can prepare viewers, not only to evaluate the new series, *Nurse*, intelligently, but also to systematically campaign for any necessary improvements.

This analysis is one part of a larger investigation of the image of nursing on television over the past 30 years. With a 20 percent sample of prime-time series with nurse characters, a research method of content analysis was used. Coding was done on research instruments developed and tested for the study. Dominant impressions of nursing, behavioral traits, and primary values of nurse characters, nursing activities, and other key variables reflective of the nurse image were analyzed. Three tools were developed, tested, and utilized in coding the content of television programs: a unit analysis tool, a nurse character tool, and a physician character tool. Coders underwent standardized training procedures and achieved an intra-rater reliability of 88.4. Measures of instrument content and convergent validity were made.

The Nurses premiered in fall of 1962 as CBS' answer to *Ben Casey* (ABC) and *Dr. Kildare* (NBC). Those old enough may recall the craze of the early 1960s, when teen-age girls wore Ben Casey smocks and the public devoured medical programming. By and large, the image of nursing did not prosper in hospital dramas—the gallant, life-saving activities of the handsome, young physician-heroes left little room for the development of nurse characters. *The Nurses*, not surprisingly, did offer the viewing public an opportunity to witness nurses at work without the domineering presence of physician characters—at least during the first two seasons of the series' life. *The Nurses*, in keeping with the proven format of health care shows, used the experienced counsellor/idealistic neophyte relationship as its fulcrum.

Main Characters

During its first two seasons, *The Nurses* followed the personal and professional lives of two nurse characters in Alden General Hospital in New York City: head nurse Liz Thorpe and nursing student Gail Lucas. Liz's experience, wisdom, and realistic view of human nature often corrected the high-minded, idealistic, frequently misguided enthusiasms of her protégé, Gail.

The character of Liz Thorpe, beautifully developed by actress Shirl Conway, provided the most consistent and positive image of all the nurse characters shown during the life of the series. Indeed, Liz Thorpe served as the linchpin of Alden General's nursing staff. In the days before "women's lib," Liz represented the best in emancipated womanhood: Feminine and compassionate, she brought a sense of authority, discipline, and professional excellence to nursing. The universal admiration for Liz by patients, physicians, and other nurses emphasized the fact that here, indeed, was the ideal nurse. Her appearance, background, and personality contributed to her appeal as a woman and protagonist of the series.

Liz's personality revealed a complex woman. She often appeared to be the eternal mother hen, clucking over the trials of young nurses and doctors. "Ma Thorpe" was forever maternally guiding Gail through the crises of youth and inexperience. The patients most in need of extra-loving care received Liz's tenderest ministrations. However, Liz's sharp tongue and acerbic wit kept her from becoming too saccharine. She did not suffer fools gladly and often lost her temper with the inefficient or the unwelcome.

Liz's main contribution to the image of nursing was her role as finder of compromises and solutions and arbitrator of disputed issues. She represented the "golden mean"—the right balance between compassion and objectivity, between involvement and distance; between idealism and pragmatism. While others about her lost their heads, she pursued the middle course—usually. Whenever she did err, it was always on the side of too much compassion, too much generosity, or too much involvement.

The series' other leading nurse character, Gail Lucas, played by Zina Bethune, had less character depth. The 18-year-old nursing student served as the show's official idealist who thought with her heart and acted on her generous impulses. Excused by her lack of experience and redeemed by good intentions, Gail blundered her way through two years as a student at Alden's hospital school of nursing and then became a staff nurse. In her starched pinafore and cap, she looked the part of the naive ingenue—big blue eyes, long blonde hair (pinned primly under her cap), and open facial expression. Young and pretty, Gail exuded girlishness, immaturity, and innocence; the character acquired a one-dimensional quality that bothered many critics and the actress herself, who once complained that Gail had no background.

Professional nursing groups and individual nurses found Gail the most disconcerting aspect of the series (3). As a student she made too many blunders to have been tolerated in a real hospital, and she rarely was seen receiving clinical instruction. At most, she learned from mistakes and listened to Liz's instruction. Gail showed poor judgment, acting in ways that second- and third-year nursing students would not. For example, in one episode, Gail—identifying a patient by name—read from the patient's chart in obvious earshot of nonprofessionals. Regardless of the seriousness of her errors, Gail emerged at the end of each show in full possession of the viewer's sympathy (although cynical viewers may have wished her fired at times), awarded because Gail was loyal to her ideals, however mistaken they may have been.

Gail's virtues, aside from her compassion and concern for others, stemmed from her stubborn insistence that truth and justice would win the day. For example, she refused to believe that she would be dismissed from nursing school because of her unprofessional handling of a particular case. After all, she said, the real issue was whether or not a mother and father were abusing their son. There was a *deus ex machina* quality to Gail's predicaments—just in the nick of time, someone or something would happen to establish her veracity or at least save her from herself. Unlike Liz Thorpe, Gail often turned to others for help, comfort, or counselling—usually to Liz.

Supporting Cast

Recurring characters on *The Nurses* included staff nurses Verna Ayres (Hilda Simms) and nursing student Kelly (Joanna Miles). These and other Alden General staff nurses who appeared in minor roles showed neither the virtuosity of Liz nor the exaggerated idealism of Gail. They appeared to be ordinary people, competent and happy in their work, but untroubled by the larger issues of life.

Verna Ayres was an attractive black nurse in her 30s who often played confidante to Liz. Occasionally, Verna took action on her own, as when she tried to persuade a married doctor to protect Liz's reputation by leaving her alone. The nursing students who shared Gail's work appeared to be happy, hard-working young women who gave little thought to the larger meaning of their careers; they seldom suffered the introspective pangs that Gail Lucas did.

In the show's efforts to explore various aspects of the human condition, the nurse characters were used not only to portray individuals but often to convey a message, not so much about nursing as about humanity in general. Consequently, many of the nurses featured displayed negative qualities or emotional disturbances. But each episode resolved the matter in such a way as to indicate that the situation was unusual in the nursing field or at least not tolerated by nursing professionals.

The non-nurse support staff provided other themes for the episodes. Romantic interest and masculine viewpoints came from young intern Ned Lowry (Stephen Brooke) and Liz's beau Dr. Anson Kiley (Edward Binns), both only semi-regular characters. The patients and staff of Alden General revealed the racial and occupational mix found in a large metropolitan area: Chinese and Pakistani doctors, black nurses and physicians, Puerto Ricans, writers, teamsters, stevedores, students, social workers, salesmen, and electricians. Although the series reflected the technical advice received from consulting nurses, the dramatic conflict emphasized moral and ethical choices rather than urgent, life-saving interventions. The series remained rather vague about specializations and staff assignments. For example, the floor that Liz Thorpe supervised housed a combination of pediatric, medical, and surgical patients. Dr. Kiley never declared a specialty. By keeping these details vague, the writers could introduce the regular cast into almost any type of health care situation.

Thematic Orientation

It was during the series' first two seasons that the nursing profession received its closest scrutiny. Although nurse characters dominated the action during the first two years, the writers did not focus solely on nursing *per se*. More often than not, stories concerned a moral or ethical issue that transcended any single profession. The stories treated racism, capital punishment, child abuse, abortion, alcoholism, death and dying, and aging, as well as a few light-hearted topics with a comic touch.

Nurse characters often became embroiled in a moral conflict that stemmed from incongruities between personal background or preferences and the responsibilities of the nursing profession. For example, a young, black nurse trying to efface ties with her ghetto background encountered professional difficulties with a black patient who challenged her motives. In another episode, an ex-alcoholic nurse jeopardized her career trying to help an alcoholic patient retain custody of her child. The nurses presented seemed in constant search of the right proportion of sympathy and concern with the right proportion of distance and objectivity. Gail Lucas was especially prone to mixing her personal feelings into professional matters, only to be straightened out by Liz Thorpe.

Thematically, the show pursued a rather consistent path as writers sought to surprise or shock viewers out of making automatic judgments about the guilt or innocence of characters based on deceptive first impressions. The hallmark of the series was a commitment to realism and social concerns. Although the resolution of the conflicts presented did not always satisfy a viewer's desire for a neat ending, in retrospect, the overall dramatic quality of *The Nurses* has not been matched in recent years by many 60-minute dramatic series and certainly not by the 1970s rash of medical-oriented shows, of which *Medical Center* and *Marcus Welby M.D.* were the most successful.

The value of *The Nurses*, however, surpasses the quality of its production in that, above and beyond the good writing, acting, and directing of the show, the series presented to the American public a rare insight into the organization, standards, and responsibilities of the nursing profession. In order to understand what made *The Nurses* such a good nursing drama, it is necessary to analyze several components of the series and compare it, broadly, to the way that other hospital dramas have treated nurses and nursing.

Comparison of *The Nurses* to Analogous Hospital Dramas

Our research into the way in which nurses have been portrayed on television during the past 30 years has generated a large number of indices by which to evaluate these portrayals. When compared to analogous hospital dramas featuring physician characters in leading roles, *The Nurses* emerges as the strongest and most positive series ever to feature nurses in regular roles (4). The routine treatment of nurse characters in most hospital dramas has been appalling. Often, nurses appear only as background scenery, fetching trays and pushing wheelchairs. When nurses do come into contact with physicians and patients, frequently the nurses are shown to be powerless, problem-prone women who cannot solve their own personal problems, much less contribute to the welfare of others.

In physician-dominated hospital dramas, it would appear to the viewer that nurses work under the direct supervision of physicians, who appear to hold the sole responsibility for hiring, firing, promoting, counselling, and otherwise intervening in nursing matters. Nurse characters are judged by how well they serve a doctor. Joe Gannon of *Medical Center* made explicit his opinion that nurses existed for the sole purpose of executing the physician's orders. Nurses sit or stand helplessly by the bedsides of patients, observing doctors do the important tasks of patient care. Furthermore, in most hospital-based dramas, physician characters provide the all important emotional support for their patients, sitting by comatose patients for hours waiting for some response or intervening in family difficulties trying to help a patient. The bulk of television nursing activity occurs behind the nurse's station, where legions of nameless nurses answer phones, pass messages to doctors, and make inscrutable notations in files and on cards.

On *The Nurses,* a totally different view of the profession was given. Many, many episodes pointed to the existence of professional nursing standards, which students strove to reach or by which errant nurses were found wanting. These nursing standards existed independent of any service to a physician. The nurses appeared to be responsible for their own discipline and for the defense of their rights and privileges. Nurses in need of counselling or reprimands usually received them from another nurse character, either a supervisor or instructor. When mistreated by physicians or patients, the nursing administrative support system intervened to protect the nurse from abuse. Nurses were problem solvers in this series rather than helpless amateurs who waited for a physician to arrive on the scene and settle matters. They helped each other with both personal and professional difficulties, and, on several occasions, nurse characters had the audacity to help and to counsel problem-prone physicians!

Nurses seemed eager to advance their profession. In addition to students studying and working to learn, older staff nurses often were shown to learn from experience or to be involved in improving nursing care and standards. The classic virtues associated with nursing—compassion, patience, self-sacrifice—were demonstrated in good quantity, but not to the exclusion of other, less romantic, qualities such as intelligence, objectivity, and articulate speech (5).

Impact on Patient Welfare

These general observations were supported by quantitative analysis. We compared *The Nurses* with other hospital dramas on certain indices of professional activity and personality traits. There was a significant difference in the positive impact on patient welfare between nurse characters in *The Nurses* and in other hospital dramas. Nurse characters on the former took a strong interest in the physical and emotional welfare of their patients and often went beyond the limits of professional obligation to provide special attention and help for individuals.

Inventory of Nursing Activities

The differences appeared significant in many areas of nursing activity, with *The Nurses* consistently demonstrating more instances of nurse characters involved in professional activities. The provision of services by nurses for a patient's physical comfort—bathing, massaging, feeding, fluffing pillows—occurred more than twice as frequently in *The Nurses*. Often, however, these important but less skilled tasks were performed by nursing students—a clear recognition of a division of authority and responsibility within the nursing staff. Thus, Gail Lucas, more often than Liz Thorpe, would be shown feeding her patients, making their beds, or bathing them. In other types of nursing activities, nurses were involved in work requiring higher levels of intelligence and responsibility than was normally assigned to nurses in other television hospital dramas.

The category of "nursing process" included all actions requiring a nurse to translate a patient's needs into a nursing intervention. When nurses were portrayed referring a patient to another health care provider or community service agency, making rounds, assessing a patient's health problem, and the like, they were coded as having demonstrated a nursing process activity.

Only *The Nurses* showed the nursing staff making rounds on a regular basis, usually at a change of shift—indicating to the viewer that the nurses maintained a constant, 24-hour-a-day evaluation of their patients and made sure that each new shift of nurses would be apprised of each patient's condition. When nurses made rounds with doctors, often a nurse would make an observation to a physician, rather than standing mute (as so often occurs in physician-dominated hospital dramas).

The category of emotional support is especially important in realizing the differences between *The Nurses* and analogous hospital dramas. Many viewers recall how assiduous Marcus Welby, Joe Gannon, Jim Kildare, and Ben Casey were in sustaining their patients' good spirits and emotional equanimity. These good doctors would spend hours solving the personal problems of their patients and sitting at bedsides waiting for patients to recover. In *The Nurses*, staff nurses provided this emotional support. Because so much hospital drama rests upon the resolution of emotional difficulties, the provider of emotional support necessarily appears all-important in a patient's recovery.

Liz spent every spare minute at the bedside of a young man dying of aplastic anemia; she monitored the ebb and flow of family and friends visiting her patients; she encouraged another nurse to help a suicidal patient to recover from his despondence; often, she would find ways in which her patients could help each other, as when she engineered a blind priest into helping a blind Jewish boy prepare for his Bar Mitzvah. Moreover, the nurses did not treat all of their patients alike. They determined that some needed a gentle, tender approach, while others profited more from a more impersonal, businesslike manner.

The most glaring distinction between nurses on *The Nurses* and those on other hospital dramas occurred in the field of professional relationships, categorized as "professional resource," and composed of both personal and professional interactions between nurses and other health care providers—doctors in particular. As noted previously, in most hospital dramas, physicians rarely consult or even listen to a nurse's opinion about a patient's condition, and physicians never turn to nurses for help with a personal problem. On the other hand, physicians often do provide emotional support to distressed nurses, who never seem to have any friends among the nursing staff. In *The Nurses*, however, not only were nurse characters shown to enjoy friendship and mutual support within the nursing staff, they also offered suggestions to physicians in a collaborative approach.

The relationships among the nurses in the series almost always expressed friendship, mutual respect, and loyalty to each other, the most important friendship existing between Liz Thorpe and Gail Lucas. But this friendship did not stand on an equal footing, since Gail clearly needed Liz's help and guidance more than Liz needed Gail's dubious contributions. The viewer suspected that Liz saw something of her own girlish idealism and enthusiasm in Gail; the older nurse never failed to save Gail from herself or from other hostile forces. Nearly every episode showed motherly Liz leading Gail from a new debacle, arm around the student's waist, comforting her with words of wisdom. At times, nurses acted as protectors of the doctors as well. In "The Imperfect Prodigy," Liz was the only champion for a brilliant but rude resident who faced expulsion. Gail also defended Dr. Lillian—in one of the two episodes featuring female physicians—who faced great hostility from a male colleague.

Respect and friendship between nurses and physicians were evident, but these relationships remained rather formal. Except for the veteran Liz, the nurses addressed physicians as "Doctor," while the doctors, in turn, addressed the nurses and students as "Miss" or "Mrs." Orders were given and taken in a mutually respectful manner; often a physician complimented a nurse or student if her handling of a given situation merited it. And physicians thanked nurses for their help, even on such minor tasks as passing a tongue blade or fetching a piece of equipment. Physicians were courteous and listened to the nurses' assessments.

Another category related to "professional resource" monitored the instances of nurses providing administrative structure for other nurses—supervision, discipline, dismissal, evaluation, promotion—and demonstrating authority over the activities of aides and orderlies. On *The Nurses,* the existence of a nursing administration appeared much more evident than in other health care series. The viewer became aware of nurses and nursing services as distinct and separate from doctors and medical services. Almost half of all instances of nurses providing administrative services in television hospital dramas between 1950 and 1980 appeared on *The Nurses* between 1962 and 1964.

Moreover, in physician-dominated hospital dramas, doctors exercised control over every aspect of the nursing staff. No hint of a hierarchical arrangement of the nursing staff was given—all nurses were equal, and there was limited evidence of less skilled employees. Alden General Hospital, on the other hand, clearly had a structure of nursing administration that bore responsibility for the control of both staff nurses and the hospital's nursing school. On only two occasions was a nurse disciplined directly by hospital administrators, and even then, nurses intervened to assist the nurse in question. Usually, however, nurses handled nursing problems. For example, in "The Barbara Bowers Story," nursing administrators closely watched a troublesome student, dismissed her from school, and eventually allowed her to return.

Besides the administrative structure, the staff nurses clearly stood on a higher professional plane than the orderlies and nurses' aides also seen in *The Nurses*. With regard to patient care, the nurse gave the orders to the support staff; there was no question of the head nurse's authority on her unit. Liz Thorpe ran her unit efficiently; she arranged staffing schedules and monitored the work of her nurses, while addressing any problems that arose. She also served as supervisor and informal clinical instructor for the nursing students on her floor.

The dimensions of nursing education are rarely explored on any hospital drama. Candy stripers and nursing students occasionally landed in the paternal nets of Joe Gannon, Ben Casey, or Marcus Welby, but viewers were never brought to any understanding of the nature of the nursing education. In *Medical Center*, set in a university hospital, nursing students appeared to be taught by physicians and "trained" in a manner reminiscent of a diploma school rather than a university. Furthermore, doctors took charge of handling nursing school matters.

Alden General Hospital ran a three-year diploma school program for nurses; *The Nurses* far surpassed other health care dramas in the depiction of nursing education activities. Few scenes of classroom instruction were shown, but often nursing students appeared carrying books, at least suggesting to the viewer that nurses learned by theoretical means as well as by practical experience. Clinical instruction on *The Nurses* was rarely shown in a formal setting, but dozens of instances of staff nurses correcting nursing students did occur. *The Nurses*, produced in the early 1960s, reflected traditional ways of educating registered nurses; there was never any mention made of nurses who possessed a baccalaureate education. (It will be interesting to see if the new series, *Nurse*, identifies the diversity of educational preparation for nursing.)

Personal Attributes of Nurse Characters

Beyond the actual activities in which nurses engaged on *The Nurses*, the producers and writers of the series presented nurse characters as strong, intelligent, ambitious women, far removed from the passive, powerless, and intellectually limited nurse characters seen in most hospital dramas. Nurse characters in *The Nurses* expressed primarily values of achievement, integrity, and desire for a better world far more often than in most health care dramas. In the other dramas, physician characters were associated with these values much more often than nurse characters. The nurse characters stood for the status quo; they seemed to revel in the application of rules and regulations, even when breaking a rule might achieve a more important goal and significantly improve the welfare of another. These nurses rarely contradicted doctors, even when the doctors seemed to be in the wrong.

On *The Nurses,* nurse characters sought to live up to their values and goals through their own actions, not merely help a physician live up to his values. Liz Thorpe personified integrity for the series. Episode after episode, the viewer witnessed her insistence upon high standards of professional service from both her subordinates and herself.

Intelligence was another attribute characteristic of the nurses in the series. Liz Thorpe talked of books, poetry, and travel; her speech was graceful and articulate. Another nurse on the program once immersed herself in the scientific literature on an experimental drug. Although conclusions she formed caused her to be dismissed for disobeying a doctor's order, she maintained a posture of honesty, integrity, and altruism—she claimed she would have done the same thing again.

While there were indications of intellectual interests, a great number of disturbed and troubled nurses did appear on *The Nurses.* This fact angered members of the nursing profession (6). At various times, Liz Thorpe encountered sadistic, ex-Nazi, alcoholic, drug-addicted, bigoted, and unmarried pregnant nurses. Despite this formidable list of undesirables, the series, for the most part, carefully maintained the positive image of the profession by emphasizing how aberrant these women were and, most importantly, how the nursing profession managed to identify and weed out undesirable people from the practice of nursing. These aberrant nurse characters also turned up on physician-oriented hospital shows, but without the presence of other, admirable nurses to balance the presentation.

In sum, *The Nurses'* greatest contribution to the image of nursing was its consistent presentation of nursing as an autonomous profession that generated its own standards and conducted its own affairs. Furthermore, the standards and values associated with nursing equalled those associated with the medical profession. The women who worked as nurses in this series actively sought solutions for both personal and professional difficulties.

Of course, there were weaknesses in the series, perhaps exaggerated now by the passing of time. The diploma school environment of *The Nurses* still emphasized practical experience more than theoretical instruction. Gail Lucas was oftentimes unbelievable in her innocence and naiveté and her mistakes of judgment might not be tolerated in real life. So many aberrant, troubled nursing characters appearing in a single hospital, let alone a single ward, did strain credibility. But when compared to analogous health care dramas, *The Nurses* remains the single, bright star of television programming with regard to the presentation of a strong and positive image of the profession.

Conclusion

In 1964, in an attempt to improve ratings, the show was re-christened *The Doctors and the Nurses* and, in effect, two male actors took over the leading roles, leaving Liz and Gail as important but secondary characters. In addition to casting innovations, the producers changed the tone of the series from an often thoughtful, discursive examination of a single issue to a more action-oriented format, with many more instances of violence, crime, and life-saving heroics featured. The network really wanted a medical show more in keeping with the enormously popular *Ben Casey* and *Dr. Kildare,* and sacrificed an original, quality drama about women and nursing to this end. This format revision did not improve the ratings significantly, and the series was cancelled at the end of the 1964–65 season.

Nurses throughout the country probably can do very little to assure the success of the new series, *Nurse.* As with every other television program, it will prosper or perish according to the iron law of the Nielsen ratings. Should the series survive, however, the producers might be susceptible to influence from individual nurses and nursing organizations, if nurse response is widespread and constructive.

The retrospective analysis of *The Nurses* provides several key issues to look for in the new series and by which to judge the image of the nursing profession. Generally, nurse-viewers should be sensitive to philosophical and professional issues rather than to technical accuracy. Whether or not a nurse character sets up an I.V. drip properly will have little impact upon the general viewer's perception of the nursing profession. The overall presentation of the nurse and her actions, on the other hand, will affect the way viewers see the profession as a whole. A brief checklist of things to consider in evaluating the program is as follows:

- Is there evidence of a nursing administrative structure in the hospital setting? That is, do nurses conduct their own personnel matters, such as hiring, firing, promoting, and disciplining?
- Are the nurse characters generally reflective of educated women? That is, do they appear to be articulate, well-read, perceptive? Is there a recognition of the variety of nurses' educational programs and of the role of advanced education for nurses?
- Are nurse characters problem solvers or do they take their problems to non-nurses, namely, to physicians?
- Do physicians and nurses interact in a collegial fashion about patient care in joint planning?
- Do nurse characters assert their rights and demand respect? Do they seek to advance themselves and their profession? Do they express altruistic, humanitarian values and act accordingly?
- Is there a professional nurse who serves as a consultant for the series? (Two registered nurses worked with the writing and production staff of *The Nurses*, one as advisor to the writers, inculcating in them sensitivity to the philosophy of nursing, the second on the set, advising the production crew on technical authenticity.)

The heritage of *The Nurses*, the past generation's singularly positive depiction of the profession, is an important one. Almost always, nurses have not been deemed important enough to hold the major roles in health care dramas. Instead, numerous primetime series featured male physicians as the principal characters and superheroes. Herbert Brodkin, the producer of *The Nurses*, was fully cognizant of the fact that writers, directors, and actors create a powerful point of view that shapes public images and ideas about nurses and their roles in health care (7). Building on this constructive tradition, the creators of the nurse dramas of the 1980s have it in their power to add to or avoid the overwhelmingly negative stereotypical and inaccurate portrayals of nurses that have characterized most television programming.

Notes

1. *Variety*, September 17, 1980, p. 58, identifies only six out of 291 made-for-TV movies doing better in the Nielsen ratings: *Guyana Tragedy: The Story of Jim Jones* (2 parts); *Kenny Rogers As The Gambler;*

Scruples (2 parts); *Carnival of Thrills; Tenspeed and Brown Shoe;* and *Aunt Mary. Nurse,* shown on April 9, earned a Nielsen rating of 24.3 and garnered a 39 audience share.

2. An introduction to research on the effect of television may be found in: G. Comstock, M. Fisher, *Television and Human Behavior: A Guide to the Pertinent Scientific Literature* (Santa Monica, California: Rand Corporation, 1975); G. Comstock, F. G. Christen, M. L. Fisher, R. C. Quarles, W. D. Richards, *Television and Human Behavior: The Key Studies* (Santa Monica, California: Rand Corporation, 1975); and G. Comstock, S. Chaffee, N. Katzman, M. McCombs, D. Roberts, *Television and Human Behavior* (New York: Columbia University Press, 1978).

Examples of studies on the portrayal of women and minorities on television are: M. L. Long, R. J. Simon, "The roles and statuses of women and children on family TV programs," *Journalism Quarterly* (1974) 51:107–10; M. M. Miller, B. Reeves, "Dramatic TV content and children's sex-role stereotypes," *Journal of Broadcasting* (1976) 20:35–50; H. C. Northcott, J. F. Seggar, J. L. Hinton, "Trends in TV portrayal of blacks and women," *Journalism Quarterly* (1975) 52:741–44; C. G. O'Kelly, L. E. Bloomquist, "Women and blacks on TV," *Journal of Communications* (1976) 26(4): 179–84; and G. Tuchman, A. K. Daniels, J. Benet, eds., *Hearth and Home: Images of Women in the Mass Media* (New York: Oxford, 1978).

3. Schorr, T., "Nursing's TV Image," *AJN,* Vol. 63:10, Oct. 1963, p. 120.

4. For the purposes of this article, *The Nurses* was compared to analogous health care dramas—series of a dramatic nature featuring physicians in leading roles. Excluded were situation comedies and action-adventure programs that featured nurses as regular characters. The series included such series as *Ben Casey* (ABC, 1961–1966); *The Bold Ones* (NBC, 1969–1973); *Doctor Hudson's Secret Journal* (syndicated, 1955); *Dr. Kildare* (NBC, 1961–1966); *Doctors Hospital* (NBC, 1975–1976); *The Interns* (CBS, 1970–1971); *Marcus Welby, M.D.* (ABC, 1969–1976); *Medic* (NBC, 1954–1956); *Medical Center* (CBS, 1969–1976); *Medical Story* (NBC, 1975–1976); *Rafferty* (CBS, 1977); *Trapper John, M.D.* (CBS, 1979–present); *Westside Medical* (ABC, 1977); and *Young Dr. Kildare* (syndicated, 1972).

5. All of these behavioral traits were found to be significantly (at the *p* <.05) more in evidence in *The Nurses* as contrasted with other health care dramas.

6. *Ibid.,* p. 119.

7. Efron, E., "Realist Faces Reality," *TV Guide,* Vol. 13:38, Sept. 18, 1965, p. 19–22.

II

The Ethical Dimension in Patient Care

8. Introduction— Dilemmas Inherent in the American Nurses' Association Code of Ethics

Bonnie Bullough and Vern Bullough

American Nurses' Association
Code for Nurses (1976)*

The Code for Nurses is based upon belief about the nature of individuals, nursing, health, and society. Recipients and providers of nursing services are viewed as individuals and groups who possess basic rights and responsibilities, and whose values and circumstances command respect at all times. Nursing encompasses the promotion and restoration of health, the prevention of illness, and the alleviation of suffering. The statements of the Code and their interpretation provide guidance for conduct and relationships in carrying out nursing responsibilities consistent with the ethical obligations of the profession and quality in nursing care.

1. The nurse provides services with respect for human dignity and the uniqueness of the client unrestricted by considerations of social or economic status, personal attributes, or the nature of health problems.
2. The nurse safeguards the client's right to privacy by judiciously protecting information of a confidential nature.
3. The nurse acts to safeguard the client and the public when health care and safety are affected by the incompetent, unethical, or illegal practice of any person.
4. The nurse assumes responsibility and accountability for individual nursing judgments and actions.
5. The nurse maintains competence in nursing.
6. The nurse exercises informed judgment and uses individual competence and qualifications as criteria in seeking consultation, accepting responsibilities, and delegating nursing activities to others.

*Reproduced with permission of the American Nurses' Association.

89

7. The nurse participates in activities that contribute to the ongoing development of the profession's body of knowledge.

8. The nurse participates in the profession's efforts to implement and improve standards of nursing.

9. The nurse participates in the profession's efforts to establish and maintain conditions of employment conducive to high quality nursing care.

10. The nurse participates in the profession's efforts to protect the public from misinformation and misrepresentation and to maintain the integrity of nursing.

11. The nurse collaborates with members of the health professions and other citizens in promoting community and national efforts to meet the health needs of the public.

The code of ethics adopted by the American Nurses' Association in 1976 is for the most part noncontroversial and straightforward. Almost all nurses would agree that they should safeguard the client's right to privacy, maintain their own competence, work to achieve high standards of care, collaborate effectively with other health care workers, attempt to expand the body of knowledge of the profession, maintain employment conditions that are conducive to good care, inform the public about hazards, and work with others for the good of society. The problems arise because of dilemmas inherent in those sections of this code where the duty of the nurse is not always clear—when there is no clear path to follow because there is right on both sides of the issue.

Human Dignity: The Right to Live versus the Right to Die

For example, the first statement in the code indicates that

> the nurse provides services with respect for human dignity and the uniqueness of the client unrestricted by considerations of social or economic status, personal attributes, or the nature of health problems.

This suggests not only that nondiscriminatory care will be provided but also that the dignity of the individual will be preserved. Unfortunately, modern science has created some situations in which the preservation of the dignity of the individual is not always possible. In the past one of the assumptions made by health care personnel was that the end, life itself, justified any means we might use to preserve it. Now scientific and technological advances have proliferated the treatment modalities that can be used to prolong life and the result is that interventions often leave painful side effects. In some cases patients can be kept alive for years in a suspended or comatose state. Should life be prolonged when rehabilitative or restorative goals are not achievable? Who determines how much suffering the patient should endure to live? What are the legal and ethical issues involved?

The answers remain ambiguous although in the past decade the legal system has been trying to sort out some of the legal issues. Forcing public attention on the problem was the well-publicized case of Karen Quinlan. The 22-year-old Ms. Quinlan lapsed into a coma from unknown causes, suffering irreversible brain damage. Her death was prevented by the use of a respirator. After several months of watching his daughter remain technically alive but in a vegetative coma, Mr. Quinlan petitioned the New Jersey Superior Court to appoint him a guardian for the ultimate purpose of withdrawing the respirator, an act that all parties thought would result in her death. The lower court denied his petition but it eventually was granted by the New Jersey Supreme Court in an opinion accepting the belief that the right to privacy included the right to decline medical treatment. Given her incompetent state, the right to speak for her could be given to her guardian. The respirator was turned off, although she did not die; at this writing she still lives (In re Quinlan, 1975, 1976).

The other well-known case is that of Joseph Saikewicz, a profoundly retarded man. His case also brings up the issue of disability. At the age of 67 Mr. Saikewicz was diagnosed as having terminal leukemia. Routine management would have been chemotherapy. There was general agreement that such treatment probably would have resulted in a remission lasting between 2 and 13 months. It also would have resulted in the usual side effects and discomfort of chemotherapy. Based on the patient's inability to understand the situation or provide informed consent, the superintendent of the state school he lived in petitioned the courts to be appointed as Mr. Saikewicz's guardian in order to decline the treatment. The courts granted that right, holding that the patient's right to privacy included a right to avoid unwarranted infringement on his bodily integrity even if that infringement would give him extra months of life (Superintendent of Belchertown State School v Saikewicz 370 NE2d at p. 419).

The effect of these two court decisions is to support the belief that it is not necessary to preserve life at all cost. Yet there are also contrary rulings. More recently, for example, a California child, Philip Becker, became the subject of a complex case involving some of the same ethical and legal issues. Philip had been institutionalized most of his life because of the mental retardation associated with Down's syndrome. He also had a congenital heart defect for which surgery was advised. For several years his parents fought a court battle to prevent such surgery because they were worried about the quality of his life if he survived them. They argued that without the intervention of modern surgical techniques nature would have taken its course and given Philip an early death. When a judge agreed with them the surgery was stopped. However, another unrelated couple who had visited Philip and brought him to their home for cub scout meetings and similar activities petitioned the court to gain custody of Philip in order to have the surgery done. In this they were successful and the cardiac surgery was performed (Will, 1981).

While these well-argued cases give some guidance, the ethical decisions nurses are called on to make relative to prolonging life seldom reach the courts. Instead the decisions are more immediate and they usually involve whether or not to give large doses of narcotics to patients with slow respirations who are in severe pain, or whether or not to vigorously resuscitate comatose patients or patients suffering from significant pain. In those states where a living will is recognized, the decision is sometimes made easier because the opinion of the patient stated at an earlier time can give guidance. Still, living wills remain rare enough that the decision ordinarily falls to the physician, nurse, and family. Sometimes a "no code" (do not resuscitate) order is given verbally but is not written, so that nurses worry about their legal liability as well as their ethical responsibility. Though nurses and physicians are very rarely punished for any failure to use heroic measures (Russell, 1975), punishment is always a possibility that nurses need to entertain.

Reporting Other Health Workers for Incompetence or Negligence

A second area of controversy in the code of ethics is contained in the third statement.

> The nurse acts to safeguard the client and the public when health care and safety are affected by the incompetent, unethical or illegal practice of any person.

This is the kind of statement that is easy to make but difficult to operationalize. Most nurse narcotic addicts or alcoholics go through a long process of deterioration before they are brought to the attention of the state board of nursing (Bissell and Jones, 1981). People hesitate to get involved. Hospitals transfer or fire nurses but hesitate to do the necessary paper work or gather the data to bring charges against them. It is perhaps in the nature of most of us to avoid policing our colleagues. The nurse who does so will often be unpopular with colleagues. Consequently, even poor nursing care is seldom reported to the supervisor. Rarely is the nurse who catnaps through most of the night shift reported. This statement in the code places an onerous but necessary duty on members of the profession.

But if it is difficult to report a nursing colleague, it is even more difficult to report a physician for neglect or incompetence. Such an action involves not only breaking old habit patterns but facing the threat of punishment by the physician-dominated health care institutions, yet physician negligence is not at all uncommon. While one of the editors of this book was a student nurse he observed a group of residents, medical students, and x-ray technicians spend 4 hours trying to insert a probe into the artery of an aged male who was half conscious and complaining of severe discomfort. The supervising professor was in and out of the area, carefully explaining where the students had gone wrong in their technique but ignoring the patient who continued to suffer. So involved were the physicians and students that they seemed to forget that the patient was a living and breathing human. The patient, who had not been catheterized, became incontinent and was very embarrassed. Then and only then did they put on a condom catheter. He was kept in an abnormal, uncomfortable position, and though he was partially anesthetized he was fearful, anxious, and moaning. Only when the nursing instructor launched a formal complaint did the group become conscious of what they were doing to the patient. If she had not been forceful enough, however, the attempted procedure might have continued for several more hours. After her complaint the medical professor intervened and quickly completed the procedure, and the instructor was not punished. While learning is important to the professionals, so is the patient, and the patient must of necessity come first to the nurse.

The third area of controversy within the code is raised by the fourth statement:

The nurse assumes responsibility and accountability for individual nursing judgments and actions.

This is a controversial position because of past norms which held the physician accountable for nursing actions. Thus this becomes as much a legal controversy as an ethical one. The changing trends in the law which highlight this issue are covered in Section V of this book. Inevitably, as nurses we will have to face making more of the difficult decisions including those with ethical dimensions. Ethics in today's world are not always absolute. Much is left to the individual and decisions are dependent on the situation in which one finds oneself. It is best to think about some of the ethical dilemmas before they happen, but the key to an effective ethical decision is to think about and know what you are and what you stand for before the need to make a decision arises.

References

Bissell L. C. and Jones, R. W. "The Alcoholic Nurse," *Nursing Outlook* 29 (February 1981):96–101.

In re Quinlan, 137 N.J. Supp 227 revd 70 NV 10 (1975).

In re Quinlan, 355 A 2d 647 (1976).

Russell, O. R. *Freedom to Die: Moral and Legal Aspects of Euthanasia.* New York: Human Sciences Press, 1975.

Superintendent of Belchertown State School v Saikewicz, Mass. 370 Ne2d.

Will, George F. "A Trip Towards Death," *Newsweek* (August 31, 1981):72.

9. Ethics of Nurse-Patient Relationships

Mila Ann Aroskar

This article discusses four possible models as bases for ethical nurse-patient relationships: priestly, engineering, contractual and collegial.

The author describes how educators can use these models in providing learning experiences that enable students to: (1) articulate and clarify values; (2) understand ethical traditions and positions as they affect decision-making; (3) think systematically and reflectively about ethical issues and dilemmas in nursing and health care.

"Many patients know more about ethical issues than nurses do," a nursing student recently told me. I had asked her why she enrolled in my course on nursing and ethical issues. Her thought-provoking remark cannot be verified with empirical data. But it might be important for nursing educators to consider its implications when evaluating curricula. Do present nursing curricula provide learning opportunities for students to think systematically about the ethical issues and dilemmas in nursing and health care which confront nurses and patients?

In a study completed in 1976, the majority of respondents from baccalaureate schools said that ethical and moral decisions were integrated in some way into every nursing course (1). However, does this answer mean that the students have the opportunity to reflect on ethical issues and dilemmas in nursing in relation to traditional ethical theories and positions? Does it mean that they articulate ethical positions and consider the pros and cons of a particular ethical stance in a given nurse/patient relationship when there is conflict over the right or best thing to do, such as assist in sterilization of a mentally retarded person or provide less than vigorous care for

Reprinted with permission: "Ethics of Nurse-Patient Relationships" by M. M. Aroskar. *Nurse Educator* 5(2):18–20, 1980.

a severely deformed newborn? Nursing students constantly observe and participate in clinical nursing practice. But do they have planned opportunities to analyze and think reflectively about what *should* be occurring in nurse-patient relationships?

This article explores available ethical relationship models and related curriculum considerations. Although there are ethical issues for nurses and nursing at all levels (individual, group, institution and community), the author focuses primarily on the individual nurse-patient relationship.

Ethical Relationship Models

Robert Veatch, a philosopher, proposes four models for looking at ethical relationships. Although he developed these models in regard to physician-patient relationships, they can also be applied to nurse-patient and nurse-colleague bonds. Veatch's models have particular implications for nursing as nurses seek more autonomy and accountability in terms of nurse-patient and nurse-colleague relationships. However, they may need modification related to the nurse's position as employee in a bureaucratic setting and the variety of roles in which the nurse engaged (patient advocate, aid to the physician, staff member, and autonomous professional).

Priestly Model

One proposed model for an ethical relationship is the frankly paternalistic "priestly model" (2). The patient comes for counsel, treatment, and comfort, and expects to cooperate with the health professional in achieving the goal of getting well. The health professional makes all necessary decisions without actively considering the patient's values. This model is generally invoked when physicians are perceived as "playing God" or the nurse says "speaking as a nurse, I definitely think you should undergo this procedure for your own good."

Of course, one can think of times when this model might be more appropriate than some of the others, such as when a patient is comatose. However, even that situation does not always mean that the health professional should be the only or primary decision maker. Health professionals do have certain expertise that enables them to make important decisions, but nothing in their background or education gives them the right to make moral decisions affecting other persons.

Engineering Model

A second model is the engineering model. Here the health professional is viewed as an applied scientist divorced from value considerations. The health professional simply presents all the facts to the patient who then makes up his own mind. For example, if physicians give patients "all the facts," nurses simply reinforce these facts without attempting to tell the patients what they "ought" to do (3). Essentially, the health professionals set aside their own codes of moral values and do what patients wish.

A major shortcoming of this model, as viewed by Veatch, is that health professionals become no more than plumbers cleaning out drains, as they service the wishes of patients. An example is the nurse who does not believe in abortion, but participates without question in carrying them out. This example also demonstrates how nurses may set aside their own values to service the system. Health professionals often find that operating under the engineering model, where they are primarily means to achieving ends, is dehumanizing. Such behavior opposes the Kantian ethic which says that a person should always be treated as an end not simply as a means. In order to deal with these difficulties, Veatch suggests another model, the "contractual model."

Contractual Model

Under the contractual model, the contract (sometimes called a covenant) between the patient and the health professional identifies general obligations and benefits for both patient and health professional (4). This model may be more familiar and even more appropriate to nurse practitioners and community health nurses than to nurses on, for example, an intensive care unit. Under this model, patients are viewed as having control over the significant decisions affecting their own lives and bodies. Both patients and health professionals are considered as ends, not simply as means to an end (the health of the patient). The aspects of care related to values are articulated and the health professional takes no major action without consulting the patient. However, the patient is aware that the health professional has the skills to make technical decisions to reach general goals that have been agreed upon. The patient, therefore, does not expect to be consulted on all the technical details of care and treatment.

Health professionals also have the right not to make a contract in the first place if it involves them in a morally abhorrent act. However, this right or option is not always accorded if it denies the patient care and treatment which is routine and acceptable or if there are no other appropriate health professionals in the area. An example is the nurse practitioner in a rural area who does not personally believe that abortion is a moral option, but is asked by a client for information about abortion alternatives.

The contractual model considers the values of both the health professional and the patient. Ryden offers an example of this model in which a nursing student identifies an ethical dilemma with a patient who needs to have a pacemaker replaced (5). The student articulates her own values and helps the patient come to a decision reflecting his own values.

Although it has many attributes, the contractual model has some obvious problems. One is that in most work settings nurses are employees rather than independent agents. Another is that many patients cannot articulate goals and values for themselves. The model also presents potential difficulties for physicians if a team of physicians, rather than a single one, is responsible for patient care. However, in spite of these difficulties, the contractual model or a modification of it, is often the most effective route to resolution of ethical dilemmas.

Collegial Model

The last model discussed by Veatch is the "collegial model" in which patient and health professional share mutual goals and act as "pals" (6). Veatch views this arrangement as highly idealistic and probably unrealistic in many situations. However, the model has potential in certain situations—particularly when a health care team and a patient are involved in reaching a decision through consensus and discussion. Such team efforts are most often found in rehabilitation and mental health care settings.

Curriculum Considerations

Each model provides a framework for the values held by the nurse, the patient, and the larger society. Examples of such values follow. Although we may not consider all of them to be positive forces, they do exist and need to be considered. They include: the individual's right to freedom and self-determination; the nurse's obligation to follow doctor's orders; the need to be truthful; the need to look at consequences of actions; the use of coercion to achieve certain ends; the responsibility and accountability of members of the profession; and the role of the nurse as a moral agent.

By incorporating discussion of the proposed models and their implications for nursing practice into the curriculum, educators provide students with the opportunity to think reflectively about nursing decisions and actions. Students can practice applying the insights thus gained to theoretical dilemmas encountered by nurses and nursing students, such as the process of obtaining informed consent. Such discussions might use an "ethical rounds" or a pre- and post-clinical conference format. Or they can be integrated into study of nursing process, development of nursing care plans, or analysis of the constraints which bureaucratic settings impose on nurses' ethical behavior.

For example, using the latter format the following question might be addressed: "What are the implications for the individual nurse as a person and for the nursing profession, of nurses consistently choosing to base relationships with patients on the engineering model, thus abdicating the nurse's *moral* responsibility?"

Setting Objectives

In teaching ethics in nursing, as in teaching any subject area, faculty first need to set objectives for the teaching/learning experience. This process will generate much discussion about the appropriateness of specific goals and objectives, for educators may fear that their objectives reflect a specific morality or religious position. Some specific suggestions of useful objectives for a course in ethics follow:

- to analyze critical issues in health care ethics.
- to distinguish between different ethical theories.
- to use ethical theories in analysis of identified ethical dilemmas in nursing.
- to recognize and articulate ethical issues and dilemmas in the delivery of nursing care at various system levels.
- to use a framework of analysis for ethical decision making in nursing practice.
- to identify implications of selected ethical approaches for nursing practice in bureaucratic settings.
- to identify values which underlie decisions and actions in ethical dilemmas confronted by nurses.

It is possible that consideration of these and other related objectives will lead to identification of conflicting faculty values in terms of the time students should spend in critical reflective thinking as opposed to the time they spend learning to apply specific skills and solve concrete problems. Although raising this question may be initially problematic, dealing with it is generally productive for faculty and students.

Meeting Objectives

Once objectives have been identified, the next step is to consider how and where they can be met most effectively in the nursing curriculum. Should this content be taught in interdisciplinary or in intradisciplinary learning settings, in courses on professionalization, or in classes on issues and trends? The author has found that selected objectives can be met in the interdisciplinary experience. Such objectives include analyzing general ethical issues and dilemmas in health care and differentiating ethical theories and approaches. However, if teaching is primarily interdisciplinary, nursing students also need concurrent or prior experiences where they discuss ethical issues and dilemmas in relation to the nursing process and the nurse's complex position in most bureaucratic settings in relation to other health professionals. Nursing students also need to have the opportunity to debate and argue stated ethical positions with other nurses. These might be positions taken by individual nurses or positions taken by the professional organization.

If the nursing curriculum requires students to take medical ethics courses offered by philosophy departments, it is important that nursing faculty identify the objectives of these courses in order to determine if and how they meet or overlap with objectives in the nursing curricula. Often such courses are more oriented to analysis of physician-patient than nurse-patient relationships.

Additional Considerations

The prior discussion offers some general consideration for looking at a present or proposed curriculum in terms of planned opportunities for students to think systematically about ethical issues in nursing specifically and in health care generally. In addition, faculty involved in this process need to consider two other factors.

First, it is important that nursing faculty identify their individual and collective strengths and weaknesses in the area of nursing and ethics. They need to ask themselves if they can effectively delineate and teach nursing problems and issues from a philosophical and ethical perspective. They need to determine whether it would be better to co-teach with a philosopher, at least in relation to some objectives. In my experience, co-teaching has been fruitful and co-teaching endeavors have received positive evaluations from participating faculty and students.

Second, discussion of how ethical situations are currently handled within the health care system, and how the nurse interfaces with that system, should be built into curriculum planning. Methods by which nurses can work together to bring about positive change in dealing with ethical dilemmas can be examined. In other words, educators should not increase students' frustration by teaching the "ideal way to do it," without also helping them to develop collegial networks that support their right to practice nursing according to the ethical standards they are learning.

Conclusion

Articulation and clarification of values, awareness of ethical traditions and positions as they affect decision-making, and planned opportunities to think systematically and reflectively about ethical issues and dilemmas in nursing and health care actually constitute only the beginning of education for nurses in this broad area. Goals and objectives can eventually reach beyond those outlined in this article as determined by providers and consumers of health care. The expansion of nursing knowledge and awareness in the area of ethics could have an enormous influence on the existing health care system.

References

1. Aroskar, M. Ethics in nursing curriculum. *Nursing Outlook*, 25:260–264, April, 1977.
2. Veatch, Robert. "Models for Ethical Medicine in a Revolutionary Age," *Hastings Center Report*, 2:5–6, June, 1972.
3. Veatch, 1972, p.5.
4. Veatch, 1972, p. 6.
5. Ryden, M. B. An approach to ethical decision making. *Nursing Outlook*, 26:705–706, November, 1978.
6. Veatch, 1972, p. 6.

10. Reporting Incompetent Colleagues II: "Will I Be Sued for Defamation?"

Jane Greenlaw

Talking about one's colleagues is a common practice in all employment settings. In the health care setting, one popular topic of conversation is evaluating and comparing the professional competencies of the various personnel.

When a nurse is aware that a colleague has made an error in judgment, or has failed to follow proper procedure, or has harmed a patient in some way, the nurse often chooses to share this information informally with other colleagues, rather than to report it through official channels. The rationale for this approach is generally that informal talking will do no one harm, while reporting through official channels may bring destructive disciplinary action upon the colleague, result in a lawsuit for defamation[1] against the reporting nurse, or both. The problems with this rationale are illustrated by a recent New York court case.

The case, *Malone v. Longo*,[2] evolved from a disagreement between two Veterans Administration nurses over a medication order. Nurse Malone interpreted an order which read "MgSO$_4$ 1cc" (magnesium sulfate) as calling for morphine, and asked Nurse Longo (an LPN) to give an injection of morphine to the patient. The two nurses have different versions of what happened next, but it is agreed that Longo, detecting the error, refused to give the morphine, Malone ultimately ascertained the correct order, and the patient received the proper medication. Later, Malone became aware that Longo had told another nurse of the incident, and warned her not to discuss it with others. This confrontation escalated to an argument in which the charge nurse intervened, sug-

Greenlaw, J. "Reporting Incompetent Colleagues II: 'Will I Be Sued for Defamation?' " *Nursing Law and Ethics* (May 1980):5. Reprinted with permission of the American Society of Law and Medicine, Boston, MA., and the author.

gesting that a report be made. The following day, the head nurse told Malone, Longo and the charge nurse to each file separate reports. The reports resulted in the placing of a letter of admonishment in Malone's official file where it would remain for six months to two years.

Malone then filed suit against Longo for defamation, seeking $12,000 in damages. The complaint alleged two specific defamatory remarks—first, that Longo told a third party, "Malone told me to give a medication that she did not have an order for, and insisted upon me giving that order," and second, that in Longo's written report was the statement, "She proceeded to tell me that I was not to question her on the doctor's orders." Prior to trial, Longo moved for summary judgment in her favor, asserting two defenses: that the remarks were true (a complete defense in most states) and that they were privileged (made in her capacity as a federal official and thus could not be the basis of a lawsuit against her even if false).

The court granted Longo's motion as to the remark contained in her report, finding that the privilege protection applied. Since Longo was directed by her superiors to make the report, it was part of her official duties. The nurse, as a federal employee, was immune from lawsuits for defamation "for acts taken within the outer perimeter" of her official duties.[3] The court explained that such a privilege was *not* an "emolument of exalted office" but rather was "an expression of a policy designed to promote effective government." As such, it extended to "lower federal officials" (including nurses). The court also concluded that there was no question that statements made in the context of a disciplinary proceeding "which the official is under a duty to complete, are within the scope of the official's duties." Indeed the court noted that refusal to file such a report when requested might itself be cause for disciplinary proceedings against the nurse.

As for the remark made to the third party, the court rejected both of Longo's claims. The defense of privilege could not apply if the remark was not made as part of her official duties. And the defense of truth was not established without a trial since Malone contended that the remark was false. It remains for a full trial to determine these issues, and to determine what damages, if any, Malone is entitled to receive.

The lesson to be learned from this case is that nurses must act responsibly when sharing information which could harm a colleague. A nurse has a duty to report, through official channels, a colleague whom the nurse reasonably believes is negligent or incompetent. But the distinction made by the court in the *Malone* case— between a remark made in the official report and one made to a third party—is an important one. Longo could not be held liable for the remark in the report *even if it were false,* because the remark was privileged. A non-federal-employee nurse, making a similar report through official channels, would probably be afforded a similar legal protection provided that the nurse was reasonable in believing it to be true—because public policy requires nurses to protect patients from negligent or incompetent colleagues.

Responsible reporting of colleague incompetence or negligence helps everyone. The patient is protected from harm. The hospital is aided in fulfilling its legal responsibility to monitor performance in order to assure good and accepted medical care for its patients. The colleague is given an opportunity to recognize possible deficiencies in his performance, as well as to respond to any charges against him in a fair proceeding. And the reporting nurse has fulfilled her duty to protect the patient.

Non-official remarks or gossip about colleagues, on the other hand, help no one and can irreparably hurt the colleague. Even if true, such remarks serve no useful purpose. If false or ambiguous, they may be considered defamatory and form the basis for a lawsuit against the irresponsible talker.

References

1. Defamation is a broad term which includes written statements, termed libel, and oral statements, termed slander. Slander lawsuits are less common since they are more difficult to prove.
2. 463 F. Supp. 139 (E.D.N.Y. 1979).
3. Barr v. Matteo, 360 U.S. 564 (1959).

11. The Consumer's Perception of Nursing Care

Russell C. Swansburg

Who are the consumers of nursing? They are adults and children of all ages; rich people and poor; people of all races and religions; people who are well and want to stay that way and people who are ill and want to regain their health. Even the providers of nursing care can become consumers of its services. Consumers and potential consumers of nursing services are children of the United States whose values will be molded by their idols, their role models, their teachers, their parents, their peers—all with whom they come in contact.

Consumers of nursing are the workers in the shipbuilding yards of Mississippi, Virginia, Pennsylvania and Maine who have been insulating ships with asbestos and who now are concerned with the possibility of developing cancer. Consumers are pregnant mothers living near the nuclear plant at Three Mile Island in Pennsylvania who wonder about the danger of radiation from the nuclear accident. Consumers of nursing are neighbors, friends, relatives, lovers, citizens and workers.

In 1975 the 93rd Congress enacted Public Law 93-641, the "National Health Planning and Resources Development Act of 1974," to finance the establishment of Health System Agencies in every state. This law states that (1) A majority (but not more than 60 per centum of the members) shall be residents of the health service area served by the entity who are consumers of health care and who are not (nor within the twelve months preceding appointment have not been) providers of health care and who are broadly representative of the social, economic, linguistic and racial populations, geographic areas of the health service area, and major purchasers of health care; (2) The remainder of the members

Swansburg, Russell C. "The Consumer's Perception of Nursing Care." *Supervisor Nurse* (May 1981):30–33. Reprinted with permission of *Nursing Management* and the author.

shall be residents of the health service area served by the agency
who are providers of health care and who represent physicians
(particularly practicing physicians), dentists, nurses and other
health professionals.[1]

The provider of health care is further defined as "a direct
provider of health care including a physician, dentist, nurse, po-
diatrist, or physician assistant . . ." or an " . . . indirect provider of
health care . . ." with a fiduciary position or fiduciary interest in
the health care industry or whose spouse receives more than one-
tenth of gross annual income from the health care industry.[2]

By law nurses and their families are included in the group
defined as providers of health care. Also, by law, the planning of
all the health care in this nation has been placed in the hands of
consumers with a proviso for nurse providers among others to
support them in their efforts to identify and provide all health
care services, including nursing care. What an opportunity for
professional nursing!

What Is Perception?

Communication is perception; sound is created by perception, the
audible aspect of it is voice. Communication and, hence, perception occurs only if the receiver (a nurse provider or a consumer of
nursing care) receives and understands sensory stimulation. This
consumer or provider must receive the message through hearing
or through nonverbal language such as gestures, environment,
cultural and social referents, feeling, smelling, seeing and tasting.
Consumers and providers learn what they are capable of hearing
in relation to their language and their experience or capacity to
perceive. Communication occurs when uttered, received and understood, not when uttered only.

Conceptualization results from perception. However, a person also must be able to conceive in order to perceive. In preparing communications, the sender must work out concepts first
and then ask the question, "Can the recipient interpret it?" The
range of perception is physiological, since perception is a product of the senses, but the limitations to perception are cultural
and emotional.

To gauge the consumers' perceptions of nursing, nurses must
assess the different perceptual dimensions of individuals and
groups. What can they see and hear and why? Because the human
mind perceives what it expects to perceive, what do consumers

expect of nurses? What do we want them to expect? People experience selective retention according to emotional association and receive or reject communication based on the good or bad experiences or associations it evokes. If nurses propagandize, consumers will become cynics. If they provide services that fit the consumer's needs, aspirations, values and goals, they will be powerful. Nurses will be most powerful if they convert aspirations, values and goals to health care as opposed to illness care.[3]

Nurses' Responsibilities to Consumers

Some nurses hold that advocacy and accountability are nurses' prime responsibilities to consumers. Kohnke, writing in the *American Journal of Nursing*, stated, "Advocacy is basic to nursing's responsibility to consumers and basic to changing the image that consumers have of nurses."[4] What is this advocacy role of nurses and how are consumers to know that nurses are their advocates? To some nurses, advocacy means that they support the consumers of nursing in terms of their needs and wishes. It means that some nurses will attempt to *support* their personal goals for nursing care and, if need be, to convert the public from being consumers of illness care to being consumers of health care.

How Nurses Perceive These Services

In an article on nurse/patient peer practice, Bayer and Brandner state that health care providers no longer should try to maintain authority over consumers but should join forces with them to achieve a more effective and satisfying system of health care. In doing so, nurses would affirm the ability of clients to work intelligently toward provision of adequate services. The authors' rationale was that "energy can be used more efficaciously to promote health for the relatively short time life offers each human being." Their approach was to assist and support clients to analyze all possible choices before making decisions. They gave examples of theoretical decision-making situations and clients' responses when asked for a suggested course of action. Although clients did not verbally express perceptions of nursing, their responses indicated a positive attitude toward nursing care. As clients' knowledge, self-reliance and self-esteem increased, their need for health care services significantly decreased.[5]

In a study of a consumer-oriented nurse-midwifery service,

Rising reported that "consumers were irate that others were determining that their needs 'were being met' when their feelings strongly indicate that that was not the case."[6] Women in this program wanted care that was personalized and family-centered. They wanted control over their own experience with care given by providers who would facilitate a safe and satisfying childbearing experience. These women are not unique. Observations of another such service in a different setting indicated that the ratio of forceps-assisted deliveries to those not assisted was 75:25 under physicians as compared with a ratio of 25:75 under nurse midwives. Why? The nurse midwives did not watch the clock. They provided the education and support that consumers say they want.

How Do Consumers Perceive Nursing Care?

A *Good Housekeeping* poll devised and analyzed by Dr. Jonathan Freedman, professor of psychology at Columbia University, recently reported that 2,000 physicians, 2,000 nurses and 2,000 readers had been surveyed at random to determine how the groups rate each other. The results are as follows: "Less than half the patients polled say they get excellent medical care from doctors and nurses and 18 percent say the care is only fair to poor. On personal aspects of care, such as warmth, concern and availability, patients are quite dissatisfied with both doctors and nurses. Only 27 percent of patients find that nurses care too much about money. Seventy-four percent of patients are dissatisfied with hospital care. Comments made by patients about nurses included 'Usually too busy,' 'Don't answer buzzers,' 'Often careless,' and 'Some try to be doctors.' Positive comments on nurses included 'Most of them are competent and they try to be courteous,' 'They know what they are doing,' and 'They're thorough.'" Freedman summarized the survey results by saying, "Despite the mystique which surrounds the whole field of medicine, everyone today feels that medical care is far from ideal."[7]

Watson reported the conclusions of a study in which patients evaluated a primary nursing project. The hypothesis tested was that patients would perceive primary nursing as more personalized than other modalities. Results showed that patients perceived that fewer nurses were needed in primary care, that nurses were friendly and prepared to sit down and talk and that they were concerned about patients' families. Communication with patients and between doctors and nurses was perceived by patients to be better in primary units. Patients made comments that indicated that their primary care nurses gave them comfort, security and better prepared them for discharge. Patients in all situations said it was much easier to approach nurses for information rather than doctors.[8]

An outraged person described two weeks of hospital care during which nurses attempted to administer medication ordered for other patients; a registered nurse deferred nursing decisions to an aide; the recovery room looked like an auto repair shop; an unskilled volunteer attempted to take blood pressures; nurses gossiped about personnel and there was horseplay outside the operating room.[9]

Robinson reported results of a 1978 survey of consumer perceptions related to nursing. The study used a marketing approach to gather data from 300 consumer respondents in two shopping areas of a Southwest metropolitan city. The first section of a three-part questionnaire was related to the consumer's conceptualization of the service provided by nurses. In answer to the question, "What service do you think a nurse could provide?", the consumers thought that nurses could provide physical care, teach you to care for yourself, explain the doctor's orders, demonstrate ways to care for others, provide information, give medicines prescribed by the doctor, do a physical exam, offer counseling, help you establish your rights as a health consumer and help you find other health resources. Consumers were asked to identify the services as ideal or actual and whether they had received these services recently.

Other questions asked were, "If there is a difference between the service a nurse provides and the services you say a nurse actually can provide, say why," "What type of help are you seeking from a nurse when you are well, have a cold or flu, are very ill?" and, "Where do you want to receive nursing assistance when you are well, have a cold or flu, are very ill?"

The report stated that consumers generally thought that nurses should confine themselves to traditional types of services such as giving physical care, administering medications and teaching patients to care for themselves. These were the services they observed nurses doing. Some believed, however, that nurses could do physical examinations, engage in patient advocacy and counseling and assist people to locate health resources. Consumers sought nursing services for information, comfort measures and monitoring activities. Some consumers did not select nurses to provide services because (1) the nurse is too busy; (2) the hospital and the physician limit the scope of nurses' activities; (3) the nurses were not prepared educationally to perform some functions. Although some nurses were prepared to offer certain services, the clients still would not seek their assistance.

This study indicates the general public's lack of understanding of the level of expertise nurses have achieved in recent years. It demonstrates the need for nurses to educate consumers of health care services so that their expectations reflect the type of care nurses are capable of giving.[10]

Students in a management class taught by this author were asked to identify consumers' perceptions of nursing. They were to use management techniques to develop philosophy, statements of purpose, primary objectives and a management plan for accomplishing those objectives. From interviews with consumers outside health care institutions, a variety of perceptions were reported. Among the positive comments reported are the following:

- "The nurse is the one who cares."
- "They provide the warmth and understanding that doctors often forget."
- "Nursing is a very demanding profession that requires a lot of study and knowledge."
- "Licensed nurses, RNs and LPNs control the quality of health care."
- "At first I hated nurses as I have sickle-cell disease and they appeared cruel and uncaring. Now I see them as caring about me and my well-being. They are there to help me."
- "I've always viewed nursing as a profession that cares about people. I've had a lot of contact with nurses due to my illness and I've been impressed with almost every nurse that I've run across. They seem to treat me as a person, an individual. Of course, I have run into a few who have a chip on their shoulders and seem to be mad at the world in general, but you meet people like that everywhere you go."
- "A nurse is a helpful person."
- "I think they're pretty competent, but maybe lacking in dedication, and that's real important. I don't want somebody taking care of me just because it's their job."
- "I never heard of nurse practitioners but if they're cheaper than doctors I'm for them."
- "The two times I have been in the hospital over a num-

ber of years . . . everyone that I have come in contact with that was an RN has been of the highest quality. Indeed, they are professionals."

- "Nurses care for ill people and serve as a link between you and the doctor. They take care of your problem."
- "Nurses have a higher level of awareness of their patients than the doctor does. I think the only reason they're subservient is because of social pressures."
- "Nurses are very kind and try to explain things to you. They are wonderful."
- "The nursing profession impresses me. They are efficient."
- "I think they are smart and nice people."

On the other hand, my student "researchers" also collected a number of less than positive perceptions of nurses and nursing care.

- "The government should regulate the health care system a little more than it does now . . . it might prevent disease and also help out those whose diseases last a lifetime. . . ."
- "Nurses are a helping hand only. Nurses are supposed to do as the physician says exactly, always. They are allowed no independent functions in my opinion. I can't imagine the nurse as a professional."
- "Nursing is the last bastion for women and a man who would go into it can't be too swift. If he was competent he'd be a physician. There is too much waste in the system and it's all caused by doctors. Nursing personnel need periodic reviews to keep up-to-date."
- "You only see a nurse once a shift in a hospital."
- "Nurses should realize that they are dealing with people and not just receptacles of malfunctioning organs."
- "Physicians control the health care system and the cost of health care."
- "Nurses take care of you for the doctor. Sometimes they are really dodoes."
- "The doctor prescribes and the nurse controls whether you get good care or poor care."
- "I don't really think nurses are very useful. They are never around when you need them. Even if they are, they always have an orderly help you anyway."
- "The nurse-physician relationship definitely is not a

partnership. Nurses are beneath doctors because they have to follow doctor's orders."
- "Nurses are damned by doctors and damned by patients. They don't have the capacity to work on their own although they probably are intelligent."
- "I think nurses should think more about the emotional needs of their patients as well as the physical needs. Patients may have family problems or other personal problems that may affect their illness or response to treatment."
- "A nurse is a woman who waits on people in the hospital."
- "The RN gives you shots and does the big important things. The practical nurse gives you water and makes the bed."
- "Doctors are in control of health care in this country. They decide what they want and make everybody do it."
- "Nurses are technical aides to the doctor and the patient."
- "A nurse is a person in a white outfit that takes my blood pressure and gives shots."
- "I think there should be more men in nursing. They can do a better job because they are stronger and won't have to call for an orderly all the time."
- "I think they are doing one hell of a lot more than I would for what they are being paid, if what I hear is true. They should be out in the community more helping people."

Proposal for Action

Average citizens, consumers, do not differentiate between professional, technical and practical nurses. They do not know, and probably don't care at this time, whether registered nurses have diplomas or associate, bachelor, master, or doctoral degrees. They clump nurses with illness, hospitals and physicians. They want nurses to meet their personal needs for physical and emotional comfort—to take care of them when they are sick. They view nurses as intelligent and necessary, but controlled by physicians.

They are well aware that costs could be decreased by more outpatient work and less hospitalization, less use of diagnostic procedures and fewer drugs. They consider physician fees too high and they attribute good care to use of technical machines. Many do not want more governmental control of health care.

To change the image that consumers have of nurses and of nursing will take some effort. First, nurses must decide how they want people to view them. Do they want to be considered as health professionals functioning both in the illness care system that exists and a wellness care system struggling to be born? Do they want to continue to play a low key role? If the choice is to change the image of nurses and of nursing, efforts to develop objectives and goals are the initial step in the process. Some goals to consider might include:

1. *Short range goals*
   • Profile the kinds of personal and professional characteristics nurses need to evidence to be effective image makers (knowledge, skills, attitudes, values).
   • Profile those nursing responsibilities that represent the desired new image.
   • Plan activities, timetables and actively work to support an organization to achieve the objectives.
   • Evaluate current nursing practice to identify deficits in communications with community groups.
   • Plan and execute improved techniques of communication with community groups.
   • Act to accomplish discharge planning.
   • Prepare a campaign to curb gossip and horseplay on the job.
   • Act to implement patient teaching plans.
   • Write objectives and plans in positive terms and use strategies that are tactful and diplomatic as well as aggressive and decisive.
   • Identify activities that will be initiated to meet each objective.

2. *Long range goals*
   • Develop programs to change the image of nurses and nursing.
   • Identify the arenas of public advocacy for health and welfare in which nurses wish to work, such as the need for improved health services for persons in jails and detention centers.
   • Establish nursing as a primary modality in all health service institutions and organizations with community education provided to support this practice.
   • Act to close unused hospital beds.
   • Act to inform the public of the nature of nursing and the necessity for nursing education.

If we do not initiate an effective plan of action, nursing will continue on its present road. This may be less risky for a time, but it will become more risky as consumers continue to gain awareness of the shortcomings of dependence upon technology to treat their illnesses and injuries. An emphasis on goals and strategies to improve the health care delivery system with plans to educate the public will improve the image and, subsequently, the welfare of nurses and nursing.

References

1. *National Health Planning and Resources Development Act of 1974.* 93rd Congress. January 4, 1975, p. 10.
2. *Ibid.* p. 27.
3. Swansburg, Russell C. *Management of Patient Care Services.* The C.V. Mosby Company, Saint Louis, 1976, pp. 261–262.
4. Kohnke, Mary F., "The Nurse's Responsibility to the Consumer," *American Journal of Nursing,* March, 1978, p. 440.
5. Bayer, Mary and Patty Brandner, "Nurse/Patient Peer Practice," *American Journal of Nursing,* January, 1977, pp. 86–90.
6. Rising, Sharon Schindler, "A Consumer Oriented Nurse-Midwifery Service," *Nursing Clinics of North America,* June, 1975, pp. 251–262.
7. Freedman, Jonathan, "GH Poll: What Nurses Think of Doctors . . . and Vice Versa!," *Good Housekeeping,* June, 1979, pp. 88, 90, 93.
8. Watson, Judyth, "Patient Evaluation of a Primary Nursing Project," *The Australian Nurses' Journal,* November, 1978, pp. 30–33, 49.
9. Anonymous, "A Consumer Speaks Out About Hospital Care," *American Journal of Nursing,* September, 1976, pp. 1443–1444.
10. Robinson, Beverlyanne, "A Study of Consumer Perceptions Related to Nursing," *Nursing Leadership,* June, 1978, pp. 14–18.

12. Peer Review: A Model for Professional Accountability

Anna C. Mullins, Ruth E. Colavecchio, and Barbara E. Tescher

Introduction

In professional practice, accountability for behavior cannot be separated from autonomy. A professional gains and maintains autonomy by demonstrating that she is answerable to the client in a public forum of colleagues and health care consumers. Nurses are, collectively and individually, accountable to their clients. Implementing autonomous professional practice, however, is a challenge to most nurses working in institutions because they are members of a bureaucracy and are not directly retained by the client. Peer review as a method for monitoring nursing practice addresses the norms required by a bureaucracy and also provides professional assessment of practice which promotes the nurse's accountability.

This article describes a working experience in a large university hospital in implementing peer review for the classification, promotion, and ongoing evaluation of professional nurses. Through the peer review process, an individual nurse's practice is critically examined through self-appraisal and validation by her colleagues according to an externally defined standard.

The phrase "peer review" was first used in medical literature to describe a physician's practice in relation to patient outcomes. If the characteristics of a professional nursing practice could be directly correlated with nursing activities, a similar approach could serve as a prototype for nursing to measure nursing practice in relation to patient outcomes. Such correlations are difficult to achieve and are seldom reported, although the nursing audit process is beginning to document some of the correlations be-

Reprinted with permission: "Peer Review: A Model for Professional Accountability" by A. C. Mullins, R. E. Colavecchio, and B. E. Tescher. *Journal of Nursing Administration* 9(12):25–30, 1979.

tween nursing activities and patient outcomes. The peer review process described here differs from the traditional approach as it attempts to identify nursing behaviors in relation to a stated standard that includes accountability, collaborative goal setting, clinical judgment, and self-initiated responsibility for continued professional growth (1).

UCSF hospitals and clinics form a 560-bed teaching hospital which employs 600 nurses. The environment supports both team and primary nursing. The Clinical Series defines four behavioral levels of competence in terms of minimal expectations and recognizes the nurse who provides direct care to patients and their families (2). In the classification of minimal behaviors for each level, consideration was given to the depth of knowledge for nursing decisions, the scope of practice, and the degree of responsibility and accountability for patient care. Each level of responsibility is inclusive of preceding levels and recommended educational and experiential qualifications are stated (3). Clinical Nurse 1 is the beginning level for clinical practice; the Clinical Nurse IV level has a corollary in the role of the clinical specialist and the person at this level carries line authority in this institution.

Staff nurses and administrators in the Department of Nursing Service chose peer review as the method for evaluating nursing staff, placing them in the appropriate Clinical Series classification, and determining their eligibility for promotion to a higher classification. A committee of nurse professionals composed of staff nurses, the Clinical Nurse IV from the unit piloting the Clinical Series, and a staff development representative, was formed to develop the review process. A staff nurse was the chairperson. Design of the system was completed in six months and peer review was implemented later.

Definition and Purposes

In defining peer review for the institution, the committee arrived at the following statement:

> Peer review is the process used to appraise the quality of a registered nurse's professional performance and is conducted by a group of registered nurses who are actively engaged in some component of nursing practice. A consumer representative also participates in the process to reflect the nurse's accountability to the client. This appraisal employs the standard of nursing practice established by the UCSF Nursing Service as described in the

Clinical Series job descriptions and conforms with University personnel policies.

The committee established the purposes of the peer review process as follows:

1. To establish an objective means for providing evaluation feedback to individual nurses
2. To recognize the individual nurse who has outstanding nursing skills and performs at a high level of clinical practice
3. To identify individual areas of the nurse's practice needing further development
4. To analyze the consistency of the individual nurse's practice compared to accepted professional standards

The Process

Candidates for peer review are (1) all nurses in the institution for initial classification into the Clinical Series (new employees are reviewed between their fifth and sixth months of employment) and (2) staff seeking promotion, for example, moving from Clinical Nurse I to Clinical Nurse II. In the near future peer review will be used for the yearly evaluation of staff as well.

Under the guidance of an assigned preceptor (a person in a leadership position on the unit) the candidate submits a written profile which documents her current work and accomplishments. After reviewing the profile, a peer review committee interviews the candidate and provides a written evaluation of the candidate's competency and a recommendation for classification to the director of nursing, who makes the final decision. The candidate and preceptor then discuss the evaluation and formulate a contract which establishes goals and accountability for achieving them.

Profile Folder Preparation

The candidate initiates the peer review process within the first five to six months of employment and must have the objectives of the preliminary employment contract. She obtains a peer review profile folder which must be completed within three weeks. The folder contains instructions about the process, a description of the candidate's responsibilities, and the necessary forms. The materials to be completed are representative of the current job level specifications of the nurse. For example, a completed profile folder for a nurse whose current classification is Clinical Nurse I would contain the following:

1.   Two Behavioral Performance Evaluation Checklists completed within the past six months: one by the preceptor, using additional resources as necessary, and the other by the candidate. The evaluation done by the preceptor must be shared with the candidate and signed by both before it is placed in the folder.

2.   Two reference letters: one written by a Clinical Nurse I, the other by someone of the candidate's own choosing. Neither letter is to be written by the preceptor.

3.   A narrative Self-Evaluation Form, which contains descriptions of short- and long-term professional goals, including a specific description of assets and areas in clinical nursing practice needing development; committee work and special projects; ongoing education within the past year; and the candidate's contribution to nursing service.

4.   Two nursing histories or assessments, each with a care plan containing a problem list and problem-oriented charting developed from the history and reflective of the candidate's work in actual, current practice.

5.   One example of current, original work reflecting the candidate's professional practice with patient care or unit organization.

The candidate is allowed four hours of off-unit time to prepare the folder. Additional time, if needed, is negotiated at the unit level. Unit leaders work closely with each candidate as she prepares for peer review, clarifying peer review procedures, and checking the profile folder to ensure its completeness. No attempt is made at this time to evaluate the quality of the candidate's documentation. That responsibility rests with the peer review committee.

When the completed profile folder is submitted, the candidate schedules an interview date with the peer review coordinator, allowing two weeks after submission of the folder for the committee to review the materials. (The peer review coordinator is an administrative assistant to the associate director of clinical practice; her role is to perform all administrative tasks and "paper work" associated with peer review.) The folder and the interview are the only data used by the peer review committee to make a recommendation concerning the candidate's classification. The interview is for purposes of clarification and elaboration of submitted materials. It is, therefore, to the candidate's advantage to make the folder as clear as possible.

The Peer Review Committee

The first peer review committee was hand-picked by nursing administrators and the Clinical Nurse IV of the pilot unit. The criteria were nonspecific but called for people who were willing to serve, who enjoyed impeccable reputations as clinicians, and who were perceived to have effective communication skills. As experience with peer review progressed, a more formalized system was developed.

Because of the number of nurses needing initial classification and promotion, there are currently two peer review committees in operation. Each committee is composed of the following permanent members:

1 Clinical Nurse I
1 Clinical Nurse II
1 Clinical Nurse III
1 nursing administrator
1 school of nursing faculty member
1 consumer

Two rotating members, representing the same job classification as the candidate, also participate in the process. For example, two rotating Clinical Nurse I representatives attend a Clinical Nurse I level interview. Alternate members for each level of classification are appointed to serve as substitutes for permanent members who must be absent for any reason.

Each committee is composed of nurses from a wide variety of specialty areas, as well as experienced peer review committee members. Although it is not always possible, every attempt is made to select rotating members who represent the specialty area of the candidate being reviewed.

Nursing administrators are appointed by the peer review coordinator in consultation with the director of nursing service or her designee. Consumers are selected from the following sources:

    1.   Interested nonnursing UCSF employees or their families
    2.   Former patients or family members who have expressed
a desire to participate in UCSF activities
    3.   Volunteers and auxiliary staff members

All committee members, with the exception of the consumers, must meet certain criteria pertaining to length of employment, satisfactory performance in current position, and interest in participation on a peer review committee. Each member agrees to serve for one year. The chairperson conducts the meetings, maintains attendance records, and writes the peer review minutes. The chairperson helps committee members formulate clear, focused, and ordered questions that will ease and enhance the candidate's presentation of self. The chairperson must be attuned to the human needs of both committee members and candidates and must demonstrate sophisticated verbal and written communication skills so that the interview process is growth-producing for the candidate *and* the committee.

Members participate in a scheduled orientation program and are expected to maintain confidentiality about committee proceedings and outcome.

The Peer Review Interview

The peer review committee members individually review the candidate's profile at their convenience during the two weeks preceding the interview and formulate questions to be directed to the candidate. Questions are intended to obtain elaboration and clarification of materials presented in the folder. Committee members particularly note inconsistencies in the documentation and tend to ask questions that help the candidate account for the discrepancies. They are also encouraged to note positive accomplishments and to comment on them during the interview. Interview questions are derived solely from the profile folder material. Gossip or hearsay reports of a candidate's performance are not permitted to enter into the interview or committee deliberations.

Committee members meet 45 minutes before each scheduled interview to share their thoughts about possible questions and topics to cover during the session.

The interview lasts 35 to 40 minutes. The candidate is invited into the room where the chairperson sets a tone of welcome and comfort and explains the interview process. The candidate may comment on the interview process or ask any questions as needed. To reduce anxiety and involve the candidate in dialogue with the committee quickly, the first question usually directs the candidate to relate her past nursing experience.

After a candidate is interviewed and dismissed the committee members reflect upon the interview and make initial recommendations. This practice helps the committee assess each candidate's performance in relation to the standard and not to other candidates who may have been interviewed on the same day.

Final recommendations for each candidate are entered on a Candidate Description and Committee Recommendations form, which provides for the following:

1. Statements about the candidate's nursing practice (acquired from the profile folder material and in the interview session)

2. Recommendations pertaining to learning needs identified by the committee or expressed by the candidate during the interview

3. The committee's recommendation for classification

The committee's recommendations are made through consensus and dissenting opinions are recorded. It is important to remember that the committee is a recommending group, not a decision-making body. The chairperson submits the profile folder and the description and recommendations form to the director of nursing (or a designee), who makes the final decision and notifies the appropriate Clinical Nurse IV.

Within 24 hours after the interview the candidate receives the profile folder and the description and recommendation form from the Clinical Nurse IV or the preceptor and reviews the recommendations. An appointment is scheduled with the preceptor within two weeks of the interview date to discuss the recommendations and to formulate a contract.

The contract is a mutual agreement between the nurse and unit preceptor stating goals for improving practice and accountability for achieving them. The completed contract is a confidential document retained in the employee's personnel file. The employee keeps a copy of the contract and the unit leader maintains an ongoing record of progress toward the goals outlined.

Staff Orientation

Staff members are prepared for the experience of peer review in a variety of ways. Although registered nurses are the only persons currently participating in peer review, the entire nursing staff (including licensed vocational nurses, unit secretaries, and nursing assistants) were oriented to the components of peer review when it was initially presented to each unit. For the initial explanation throughout the institution, a nursing administrator, the Clinical Nurse IV for the unit, and nurses from other units who had experienced peer review participated in a meeting in which the process was discussed in depth.

The representative from nursing administration offered a systems view. She is responsible for the entire review process, and her presence communicated the department's commitment to peer review. The Clinical Nurse IV works closely with staff members throughout the orientation and during preparation for review. Staff members who have experienced the review process were available to "tell it like it really is."

Staff members were encouraged to read copies of the peer review process that are available on the unit. After a time interval (usually a week) that enabled the staff to digest the process and formulate additional questions, the Clinical Nurse IV met again with staff for continued discussion.

Individual staff members were then given copies of the forms used in peer review. They were taught how to complete the forms and informed as to how the peer review committees use the material. Presenting examples of questions asked by the committee during the interview seemed to alleviate some concern about the experience. An explanation of the peer review process is now part of the orientation for all new nursing staff.

Peer Review Committee Orientation

Peer review committee members are oriented each year to their role and function by participating in a workshop that provides both didactic and experiential learning. The didactic material includes exploration of historical and theoretical bases for the concept of peer review, and an overview of the specifics of the process. Participants are encouraged to express feelings that arise during the discussion. The idea of peer review, taken in the abstract, is generally perceived as positive; however, the reality of the process often produces anxiety and conflict. The issues of accountability, autonomy, responsibility, and authority, whether stated or implied, evoke some degree of anxiety in everyone, regardless of previous experience with peer review. Nursing service personnel (Clinical Nurse IVs, former peer review committee chairpeople, and some nursing administrators), who are the faculty for the workshop, must be prepared to help participants resolve the conflicts and reduce anxiety. Some people identify with the as yet hypothetical review candidate and recall instances in which *they* were judged and perhaps found wanting. Many share a perception of past evaluation experience as a negative experience that did not seem to differentiate performance evaluation from personal worth. Others may reflect on their own practice and silently evaluate themselves in relation to some mythical ideal. Still others become very concerned about "power" and "responsibility for someone's career." These concerns are often signaled by questions such as, "What if our recommendations are not accepted?" "What if we make a mistake?" "What if somebody on the committee doesn't like the candidate?" These issues must be worked through for people to "get on with the job" in a cognitive sense.

Faculty for the orientation workshop must serve as role models for committee members. As more people gain actual peer review committee experience, it is useful to invite some of them to participate as faculty assistants in subsequent workshops.

The experiential component of the workshop is the simulation of an actual peer review, including review of typical documentation submitted by a Clinical Nurse I candidate, formulation of questions for use during the interview, a role-play of the interview, and construction of recommendations for appointment. Although it is tempting to use materials from a "real" peer review, documentation used for the workshop must be fictitious, since the use of actual documents would violate rules of privacy. The development of a credible set of fictitious documents, though time-consuming and difficult, is crucial to the success of the learning experience.

The simulated review is done in small, faculty-led groups that are similar in size to those of the actual peer review panel. Experienced committee members can be used effectively as coleaders for these groups, but they should not be expected to assume sole leadership responsibilities. Participants are guided through a careful documentation review and formulation of questions for the interview. The role of the candidate should be played by a person who is familiar with the documentation, and not a member of the faculty or a workshop participant. Faculty must be free to observe and make notes about the interview process for subsequent group discussion, and participants need the experience of "being on the other side of the table."

After the simulation interview, all the groups assemble to share their reactions to the experience. Faculty clarify further elements of the process and share their perceptions of the simulated interviews.

A need for a second-level orientation for committee chairpersons was recently identified. The chairpeople usually benefit from additional learning experiences that focus on the specific skills required for group interview. Among them are questioning skills, anxiety reduction strategies, set, and closure (4).

A reference module and 15-minute videotape of a simulated review have recently been developed as additional learning resources (5). Staff members verbalized a need for assistance with reference letter writing, self-evaluation, and self-presentation skills, and the reference module was designed to fill this need. It serves as a guide to preparing a profile folder and also helps prepare individuals for the experience of peer review. The materials will be used as part of the orientation for all new professional staff, as a component of the peer review committee orientation, and will be available to staff members of units preparing for Clinical Series classification. Plans are under way to share the reference module and videotape with other departments in the institution in anticipation that other administrative directors will become interested in these nursing service activities.

Problems and Changes

Institution of the peer review process has had a significant impact on both individuals and the system. Although strategies for implementation were carefully devised on paper, there were unanticipated mechanical and procedural problems. For example, insufficient time was allotted for candidates to complete their documentation. Peer review folders were often submitted late and the entire peer review process lacked coordination. Administrative and clerical support services were inadequate to handle documentation of materials and coordinate time schedules for candidates and review committees. These problems were resolved by assigning a departmental resource person, who is an administrative assistant, to coordinate the peer review process. Although the solution seems obvious and simplistic, cost constraints could not be dealt with effectively until the problems became intolerable and, more important, until the process of peer review became part of the value system of the organization.

Candidates experienced apprehension and concern related to preservation of self-image. Because the new peer review committees were inexperienced in developing questions and writing summaries and recommendations, candidates were often kept waiting for the interview to begin and for recommendations to be communicated. Once the committee members and candidates mastered the process, and the procedural and mechanical support system improved, these difficulties subsided.

Many candidates expressed concern that part of the peer review committee's assessment of their professional ability included an evaluation of how the candidate presented herself in the interview. These individuals were helped to understand that presentation of oneself is important in the current, professional world, and were assured that they *could* present themselves in a professional manner. Some negative reactions arose because a few candidates were not recommended for higher classification by the peer review committees. When candidates were not classified at the level they desired, their nursing colleagues often rallied to attack the process instead of looking objectively at the candidates' performance. Confidentiality compounded the problem, since only the candidates were at liberty to discuss the peer review process; peer review committee members were not.

As the peer review process becomes more familiar to more people, and as staff members become convinced that the process is essentially positive, these kinds of reactions diminish. Currently, unhappy candidates either go directly to the appropriate committee chairperson or to their Clinical Nurse IV for clarification and explanation. Dissatisfied candidates can initiate an appeals process.

Peer review committee members also experienced their share of anxiety and apprehension. Some had difficulty reading and making sense out of the documents submitted and had further problems relating the documents to the interview. At times committee members did not question a candidate about a particular area but made recommendations from data in the folder. In time, and with guidance, they developed the ability to acknowledge discrepancies directly to a candidate during the interview rather than simply recording them later. As mentioned previously, committee members developed personal anxieties because of their sensitivity to the candidates' need for understanding and acknowledgment. A conflict arose from their need to be humane while attempting to render an objective performance appraisal.

Nursing administration committed considerable time, effort, and money to initiating the peer review process. Planning and implementation of orientation sessions for peer review committees and nursing staff required considerable financial investment. Facilitation of the initial peer review sessions by top-level personnel was time-consuming, as were the one-to-one discussions with employees who were unhappy with their peer review results. However, as knowledge and experience with the process have increased, many of the cost factors have been minimized. The early procedures were somewhat overelaborate and have since been simplified without losing the essential thought or intention.

Initial classification on the pilot unit began with the lowest level (Clinical Nurse I). It later seemed more appropriate to classify the top levels of the Clinical Series first (Clinical Nurse III, IV) to demonstrate commitment by unit level leadership to both the Clinical Series and the peer review process and to provide unit leaders with firsthand experience to assist other staff members through the same process.

Based upon this experience, we suggest that a nursing organization contemplating the initiation of such a review process consider several questions:

1.   What are the risks associated with implementing a process for which the outcomes are largely unknown?
2.   Once the organization is committed to the implementation of peer review, what alternatives are available if the review process is not suitable?
3.   Given that confidentiality is an issue, what, if any, should be the feedback mechanism between peer review committees and the various departments in the institution?
4.   What responses can be anticipated from other disciplines within the institution?
5.   Can the expense of initiating such a process be justified?

Fortunately, the timing for peer review implementation appeared to be right for UCSF nursing service. Several thoughtful risk-takers in the department believed that unknown outcomes could be managed, and many staff members were excited about the prospect of a new evaluation system. The new protocol was not cast in concrete and could be altered, or even dropped, if warranted. The significant change in the evaluation process is perceived by most to be healthy. Everyone concerned feels that peer review addresses the issues of accountability and autonomy and has enhanced nursing practice within the department. We acknowledge that beliefs and judgment about the benefits of any peer review system must be substantiated by stringent research related to cost-benefit ratios, nursing practice outcomes, and effects of the professional esteem of the nurses involved. This research is part of the future plans for UCSF service.

Notes

1. Colavecchio, R., Tescher, B., and Scalzi, C. A clinical ladder for nursing practice. *Nurs. Admin.*, 4(5): 54–58, 1974.
2. Tescher, B., and Colavecchio, R. Definition of a standard for clinical practice. *Nurs. Admin.*, 7(3): 32–44, 1977.
3. Colavecchio, R., Tescher, B., and Scalzi, C., 1974, p. 55.
4. De Tornyay, R. *Strategies for Teaching Nursing.* New York: Wiley, 1971.
5. The reference module and videotape of a simulated review are available to individuals interested in implementing the peer review process. Please contact Anna C. Mullins for details.

III

Nurse Practitioners and Other Specialists

13. Introduction—
The Developing Nursing Specialties

Bonnie Bullough and Vern Bullough

The growth of a knowledge base in any field traditionally has been associated with greater and greater specialization. In almost every field of knowledge, there are more subfields of specialization today than there were 20 years ago, and if present trends continue, there will be more 20 years from now than there are now. One of the reasons for this trend is the expanding knowledge base. As knowledge in a field expands it becomes difficult for any one person to encompass it. Thus we have the paradox that people in a field such as history focus on narrower and narrower parts of history. Doctoral students now not only specialize in American history but in various portions of American history such as the early national period of American history or history of women in America. Though many of these individuals could probably teach a survey course in American history if they were forced to do so, they know almost nothing about ancient, medieval, or modern history in Europe, Asia, or Africa except as it impinges on their area of expertise.

What is true of history is even more true of medicine. Periodically a wishful desire is heard to return to the age of the general practitioner, that semimythical person who treated or mistreated everyone the same. Programs have even been created to establish new kinds of general practitioners, such as the internist programs of 30 years ago and the family practice programs of today, but usually the graduates of these programs soon develop specialties. In fact, the whole basis of medical progress has been dependent on the growth of specialization. It is the specialist who sees enough cases in the same category to make generalizations about the kind of illness he or she is seeing. It is also by handling a number of cases of similar types that the specialist gains the necessary expertise to deal with what he or she is seeing. This is not to say that specialization is always good for the patient, for the specialist, or for society. From the patient's point of view one of the problems with specialization is the fragmentation of care; a cardiologist treats a patient for his heart problems, ignoring everything else, including some of the regimens prescribed by the neurologist or urologist. The patient at times needs an advocate, a general protector to coordinate the uncoordinated ministrations of the specialist.

Nursing, though it has always had some specialists, was primarily a generalist occupation until the 1950s. Before that time nurses who wanted to improve their techniques in a special area often took a "postgraduate" course at one of the major hospitals in such fields as fever nursing, pediatrics, or operating room technique. These programs for the most part utilized an internship format and put a heavy emphasis on experiential learning rather than classroom education. Only a few specialists were recognized as demanding either more education or more technical skills than those which could not be learned on the job. Four such nursing specialties come to mind, two of them requiring college degrees as entry, something that few nurses had until the last 20 years, and two requiring an extensive practicum. The two educationally dependent specialties were public health nursing and nursing education while the two requiring practicums were anesthesia and midwifery. In a sense it was unfortunate that the preparatory backgrounds for the two groups of specialists were so different since organized nursing, in its effort to upgrade itself by requiring more and more formal education, tended to look down on the nurse whose theoretical training was limited, and it has only been in the last decade that technical specialties are being effectively integrated into collegiate nursing programs. The history of the development of anesthesia as a nursing specialty presented and analyzed by Ira Gunn in this section demonstrates the problems of such a specialty.

Nurse Midwifery

The development of nurse midwifery is similar to that of nurse anesthesia. Although midwifery is as old as nursing—and, in fact, the roles often have been interchangeable in the past—the trained midwife developed with the trained nurse. In most countries of the world midwifery was part of the basic nursing program, but this was not so true for the United States because the medical profession was determined to dominate the whole field of obstetrics. This meant that American nurse midwives were usually able to practice only in those areas where physicians were unavailable or unwilling to serve. Emphasizing this official exclusion of nurses was the Sheppard-Towner Act of 1921 which, while assigning public health nurses the task of working with and training lay midwives, assumed that nurses themselves were not to practice midwifery. Instead, the legislation aided the phasing out of lay midwives and encouraged their replacement by physicians (Bullough and Bullough, 1978).

Because of such attitudes, it was not until 1932 that the first American school of nurse midwifery, associated with the Maternity Center of New York City, was founded. It was at this school that most of the early American nurse midwives received their training, although many of the Maternity Center graduates were prevented from practicing as midwives and had to content themselves with serving as teachers or working in hospital maternity units (Olsen, 1974). Such exclusion continued despite the fact that research evidence indicated that lives could be saved by nurse midwives. This was documented in the 3-year demonstration project in California's rural Madera County, where two nurse midwives were employed by the county hospital to manage normal deliveries. They gave prenatal care, attended labor and delivery, and managed the care of the mothers and infants in the postpartum period. During the span of the project (1960–1963) prematurity and neonatal mortality rates among the patient population fell significantly. Yet when the project sponsors sought to institutionalize the practice and secure a change in the state laws which would have allowed nurse midwives to continue practicing, they were unsuccessful because of opposition from the California Medical Association. The year after CMA opposition forced the cancellation of the project the neonatal mortality rate went from the project rate of 10.3 to 32.1 per 1,000 live births (Levy et al., 1971). Finally, in 1974, the California Medical Association withdrew its opposition and the law was changed to allow nurse midwives to practice in that state. As can be noted in Table 26–1, the majority of the states now allow nurse midwifery.

Clinical Specialists

The stratification of the nursing role and the replacement of the nurse with the nursing team which occurred primarily in the post-World War II era had some far-reaching consequences for the profession. The nurse with the most education was moved away from the bedside and into patient care coordination or administration. While hospitals supported this change because of the cost-saving factor, nurses were concerned because it fragmented and depersonalized patient care. Consequently, solutions to this problem were sought. One proposed mechanism was the development of a masters level clinical specialist who could give skilled nursing care to selected groups of patients and serve as a teacher and role model for staff members with less formal education.

The expansion of graduate education for nurses made this proposal a real possibility. The expansion was stimulated by the nurse training act of 1964, which strengthened nursing education at all levels but earmarked traineeships and special developmental funds for graduate education. In response the nursing schools established master's programs or expanded existing programs and made clinical specialization the focus of the expansion (Kalisch and Kalisch, 1978).

Probably the most effective of the early clinical specialties was the one in psychiatric nursing. Psychiatrists, who had already coped with the entry of social workers and clinical psychologists in their domain, saw no reason to exclude psychiatric clinical nurse specialists. In other areas, where the social and psychological problems of patients had often been ignored, the work of the clinical specialist often went unnoticed or was simply regarded as an additional task. In either case the specialist's focus constituted no threat to the medical staff, who regarded it as peripheral to the patient's major diagnosis and the physician's work role. Though hospitals encouraged nurses to pay attention to the social and psychological needs of patients, they did not pay nurses for doing so and the result was an added burden to the dedicated nurse. This administrative failure forced clinical specialists to modify their role and take on greater administrative and teaching responsibilities or move in the direction of the nurse practitioner and take on functions traditionally in the medical domain. This melding of the roles of the clinical nurse specialist and the nurse practitioner has enhanced job opportunities in many areas. There is now a blurring of the distinction between the nurse practitioner and the clinical specialist.

Acute Care Nurses

The most successful of the hospital-based specialists in terms of the job market are not, however, clinical specialists. Rather they are the nurses who staff the acute coronary and other intensive care units. Although few have graduate education, these nurses are responsible for monitoring patients' conditions using complex equipment, making on-the-spot, life-saving decisions, and acting on those decisions. There is often no time for physician consultation before action is taken. It is clearly an area where strong educational preparation is needed, but the mainstream of graduate nursing education has not focused on this area to any significant degree. The reasons behind this apparent paradox are complex but probably relate to a belief system held by some nurse educators that highly technical tasks are somehow easier than nontechnical ones. Thus, the patient who is in the midst of a physiological and psychological crisis is left to nurses with "technical" preparation while the patient who is on the road to recovery is given the services of a master's level clinical nurse specialist. Noting this paradox, the Division of Nursing of the Department of Health and Human services recently funded a few demonstration projects to strengthen education for acute care. This is a small beginning but it is an area which can be expected to expand.

Nurse Practitioners

Probably the largest and most publicized of the emerging specialty groups are the nurse practitioners. While the definition of the nurse practitioner is an evolving one, it clearly overlaps with the role of physician. One of the candidates for serving as the first nurse practitioner is Barbara R. Noonan, who started seeing patients in the Medical Nurse Clinic at Massachusetts General Hospital in 1962 (Noonan, 1972). She was not typical, however, because most of the early practitioners as well as the early training programs specialized in pediatric rather than adult care, probably because of the strong support of the pediatricians and the American Academy of Pediatrics. In 1963 Siegel and Bryson reported the experimental use of public health nurses in an expanded role in northern California clinics (Siegel and Bryson, 1963). A 4-year controlled comparison of prenatal and infant supervision by nurses and physicians was completed in 1967 by the Montefiore medical group in New York City. They reported that the care delivered by nurses was safe and well accepted by patients and physicians (Seacat and Schlachter, 1968). The first formal training program was started in Denver in 1965 by Henry K. Silver and Loretta C. Ford and it was from this group that the term nurse practitioner evolved (Silver et al., 1968).

Research about nurse practitioners has reached voluminous proportions. Their ability to deliver care that is safe, thorough, effective, and satisfactory to physicians and consumers has been well documented (Sackett et al., 1974, 1977; Sox, 1979; Andrews and Yankauer, 1971). In addition, they are also able to help patients to better understand their illnesses, so that adherence to treatment regimes is improved when there is a nurse practitioner on the team (Sullivan, 1982; Ramsay et al., 1982; Watkins and Wagner, 1982). These studies, which document the communication function of nurse practitioners, suggest that the nurse practitioners are becoming more like clinical nurse specialists. As the nurse practitioner role matures its roots in nursing become more evident; patient communication and support services are emerging as crucial elements in the practitioner role. As indicated in the above section, the clinical specialists are taking on more assessment and treatment functions so their role is often similar to that of practitioners. The gap between the two specialties seems to be narrowing.

The longitudinal study of nurse practitioners sponsored by the Division of Nursing of the Department of Health and Human Services also points up some interesting trends. For that study cohorts of nurse practitioners from the classes of 1974–1975, 1975–1976, and 1981–1982 have been studied during and after their educational programs. While the data from the 1981–1982 cohort are still being published, the overall picture indicates that the role is now well accepted, that it has expanded the ability of the health care delivery system to reach the population in need of primary care, particularly the disadvantaged segment of the population. There is clearly a trend to lengthen the preparation of nurse practitioners as the early certificate programs close and master's degree programs open. The early focus on pediatrics and other "women's" roles has broadened to include all of the major patient care specialties (Sultz et al., 1976, 1978, 1979, 1980). It will be interesting to see how well the movement can survive the impact of the GMENAC Report, which is discussed in this section.

References

Andrews, P. M. and Yankauer, A. "The Pediatric Nurse Practitioner: Growth of the Concept," *American Journal of Nursing* 71 (March 1971):504–506.

Bullough, V. L. and Bullough, B. *The Care of the Sick: The Emergence of Modern Nursing.* New York: Prodist, 1978, pp. 147–148.

Kalisch, P. A. and Kalisch, B. J. *The Advance of American Nursing.* Boston: Little, Brown, 1978.

Levy, B. S., Wilkinson, F. S., and Marine, W. M. "Reducing Neonatal Mortality Rate with Nurse-midwives," *American Journal of Obstetrics and Gynecology* 109 (January 1, 1971):50–58.

Noonan, B. R. "Eight Years in a Medical Nurse Clinic," *American Journal of Nursing* 72 (June 1972):1128–1130. Reprinted in *Expanding Horizons for Nurses.* Edited by B. Bullough and V. Bullough. New York: Springer, 1977, pp. 34–38.

Olsen, L. "The Expanding Role of the Nurse in Maternity Practice," *Nursing Clinics of North America* 9 (September 1974):459–466.

Ramsay, J. A., McKenzie, J. K., and Fish, D. G. "Physicians and Nurse Practitioners: Do They Provide Equivalent Health Care?" *American Journal of Public Health* (January 1982):55–57.

Sackett, D. L., Spitzer, W. O., Gent, M., Roberts, R. S., et al. "The Burlington Randomized Trial of the Nurse Practitioner: Health Outcomes of Patients," *Annals of Internal Medicine* 80 (February 1974):137–142. Reprinted in *Expanding Horizons for Nurses.* Edited by B. Bullough and V. Bullough. New York: Springer, 1977, pp. 55–66.

Seacat, M. and Schlachter, L. "Expanded Nursing Role in Prenatal and Infant Care," *American Journal of Nursing* 68 (April 1968):822–824.

Siegel, E. and Bryson, S. L. "Redefinition of the Role of the Public Health Nurse in Child Health Supervision," *American Journal of Public Health* 53 (June 1963):1015–1024.

Silver, H. K., Ford, L. C., and Day, L. R. "The Pediatric Nurse-Practitioner Program," *Journal of the American Medical Association* 204 (1968):298–302. Reprinted in *Expanding Horizons for Nurses.* Edited by B. Bullough and V. Bullough. New York: Springer, 1977, pp. 39–48.

Sox, H. C., Jr. "Quality of Patient Care by Nurse Practitioners and Physician's Assistants: A Ten-Year Perspective," *Annals of Internal Medicine* 91 (1979):459–468.

Sullivan, J. A. "Research on Nurse Practitioners: Process Behind the Outcome?" *American Journal of Public Health* 72 (January 1982):8–9.

Sultz, H. A., Zielezny, M., and Kinyon, L. *Longitudinal Study of Nurse Practitioners, Phase I.* Washington, D.C.: U.S. Government Printing Office, March 1976.

Sultz, H. A., Zielezny, M., Gentry, J. M., and Kinyon, L. *Longitudinal Study of Nurse Practitioners, Phase II.* Washington, D.C.: U.S. Government Printing Office, September 1978.

Sultz, H. A., Henry, O. M., and Sullivan, J. *Nurse Practitioner USA.* Lexington, Mass.: Lexington Books, 1979.

Sultz, H. A., Zielezny, M., Gentry, J. M., and Kinyon, L. *Longitudinal Study of Nurse Practitioners, Phase III.* Washington, D.C.: U.S. Government Printing Office, May 1980.

Watkins, L. O. and Wagner, E. H. "Nurse Practitioner and Physician Adherence to Standing Orders Criteria for Consultation or Referral," *American Journal of Public Health* 72 (January 1982):22–29.

14.   The GMENAC Report: An Opportunity for Nursing

Fay Whitney

Opportunity is often fashioned from the fragments of disaster. The Chinese have created the symbol "crisis" from the elements of opportunity and disaster. This representation has been used to illustrate methods of looking at situations which may appear to be either fortuitous or enigmatic and deciding how to approach them. A perception of whether the cup is half full or half empty has been used to define the difference between an optimist and a pessimist. In all of this, what we look for in our lives are chances to make a difference, visions of how to proceed in difficult circumstances, and ways to justify our particular choices when dynamic options are presented to us.

True opportunities do not often address themselves directly to us. They come clothed in threat, surprise, confusion, and incomplete information. They are often presented as unopposable facts, *fait accompli, raison d'être*, and signs of the times. They are greeted with a mix of resignation, fright, indignation, anger, and enthusiasm. Sometimes we never see them for what they are. Often, when we do, we cannot summon the forces to respond positively to their dynamism and move productively forward with them. The last 15 years, which produced nurse practitioner issues, have been full of opportunity and crisis. For a while the nursing establishment did not support the nurse practitioner movement. Now, nursing has decided to take nurse practitioners seriously, to

Thanks are expressed to Dr. Bruce Dearing, Professor of Humanities, SUNY, Upstate Medical Center, for his critique of the manuscript.

be grateful for the visibility in the health care arena they have provided, to commend them for their focus on patient care and health delivery in the broader sense, and to applaud them for the courage and persistence they have shown in the face of more opportunity than they have sought. Concurrently, it appears that the medical profession, in the form of the GMENAC Report, has struck a strong blow against future use of nurses in primary care.

Preliminary reports from the Graduate Medical Education National Advisory Committee (GMENAC) were published in an interim report in the fall of 1979, and a final report September 30, 1980. The report recommended that in light of an anticipated oversupply of physicians in 1990, it would be wise to curtail further expansion of programs to prepare nurse practitioners, physicians' assistants, and midwives. For many, this seemed like a critical blow, a threat to the future of nursing in primary care, and definitely a setback in the forward movement of nursing's evolving role in health care.

But, to some of us, it is seen as an opportunity, a chance to set the record straight and to attack the notion that physician head count is the only feasible measure of the health care system and its efficacy. The report is an invitation to do something positive to show the crucial importance of nursing services in the health care industry, to help define and shape the future of health and planning in this country. The authors of the GMENAC Report saw it as a vehicle to generate controversy and response. They called it "an experiment in policy development through collaboration between the private sector and the government working in open public forum" (GMENAC, Vol. 1). It seems to me that nurses can be no less foresighted.

This paper will examine the report, the history of its development, its recommendations in general, and the implications of those recommendations for nursing. An analysis of what the author sees as the opportunities it presents and an agenda for seizing them will be included. Throughout, the theme will be fashioned after this philosophy; in the guise of a crisis, you have handed me a gift, the opportunity to create and build. From the sands of concern and the wash of misunderstanding, I will build you a fortress from which we can shape together a future that will serve the very substance of humanity.

Background of the GMENAC Report

History

Patricia R. Harris, Secretary of Health and Human Services, received a report of September 30, 1980 which summarized in seven volumes the work of the Graduate Medical Education National Advisory Committee (GMENAC) from April 20, 1976, when it was established by that office, until the submission of the report. Chartered on April 20, 1976, rechartered May 1978 by Secretary Califano and March 1980 by Secretary Harris, the committee was charged to advise the secretary of (1) the numbers required in each medical specialty to bring supply and needs into balance, (2) ways to improve geographic distribution of physicians, and (3) mechanisms to finance graduate medical education. Suggestions for implementation of the advice and recommendations of GMENAC were to be formulated. It was to be primarily a manpower planning group. The committee reported that it had developed methodology for estimating physician supply, and requirements for general health services and specialties. They felt they were instrumental in developing new concepts relating to manpower and underserved areas based on population needs rather than population figures. They recommended methods for determining impact of services in many areas. They developed panels of experts in four fields. They used private and public sectors to explore the depth of their charge and to form cooperative relationships between the two sectors. Research needs were discovered and suggestions for specific kinds of methodology and areas of inquiry were defined. GMENAC developed 40 general recommendations in the areas of their charge. Each expert panel generated statistics and subrecommendations in answer to their individual charges. It was a large undertaking and seriously attended to by the members.

GMENAC Planning Group

The composition of the planning group and the relation of the private and public sectors to the development of the final report is best seen in a schematic representation from the summary of the report (Figure 14–1) (GMENAC, Vol. 1, p. 43).

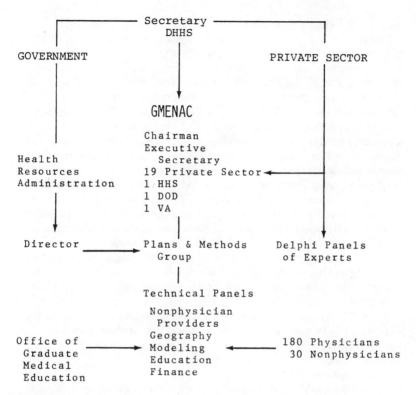

Figure 14–1   Structure of GMENAC.

Early Work

The committee found that the data base for its planning effort was inadequate. Three major thrusts were begun to overcome the limitations problem: (1) refinement of data through literature searches, expert testimony and hearings, and standardized data bases such as statistical data from the National Center for Health Services Research, (2) modification of existing models and development of new models for forecasting physician supply and needs of the public, and (3) constitution of technical panels to study specialty determinations and geographic distribution.

GMENAC developed an unique, adjusted need-based approach to project and determine how persons would seek specialty physician services. Although the model will not be covered in detail here, it is interesting as a planning tool and should be studied by those interested in this effort.

The physician requirements model, which was developed as a mathematical model, used a baseline of 1978 supply, added U.S. and foreign medical school graduates from 1978 to 1987, and the residents' contribution to practice (figured at .35 of one physician service unit), considered a complicated "residency choice specialty-specific component" to project how many physicians would be choosing each specialty by 1990 and arrived at a projected number of physicians to be available by 1990. The year 1990 was used because of the need to forecast 10 years in advance in order to address the 8- to 10-year turnaround time presumed to be needed to effect change in medical education. Present manpower statistics, findings of the technical panels, and literature searches were used to develop the numbers which were used in the Delphi probe technique which produced projections for 1990. This technique has often been criticized for number-crunching aspects, nonappropriate manipulation of variables, and oracle guesswork. The deficiencies of the methodology were conceded by the committee rather than ignored and taken into account in its recommendations. Narrative additions to the recommendations derived from the numbers produced were added in the reports, which did consider some of the variables not earlier taken into account.

A total of 40 summary recommendations emanated from the committee in the final report. Each technical panel produced recommendations which were written in separate reports and are part of the final seven volumes. All recommendations were voted upon by the GMENAC.

When one reads the entire report, one cannot help feeling that a very thorough job was attempted and that the spirit of open inquiry was embraced. A great number of recommendations which were presented could be validated from material that was examined and considered. Experts in areas of health care delivery, manpower preparation, the professions, and allied fields were consulted. What, then, was the negative effect that GMENAC has had? Why has it evoked such a protest in nursing? In answering these questions, it is timely to look at the report recommendations and the impact they have had since September 30, 1980.

The Recommendations

GMENAC developed 12 categories of recommendations encompassing the 40 recommendations offered in summary. They addressed the original charge of the committee as outlined in the introduction. These recommendations arose from the technical panels, the Delphi probe results, and consensus of the GMENAC members regarding their appropriateness and validity. One of the panels that was constituted was a nonphysician health care provider technical panel. It was this panel and its recommendations which created such a stir in the nursing community, and to which we will pay the most attention.

The primary finding of the 3-year study was that the projected surplus of physicians in the United States could reach 70,000 by 1990! This projection was surprising to the public and the medical community because it was contrary to initial impressions in the 1960s that a shortage of physicians existed. At that time foreign medical schools were asked to gear up for increased applicants and foreign medical graduates were imported freely to fill the residencies in our country. The familiar maldistribution and limited access to physicians were ascribed to a dearth of physicians, and "physician substitutes" were called for.

However, other less publicized projects have also shown an anticipated surplus. The Bureau of Health Professions (HRA) (formerly Bureau of Health Manpower), estimates that between 23,000 and 51,400 physicians will be in surplus by 1990. The Manpower Supply and Utilization branch of HRA estimates an excess of 50,000 (Scheffler et al., 1979). The National Academy of Sciences has also warned that NPs and PAs should be curtailed because of an anticipated surplus of physicians in practice (Miike, 1979).

Second, the committee used its mathematical specialty model to ascertain that there would be shortages in some specialties and surpluses in others. Cautioning that there could be a wide margin of error in their model, surpluses were noted in urology, orthopedic surgery, ophthalmology, thoracic surgery, infectious diseases, ob/gyn, plastic surgery, nephrology, rheumatology, cardiology, endocrinology, neurosurgery, and pulmonary medicine. Near balances were seen in hematology/oncology, dermatology, gastroenterology, osteopathic general practice, family practice, general internal medicine, otolaryngology, general pediatrics, and related subspecialties. Shortages were projected in child psychiatry, emergency medicine, preventive medicine, and general psychiatry.

The report addressed the need to consider the geriatric population (expected to reach 35 million by 2003), and the impact of this population on general internal medicine and family practice as a possible area of unmet needs. Recommendations to reduce entering class size a minimum of 10 percent by 1984, restriction of entry of foreign medical graduates to U.S. medical schools and a mandate to look at the training and role of nonphysician providers in the projected oversupply of physicians were derived from the model.

The Nonphysician Technical Panel

The technical panel to study nonphysician providers was constituted and charged with responsibility for projecting physician needs and developing recommendations in response to this projection. Early reports relating to the recommendations of this panel often evoked the question, "What is a committee who is looking at physician supply doing making recommendations about nonphysicians?" As one friend was overheard saying, "Focusing on physician supply as a way of measuring health in the nation is like counting gas stations in order to assess the energy crisis."

Not surprisingly, nurses and other health providers became indignant about the arrogance of one profession determining the need for other professionals. Many distrusted the figures in the wake of the disastrous miscalculation of the nursing surplus by the Carter administration in 1979. The reaction of some mirrored Nicholas Lemann's comments in his chapter "Let the Nurses Do It."

> Having been to medical school seems to affect one's income a lot more than it affects one's ability to treat patients effectively . . . the flaw in Flexner's perfect vision is that the fit is loose; it's possible to do the job without having had the schooling, and to have had the schooling and not be able to do the job. Seventy years ago, when the professions were new, that was a minor point. Now that they have M.D.'s control of most of our services and a good portion of our money, it isn't so minor any more (Lemann, 1981).

Most felt that the definition of health care was broader than that of physician-illness orientation and that the GMENAC report had, at the very least, missed the point that the American public is seeking a new kind of health care in the 1980s. It would certainly be more inclined in that direction by 1990. For many, the recommendations reflected an illogical train of thinking, decisions based on faulty information and either a naive understanding of health care delivery in our century or a blatant display of monopolistic thinking.

Considering the political and economic power of physicians, nurses felt that the "docs" had leveled a blow at nursing's midsection through GMENAC. As nursing was gearing up its educational systems to meet the primary and preventive health needs of its patients, it was feared that programs and the funding for such efforts would be further eroded and curtailed. Already squeezed in ability to command money for research, education of professionals, and third party reimbursement, the profession of nursing feared it would be strangled in its efforts even to exist. It was a feeling of flying backward in time, to a role where the dictates of the medical profession were the rules of the land. Fear, frustration, and hopelessness were echoed in the cries of the nursing profession, patients, and those who cared about the future of health care in our nation.

Hostile feelings within nursing were also aroused. The report clearly defined nurse practitioners as physician substitutes doing delegated tasks under medical supervision, an image long fought by nurse practitioners and long used as the wedge within the nursing ranks to disclaim the nursing role of the NP and to isolate the NPs from their own colleagues. It seemed that the conflict over nurse practitioners within nursing had only just been smouldering. Now, it was rekindled.

The summary recommendations directly relating to NPs, PAs, and midwives were listed under "The Requirements for Nonphysician Health Care Providers Should Be Integrated into Physician Manpower Planning." The section began:

> GMENAC concluded that nurse practitioners (NP's), physician assistants (PA's), and nurse-midwives (NMW's) make positive contributions to the health care system when working in close alliance with physicians. The committee supports the practice of nonphysician providers under the supervision of physicians, but does not endorse the concept of their practicing independently. Nonphysician providers can enhance patient access to services, decrease costs, and provide a broader range of services. Certain consumers prefer the nonphysician provider (GMENAC, Vol. 1, p. 27).

• *Recommendation 1:* Extensive research on the requirements for NPs, PAs, NMWs, and other nonphysician providers should be undertaken as soon as possible. Special attention must be given to the effect of a physician excess on their utilization and to the benefits these providers bring to health care delivery. These studies should consider the full range of complementary and substitute services.

• *Recommendation 2:* Until the studies in Recommendation 1 have been completed, the number of PAs, NPs, and NMWs in training for child medical care, adult medical care, and obstetrical/gynecological care should remain stable at their present numbers. Delegation levels recommended by GMENAC for 1990 are: in obstetrics/gynecology 197,000 of the normal uncomplicated deliveries (5 percent of all deliveries), 7.1 million maternity-related visits (20 percent of the obstetrical case load), and 7.5 million gynecological visits (18 percent of the gynecological case load); in child care not more than 46 million ambulatory visits (16 percent of the child ambulatory case load); and in adult medical care not more than 128 million ambulatory visits (12 percent of the adult medical ambulatory case load).

Another section (D) related to "The Laws, Regulations, and Programs Pertaining to Nurse Practitioners, Physician Assistants, and Nurse Midwives." It began:

> The State laws and regulations governing licensure of non-physician providers including supervision by physicians, ability to write prescriptions, reimbursement for services, and services performed in medically underserved areas are inconsistent and often contrary to policy objectives. State regulation, which is relatively new, has been devised to meet local needs and to respond to local political processes. The variations and inconsistencies among the States seem to interfere with the nation's objective to provide equal access to high quality health services for all Americans (GMENAC, Vol. 6, pp. 3, 6).

The recommendations under this area were:

• *Recommendation 2:* State laws and regulations should not impose requirements for physician supervision of NPs and PAs, beyond those needed to assure quality of care.

Supportive Recommendations

a. State laws and regulations should be altered as necessary so that a PA or NP working under appropriate physician supervision can independently complete a patient encounter for conditions which are deemed eligible.
b. The states should provide PAs, NPs, and NMWs with limited power of prescription, taking necessary precaution to safeguard the quality of care, including explicit protocols, formularies, and mechanisms for physician monitoring and supervision.
c. At a minimum, PAs, NPs, and NMWs should be given power to dispense drugs in those settings where not to do so would have an adverse effect on the patient's condition.
d. States, particularly those with underserved rural areas, should evaluate whether the laws and regulations pertaining to nonphysician practice discourage nonphysician location in these areas.

* *Recommendation 3:* The requirements of third party payers for physician supervision should be consistent with the laws and regulations governing nonphysician practice in the state.
* *Recommendation 4:* Medicare-Medicaid, and other insurance programs, should recognize and provide reimbursement for the services by NPs, PAs, and NMWs in those states where they are legally entitled to provide these services. Services of these providers should be identified as such to third party payers and reimbursement should be made to the employing institution or physician.
* *Recommendation 5:* NPs, PAs, and NMWs should be eligible for all federal incentive programs directed to improving the geographic accessibility of services, including the National Health Service Corps Scholarship Program.
⊁ * *Recommendation 6:* Graduate medical education should be constructed to give residents experience in working with PAs, NPs, and NMWs to ensure that these physicians will be prepared to utilize nonphysician services.

Other recommendations affecting nursing are sprinkled throughout the Report. They will be considered in our final discussion.

Nonphysician Provider Technical Panel

Originally, the panel was constituted to describe the "state of the art" of the work of nonphysician providers. Early in their discussions, nonphysician providers were defined as "individuals who are trained to provide services traditionally provided only by physicians." Following an extensive literature review and review of major data sources relating to manpower statistics and professional standards and criteria, the panel produced an interim report (1979) which convinced GMENAC that the role of nonphysicians in the delivery of primary care was viable and active. GMENAC then decided to expand the role of the panel and to make recommendations regarding the impact of nonphysician providers on the supply of physicians.

Members of the committee include:

Hertzog, Francis C., Jr., M.D.
Chairman, Board of Directors
Memorial Hospital Medical
    Center
University of California at
    Irvine
Long Beach, California

Magen, Myron S., D.O.
Dean and Professor of
    Pediatrics
Michigan State University
College of Osteopathic
    Medicine
East Lansing, Michigan

O'Rourke, Karen G., R.N.,
    M.S.
National Representative
Federation of Nurses and
    Health Professionals
AFT/AFL-CIO
Washington, D.C.

Spurlock, Jeanne, M.D.
Deputy Medical Director
American Psychiatric
    Association
Washington, D.C.

Taylor, E. Lee, M.D.
CDR, MC, USN
(Ex Officio)
Director, Medical Corps
    Programs
National Naval Medical Center
Bethesda, Maryland

Trevino, Margarita C., R.N., M.S.
Nursing Director
Community Health Centers of
    Dallas
Dallas, Texas

Wilson, Almon C., M.D.
RADM, MC, USN
(Ex Officio)
Commanding Officer
Naval Health Science
    Educational and Training
    Command
National Naval Medical Center
Bethesda, Maryland

Carbeck, Robert B., M.D.
    (Convener)
Executive Vice President
Catherine McAuley Health Center
Ann Arbor, Michigan

It is important to note that the nonphysician panel arrived at decisions and assumptions relating to NPs, PAs, and NMWs. Some of these assumptions and decisions are noteworthy because they distort and change the meaning and impact of the recommendations on the nursing profession.

First, although they stated that they recognized the *complementary functions* of nonphysician providers, the focus of this study was *only* on *substitution potential*. The panel was not interested in looking at personnel who had no shared functions with physicians. They recognized that physician supply was not affected, nor was the care of patients, by the impact of the complementary roles of nonphysician providers.

Second, they placed nurse practitioners and physician assistants in the same category (dependent on physician delegation for their role). Contrarily, they pointed out that "although physician assistants practice only as dependent providers, the nursing profession has traditionally been regarded as having an independent sphere of practice, owing to its unique body of nursing knowledge" (GMENAC, Vol. 6, p. 44). They further recognized that there was disagreement between professions about whether particular activities were in the domain of nursing or medicine, the so-called grey area of practice. They stated that nursing needed to define more clearly the boundaries of its practice, the types of patients seen, the services provided, the outcome of their intervention, and the legal status of the providers. Later in the report the exact same recommendation was made regarding physicians.

Third, an overriding principle of the report was that the services considered in the model used were *medical services*. As such, they were to be provided by nonphysician providers only under the supervision of the physician, as *delegated tasks*. Distinct nursing functions were never addressed by the panel. The delegation of medical tasks to nurses is an old methodology for expanding physician services and has been used for years in the ongoing delivery of health care. What has been at issue following the report are those acts which medicine claims and for which they may not be the omnicompetent providers. Nurse practitioners do not practice medicine. They do not because they are not legally able to do so and because they are not trained to be physicians. The services they provide are nursing services, some falling in the grey zone, and some definitely delegated tasks, not only of physicians, but of pharmacists, physical therapists, dieticians, and social workers.

It is clear, when the report is read carefully, that the

GMENAC recognizes the impact on health care that nonphysician providers have in the areas of adult health, maternal and child health, psychiatry, emergency medicine, anesthesiology, emergency care, and other primary and preventive care services. What the report clearly says is that nursing does, indeed, have a unique practice. What we must do is define it, refine it, and own it.

Last, the definitions presented in the report of nurse practitioners and midwives in primary care do not include adequate terminology dealing with functions. There are several inconsistencies of definition in the report regarding nursing practice that strike the careful reader of the document as illogical when considering the final recommendations of the committee as they impact on nursing. One cannot lump nurse practitioners together with physician assistants when their definitions of function differ in such significant ways. Nurses *are* independently licensed professionals, and although they do perform some delegated functions, the majority of their practice is based on a body of nursing knowledge and their licenses do not require them to be directly supervised by physicians in that practice.

It is a curious habit of thought which labels shared acts of practice as traditional to one of the professions alone. It is the same habit of thought that allows medicine to encroach on every other profession, by virtue of open-ended practice acts which allow all physicians to do all things to all patients, regardless of their training, but seeks to limit by law and tradition other professionals who have both the training and the skill to perform acts which medicine chooses to label as its own. Tradition is understandable, but change is inevitable.

Supportive Recommendations

The GMENAC Report, in the summary of the nonphysician provider panel, Recommendation 13, reads, "State laws and regulations should not impose requirements for physician supervision of NPs and PAs, beyond those needed to assure quality of care." Subrecommendations relating to function, prescriptive powers, and use of nonphysician providers in rural areas were also addressed. In citing Weston's paper which relates to the location, or lack of it, of nonphysician providers in areas of need because of restrictive laws relating to practice, the panel suggested that relaxation of the laws currently in force would result in increased service accessibility

(Weston, 1980). Since this is a first priority identified by the GMENAC in its introductory remarks, they lamented the present restriction of practice. GMENAC had concern about the charade of reimbursement policies which require that physicians be present periodically for agencies to receive reimbursement, but in actuality are only "stop-in visits" which make work done by NPs, PAs, and NMWs "look as if the physician is the provider" (GMENAC, Vol. 6, pp. 42, 45). They encouraged federal expenditure for incentive programs (training, scholarship, etc.) for NPs and PAs which would encourage accessibility of services by these providers to underserved geographic areas to be continued and reinforced.

Unlike the negative and restrictive nature of the general recommendations which were widely publicized, these recommendations recognize the disincentives to practice, point out the cumbersome and often manipulative methods used in practice to provide services to patients in less desirable locations and of less desirable status, and recommend that NPs and PAs be encouraged by the government to practice where their services are needed. In short, they recognize the contributions of these providers and the barriers to their use in present health delivery.

Problems of insurance companies were addressed and it was recorded that four major insurance companies and many smaller companies now reimburse nurse midwives and PAs for "in name" reimbursement.* These providers pay the same rate for the same service, regardless of whether or not it is provided by the midwife or M.D.

Recommendation 14 of the panel report stated that Medicare, Medicaid, and other insurance programs should recognize and provide reimbursement for the services provided by NPs, PAs, and nurse midwives in those states where they are legally entitled to provide these services. Services of these providers should be identified as such to third party payers and reimbursement should be made to the employing institution or physician (GMENAC, Vol. 6, p. 47).

Although there should be strong debate over the validity of reimbursement of physician services to physicians, and the services of others only to the employer or, worse yet, the physician, this recommendation *clearly* recognized the antiquity of the present system of lack of reimbursement for services nonphysicians

*This information was listed as a personal communication. The major companies listed were Traveler's, Continental, Mutual of Omaha, and Hartford.

provide. The panel further recommended that physician supervision requirements imposed by the third party payers should be consistent with law relating to practice in the states.

There is opportunity in these recommendations to raise appropriate questions about present procedures that limit practice, or require fraud and manipulation, and that really limit access to qualified providers. It is a big step forward and should be seized with all speed and enthusiasm by nurses across the states as one more argument for change in the present system.

One of the most positive aspects of the panel report is found in the section titled "IV. Expanded Charge." In this section (GMENAC, Vol. 6, p. 14), the panel addressed the question, "Given a situation of adequate physician resources, *what other reasons might there be for supporting nonphysician providers in these specialties?*" A second question of whether or not the "delegation" level which was projected could be reached was also asked. The panel adopted the following principle:

> Even in the event that there is an adequate number or a surplus of physicians in a particular specialty, the use of nonphysician providers (NPs, PAs, or nurse midwives) may be supported for one or more of the following:
> 1.   When they increase the accessibility of services.
> 2.   When they decrease the costs or expenditures associated with health care delivery.
> 3.   When they are the providers of choice for some consumers.
> 4.   When the utilization of nonphysicians increases the quality of service (i.e., services provided by a team composed of a physician and a nonphysician are superior to those which a physician working alone could provide).

These criteria obviously refer to judgments as to how care should be delivered. "Access to services, control of inflation, and optimization of health status had been cited in the Interim Report as national health objectives which GMENAC would observe in its recommendations" (GMENAC, Vol. 6, p. 15).

Implications, Analysis, and a Call for Action

Health care services and institutions are in crisis. There is no doubt that the notions of cost containment and health care as a right must be reconciled, that innovation and new health care delivery designs must be adopted by 1990. The danger is that we will continue to increase technology, use health personnel in traditional ways, and continue to look at health care as illness care alone. The opportunity expressed in the rather wholesome and carefully considered outlook of the GMENAC lies in the ability of nurse practitioners and the entire nursing profession to tackle head-on four areas just outlined as reasons for the continued need to support nonphysician providers and show, through research, hard numbers and simple patient preference in the marketplace those things which we often claim, but fail to prove in quantitative ways. The in-depth literature review undertaken by the panel still leaves many areas of research open and appropriate documentation of the impact of nursing in the four areas described is still lacking.

Nursing has the opportunity to leap out of its state of quiet desperation and anonymity. We need to imitate the courage of those nurses who have put themselves in the marketplace, grappled with interdisciplinary primary care delivery, fought to change restrictive laws which govern their practice, and gathered preliminary data which suggest that the impact of nonphysician health providers is real, important, and accepted. Only failure to grasp this opportunity can blunt the entire forward movement of nursing in the next decade. If nursing fails to respond to so clear a request and need, it will not be the GMENAC Report which can be blamed.

Projections and Figures

The statistics in GMENAC project that by 1990 there will be 39,000 trained NPs. They will be seeing 2.5 percent of all ambulatory visits by adults and 34.6 million child care visits per year. Nurse midwives will number between 4,000 and 5,000; be participating in 197,600 deliveries, seeing 2.8 million prenatal/postpartum patients and an additional 2.8 million patient visits for primary care needs. Ob/gyn nurse practitioners are expected to cover 7.8 additional visits. That totals over 5 percent of obstetrical and gynecological care (GMENAC, Vol.1, p. 99). More documentation of patient contacts and service provided in other areas is needed.

Among other recommendations in the summary report of import to nursing, number 16 calls for recognition of the need for a different organization of health care delivery. Nurses can help shape that new organization.

In every part of the GMENAC Report there is opportunity to make a difference. It is necessary to overlook some of the semantics, overcome some of the hostility of being evaluated against our will, shake off the easy reaction of discounting its worth or impact, and face the reality that much of what was done was excellent. There is a research agenda to be attended to, inconsistencies to be addressed, misconceptions to be corrected, and some soul searching to be done. The charges are clear:

1.   Increase research to document impact, cost effectiveness, and retention of nurses in the primary care sector and other practice arenas.

2.   Explain our services, document them, separate them, if need be, but do not leave them for others to define.

3.   Get practice and reimbursement legislation straightened out. If the practice act is restrictive, liberate it. If it is inconsistent, clarify it. If someone else is trying to determine it, wrest it away from them. But do not sit by and let things happen, sighing and whining about our lot.

4.   Create new opportunities for nurses in education, service, and planning. Decide on *how* to produce nurses for primary care and other needy fields rather than argue about *whether* they should be. There is no need to knuckle under to the recommendations of another profession—unless you have no idea where you want to go yourself or how to get there.

GMENAC harped on *delegation* of duties. There is a difference between *accepting* accountability for services you can provide and being *delegated* services that are now provided by others. The difference is whether the service is a referral to a valid practitioner or passing off one's own responsibilities to another. We all do some of that from time to time, but basically what one does is not as important as why she does it and how accountable she is for it. Nurse practitioners have often seized the opportunity to do a delegated task only to turn it into accepted nursing practice.

If we are less afraid of turf and more sure of what it is we can do well, we will not shudder at such reports as the GMENAC, but will look to them as an opportunity. It is a rich report. It is a successful report. It accomplishes what it states in its final paragraph, "The Report will be successful if it generates controversy, and improvements" (GMENAC, Vol. 1, p. 99). We know that it has done the former. Whether it does the latter is yet to be seen.

Whether we take the opportunity to be part of that success as nurses is a function of whether we have a vision of what part we can play, feel the exhilaration of new challenges, and, most important, feel the confidence of our ability and the commitment of our profession to make it happen.

References

Lemann, N. "Let the Nurses Do It." In *The Nation's Health,* edited by P. Lee, N. Brown, and I. Red. San Francisco: Boyd and Fraser, 1981, p. 223.

Miike, L. "The Future of New Health Practitioner," *Family and Community Health* (1979):65–68.

Scheffler, R.M., Yoder, S.G., Weisfeld, N., and Ruby, G. "Physician and the New Health Practitioners: Issues for the 1980's," *Inquiry* 16 (1979):195–229.

Summary Report of the Graduate Medical National Advisory Committee, Vols. 1–7, September 30, 1980, HRA Publications (HRA 81-651-657).

Weston, J. L. "Distribution of Nurse Practitioners and Physician Assistants: Implications of Legal Constraints and Reimbursement," *Public Health Reports* 95 (May/June 1980):253–258.

15. Professional Territoriality and the Anesthesia Experience

Ira Gunn

The central issues with regard to nurses functioning in expanded roles are usually fought out in the arenas of the legal definitions of medicine and nursing, including the legal relationships between physicians and nurses who choose to practice collaboratively. This professional conflict in reality has less to do with protecting the public, the purpose of legal practice acts, than it does with protecting medicine's professional turf. Essentially, interprofessional conflict often has as its basis the biological phenomenon of territoriality that finds translation in the human social experience of individuals, groups, or nations as they strive for status, power, and wealth. While aggressive behavior is characteristic of territorial conflict, survival in our age is seen as being dependent on the development of a society in which conventional competition is substituted for territorial warfare, a society in which people learn to cooperate and communicate because the alternative is to destroy themselves (Storr, 1970).

State health practice acts preclude conflicts from being resolved through conventional competition within the health care arena, so the territorial warfare is moved to their legal and legislative sources. The historical conflict between nurse anesthetists and anesthesiologists demonstrates the nature and extent to which professional territorial conflicts can be taken. This chapter reviews this conflict and addresses a rationale which has potential for the resolution of such conflicts between medicine and nursing.

The development of the clinical specialty of anesthesia for nurses has its roots in three significant events of the nineteenth century which provided the impetus for today's modern era of health care. These events were (1) the demonstration of the anesthetic properties of ether, chloroform, and nitrous oxide, (2) the invasion of health-related institutions, including the hospital, by women demanding improvements in institutional housekeeping and care of the infirm following the Crimean War in Europe and the Civil War in the United States, and (3) the incontrovertible evidence demonstrated by Robert Koch of the pathological role of organisms in human and animal diseases and surgical sepsis. These three events demonstrated (1) that patients could undergo required surgical intervention without pain, making surgery more feasible and acceptable, (2) that women, as nurses, had a major and viable role in health care requiring a sound educational base, and (3) that sepsis could be controlled and did not have to be the major scourge producing morbidity and mortality following surgical intervention (Thatcher, 1953, pp. 27–46).

Anesthesia, being considered an ancillary service in the nineteenth century, did not generate much enthusiasm on the part of physicians to engage in its practice on a regular basis. Thus surgeons began to utilize whoever was available—the general practitioner, the house officer, the medical student, or the nurse. The dissatisfaction with this service, as provided by the occasional anesthetist, led some surgeons in the United States to turn first to the Catholic Hospital Sisters for help in this matter and then to the trained nurse. This perhaps was inevitable since the status of women and nurses ranked with that of the anesthetist at that time. "The apparent need was for anesthetists who would (1) be satisfied with the subordinate role that the work required, (2) make anesthesia their absorbing interest, (3) not look on the situation of anesthetist as one that put them in a position to watch and learn from the surgeon's technique, (4) accept comparatively low pay, and (5) have the natural aptitude and intelligence to develop a high level of skill in providing the smooth anesthesia and relaxation that the surgeon demanded" (Thatcher, p. 53).

Credit must be given to the surgical team of the brothers Mayo (William J. and Charles H.) and their nurse anesthetist, Alice Magaw, for much of the evidence that gave broad-spread impetus to the utilization of nurses in this field. Early in its history, St. Mary's Hospital in Rochester, Minnesota became a demonstration place for observing outstanding surgical skill. What also impressed these visiting surgeons was anesthesia being administered by Miss Magaw in such a manner that it "satisfied the demands of the surgeon while providing the ultimate in comfort and safety for the patient" (Thatcher, p. 57).

It is interesting to note that while the "anesthetic death furor" of the 1890s was still being heard, Alice Magaw published an article in the *St. Paul Medical Journal* in 1900 reporting 1,092 anesthetic cases using an open-drop technique "without an accident, the need for artificial respiration or the occurrence of pneumonia or any serious results" (Thatcher, p. 59). In 1906, she published in *Surgery, Gynecology and Obstetrics* 14,000 cases "without a death directly attributable to the anesthesia" (Thatcher, p. 59).

These publications and the growing respect for nurses in this field in the United States demonstrated the need for education in anesthesia as well as the efficacy of nurses administering anesthesia. Initially, nurses were trained by surgeons; then nurses were sent where other nurses were practicing anesthesia to learn this skill. In 1909 the first true postgraduate course in anesthesia for nurses was established at St. Vincent's Hospital, Portland, Oregon. By 1914, three others had been established: St. John's in Springfield, Illinois, New York Postgraduate Hospital in New York City, and Long Island College Hospital in Brooklyn. These courses were 6 months in length and included instruction in anatomy, physiology, and pharmacology as well as training in the administration of the commonly used anesthetic agents.

World War I not only generated a proliferation of nurse anesthetist educational programs, but demonstrated to the world the competence and capability of these individuals. It also brought together a small cadre of U.S. physicians who had caught a vision of the potential of the field for medicine and who determined that they would make anesthesia an all-physician service.

Methods utilized by these physicians to eliminate nurse anesthetists from the field of anesthesia during the period 1917–1925 included the following:

1.   Defining anesthesia by professional proclamation as the practice of medicine.

2.   Requesting legal interpretations of medical and nursing practice acts of attorneys general in an attempt to get an opinion declaring that nurses could not legally administer anesthesia.

3.   Seeking amendments to the medical practice acts, restricting the administration of anesthetic agents to physicians.

4.   Passing resolutions endorsing boycotts by medical societies, such as one in Kentucky which made the employment of a nurse (or nonphysician) a violation of the professional code of ethics stating "the profession should not refer cases to hospitals where nurses are allowed to give anesthetics, and that hereinafter no member who violates the law and ethics shall be considered in good standing in this Association" (Thatcher, p. 115).

This action in Kentucky brought about the immediate filing of a test case in the courts by Louis Frank, a Louisville surgeon, and his nurse anesthetist, Margaret Hatfield. Dr. Frank insisted that the state board of health be partner in this suit within the courts. While they lost their first hearing in the circuit court, the case was appealed. The judge hearing the case in the court of appeals ruled in favor of Dr. Frank and Miss Hatfield and his legal opinion as written in 1917 bears repeating in 1982:

> [These] laws have not been enacted for the peculiar benefit of the members of such professions, . . . but they have been enacted for the benefit of the people.
>   . . . While the practice of medicine is one of the most noble and learned professions, . . . Neither should such a construction be given to it as to deprive the people from all service, . . . (Thatcher, pp. 115–116; Frank et al. v. South et al.: Kentucky Rep. 175).

Despite this decision, the physician anesthetists continued their challenges. However, in 1919, through the efforts of Dr. George Crile, a noted Cleveland surgeon, whose principal nurse anesthetist was Agatha Hodgins, the Ohio Legislature passed an amendment to the Medical Practice Act, which stated:

> Nothing in this chapter shall be construed to apply to or prohibit in any way the administration of an anesthetic by a registered nurse under the direction of and in the immediate presence of a licensed physician providing such nurse has taken a prescribed course in anesthesia at a hospital in good standing (Thatcher, p. 116; "Bill to Legalize," 1919).

While this is the only example in the United States where the nurse anesthetist is recognized in the Medical Practice Act of a state, it spelled out a doctrine which fairly well holds to today. Physician, in most instances, has been interpreted to include physicians, dentists, osteopaths, and others who by law are permitted to authorize anesthesia.

The ability of the nurse anesthetists to withstand the challenges of the physician anesthetists was in no small measure due to the support of surgeons and hospital administrators. It might well have been this alliance, forged in adversity, that fostered to some extent the schism between the mainstream of the nursing profession and the nurse anesthetists.

It should be recognized that it was in the first two decades of the twentieth century that the nurse anesthetist's position within the hospital nursing hierarchy was beginning to be established differently from that for other nurses. There were two principle modes of employment: (1) employment by a hospital "subject to general control of the Superintendent (Administrator), and as to House Rules to the Matron and Chief Nurse" (Thatcher, p. 83), and (2) employment by a surgeon whereby the nurse anesthetist became his office nurse and nurse anesthetist. The midwestern and northeastern sections of the country seemed to prefer the first arrangement, while the south preferred the latter. There is evidence that some nurse anesthetists at this time were working on a fee-for-service arrangement in California during this period.

In essence, what had evolved by 1920 was a clinical nurse specialist:

1.   Who required additional education beyond that afforded in the generic nursing program.

2. Who was responsible and accountable for her professional practice to someone other than the matron or chief nurse.

3. Whose remuneration for services was better than that for most other nurses.

4. Whose competence was so significant for the times that it won the respect of the surgeons and led to the development of collegial relationships, often affording the nurse anesthetist more autonomy than her other nursing colleagues enjoyed.

5. Who engaged in early clinical research and descriptive studies, publishing their findings in nursing and medical journals as primary authors.

6. Whose services evoked continuing debate as to whether they could be performed legally by a nurse.

The social and professional status of the nurse anesthetist within the hospital system provided the basis for the schism between nurse anesthetists and the mainstream of nursing which was formalized with the establishment of a professional specialty organization, the American Assocation of Nurse Anesthetists (AANA), following the failure of the American Nurses' Association (ANA) to develop a section for nurse anesthetists and office nurses within its structure in 1930.

Certainly the lack of success in gaining recognition in ANA and the revitalization of the attacks on nurse anesthetists by physician anesthetists during the Great Depression made nurse anesthetists feel exceedingly vulnerable and thus the climate was ripe for organization. The young organization made one more attempt at alignment with the ANA in the same manner as had the Red Cross, the National Organization of Public Health, and the National League of Nursing Education, and once again their proposal was turned down. While both the ANA and the leaders of the new organization must share responsibility for the failure of negotiations for alignment, nurse anesthetists did not fit the mold that some nursing leaders had for the profession; they represented change and an expansion of role which the profession was not ready to recognize, and in some instances is still not ready to do so.

The revitalized attack by physician anesthetists concerning the legality of the nurse anesthetist took the form of a test case in California filed in 1933. Essentially, the arguments by these physicians sound similar to those heard today with reference to the practice of nurse practitioners: (1) that the service constituted a medical act rather than a nursing one, (2) that the physician rather than the nurse must assume ultimate responsibility for the service (considering the status of the captain-of-the-ship legal doctrine prevalent in those days, this argument was probably more valid then than it is today), (3) that medical education, rather than nursing education, was the more appropriate background for the specialty, and (4) that if nurses wanted to practice medicine, why didn't they go to medical school?

The prelude for this case took place in 1928 when physician anesthetists, working with the California Board of Medical Examiners passed a resolution that "inasmuch as the administration of anesthetics by persons not licensed under the Medical Practice Act constituted a violation of said Act, the Secretary of the Board of Medical Examiners . . . is hereby requested to give notice . . . in order that physicians, surgeons and hospitals may govern themselves accordingly" (Thatcher, p. 132). The nurse anesthetists then sought an attorney's general opinion on the matter. Dated January 1931, the opinion confirmed that there was nothing in the law which precluded nurses from administering anesthesia. In 1933, another opinion was issued by the attorney general of California to the secretary-treasurer of the Board of Medical Examiners ruling that "a registered nurse may administer drugs or an anesthetic to a patient. But, she must not attempt to prescribe for the patient" (Thatcher, p. 140).

Failing in their efforts to get an opinion from the attorney general favorable to physician anesthetists, the physicians working within the framework of the Los Angeles Medical Association filed the test suit seeking an injunction against Dagmar Nelson, a nurse anesthetist, requesting that she be permanently enjoined from administering anesthesia because she did not possess a medical license. This case was taken through each step of the state judicial system and in each instance the ruling was in favor of the nurse anesthetist.

Again, the essential support for nurse anesthetists during this challenge had come from surgeons and hospital administration rather than from organized nursing through the ANA. As a part of Nelson's defense, the young specialty organization was able to file a brief in *amicus curiae* in support of Nelson and all nurse anesthetists. While an adverse ruling in California would not have had the effect of law outside of California, it would have set an undesirable legal precedent which could have rebounded to other states.

The persistent challenges to the legality of nurse anesthetists over this first third of a century was only the forerunner of challenges to come. While no other court cases were filed, there were continued requests for attorney general opinions, one of which finally was favorable to physician anesthetists in the State of Indiana. There were also attempts to pass restrictive legislation in both New York and California, both of which failed.

Immediately following World War II, many young physicians who had been exposed to anesthesia as a part of their military service provided opportunity for the physician specialty to be expanded. At this time, a new tactic was employed to force the nurses out of the field. This tactic consisted of the use of the lay press, both newspapers and popular magazines, in an attempt to discredit the nurse anesthetist in the eyes of the public. This campaign in a sense backfired when the Southern Surgical Association, the American Medical Association, and the American College of Surgeons all passed resolutions deploring such tactics and expressing support for nurse anesthetists. The one adverse effect that this effort did have was the discouragement of many qualified nurses from entering the specialty. The irony of this tactic in the late 1940s was that there was only one-third of the trained anesthesia personnel needed to fill hospital vacancies.

The campaign against nurse anesthetists by selected academic anesthesiologists who were involved in setting up medical residencies in this specialty took the form of orienting nursing faculty, who were involved in baccalaureate nursing education, that anesthesia was the practice of medicine, a specialty into which nurses should not be admitted. The degree of willingness on the part of nursing educators to accept unquestionably such physician dogma is a paradox within itself, particularly in view of the failures that anesthesiologists had encountered in attempting to get nurse anesthetists declared illegal as well as those directed at legislating them out of the field. The only reasonable explanation can be found in the depth of the schism between ANA and AANA and the fact that the war had done little to stimulate thinking about new or different roles for nursing. But the effect of this was to leave nurse anesthesia education outside the mainstream of nursing education, a situation which today is reflected in only four graduate programs to prepare nurse anesthetists existing within schools of nursing. Other such programs exist in schools of allied health, schools of medicine, basic science departments, and so on.

In the 1950s and early 1960s, physician opposition took the

form of professional codes of ethics in which anesthesiologists who participated in the education of nurse anesthetists or who worked with nurse anesthetists could be censured by the professional society if the physician belonged to it. Probably the only thing learned by this experience was that you could lose members through censure, but you did little to prevent a practice. In fact, many prestigious anesthesiologists involved themselves in the education of nurse anesthetists during this period.

By the early 1960s it had become obvious that anesthesiology (physician) leaders were beginning to recognize that the goal of having all anesthesia administered by qualified physician anesthetists was unrealistic (Bendixen, 1967; Dripps, 1962). In 1965, the National Institute of General Medical Science of the National Institutes of Health held a conference on the "Crisis in Anesthesia Manpower." Even though nurse anesthetists were administering 46 percent of the anesthesia in the country at that time, whereas anesthesiologists administered only 39 percent, nurse anesthetists were not invited to participate. In 1967, *Clinical Anesthesia* devoted a major part of its second volume to anesthesia manpower problems. While there were articles supportive of nurse anesthetists and others equally opposed, it was noted that by this time 50 percent of the anesthesia residents were graduates of foreign medical schools, a figure that rose to near 60 percent by the mid-1970s.

In 1964, an attempt to improve the relationship between organizational ASA and AANA resulted in the formation of a liaison committee. In 1969, C. R. Stephen, an anesthesiologist, commented: "Progress has not been rapid, but the dialogue has enhanced understanding" (Stephen, 1969).

In 1972, a joint statement pertaining to the qualifications of persons administering anesthesia was released by AANA and ASA. The statement did recognize the CRNA as an appropriate anesthesia care provider and conceded "that the ideal circumstances of qualified anesthesiologist and nurse anesthetists working together as an anesthesia care team may not be totally possible in the future" ("Joint Statement," 1972). The maldistribution of anesthesiologists is a major factor which precludes such an ideal. Despite this factor, and in the midst of the next exacerbation of this historical conflict, ASA withdrew its support for this joint statement and to date the two organizations have not been able to agree on a replacement.

The last major challenge by the ASA to nurse anesthetists

came in the years 1974–1978, with an attempt to take over the credentialing mechanisms for nurse anesthesia education and the nurse anesthetist accreditation and certification. It was at this time that the U.S. Office of Education (USOE), which had recognized the AANA as the accreditor for nurse anesthesia education in 1955, published a major revision of its criteria for nationally recognized agencies. Since the accreditation mechanism had been tightened up in anticipation of these changes, the challenge was unsuccessful.

The second provocation to AANA was a letter written to the Senate Finance Committee, which was reviewing Medicare legislation for amendment, suggesting that the CRNA should be included in the law as being eligible for direct reimbursement from Medicare. Because of this nurse anesthetists were not included in the legislation.

Perhaps one of the reasons nurse anesthetists have such a strong specialty organization is that adversity forges strong bonds, and there were hardly any periods of time in the first 90 years when they were allowed to relax and become complacent. Despite the expenditure of energies in meeting all of these physician challenges, the AANA did find time to develop its certification program in 1945, its accreditation program in 1952, a voluntary sustained professional excellence program based on continuing education credits in 1968, and a mandatory recertification program in 1978. In light of the association's many achievements, its failure to initiate the move of nurse anesthesia education into academic setting until the early 1970s has been a puzzlement.

Expanded Roles and Professional Territoriality

The expanded role movement within nursing is often dated to coincide with the emergence of the nurse practitioner movement in the 1960s. In reality, expansion of nursing roles has been the history of modern nursing since its advent in the nineteenth century. But such expansion has most often been a function of filling vacuums within health care rather than aggressive behavior seeking new or expanded territory. It is for this reason that territorial conflicts have often been absent at the time of the inception of the role, but emerge when it becomes attractive or desirable to other professions, or when economic or ego threats are perceived by a group.

At the heart of the issue of role expansion is the perceived territorial conflict between medicine and nursing: What constitutes medical practice? Nursing practice? What is the relationship between the two and how do they change over time?

The philosophy most accepted within AANA, and which it believes has the most potential for resolution of role conflict, is that medicine and nursing, while being separate and distinct professions, do not have mutually exclusive practices. It has accepted the position of Dorothy Johnson that professions are identified and differentiated on the basis of their central purpose for being.

> Whatever "it" is, there is ample reason to believe "it" does not change with age, or geographic setting, or medical diagnosis, anymore than law, medicine and teaching change with such variables. Certain activities may change, the problems encountered in practice may differ in degree or even in kind, but the central purpose of the profession and the reason for its being does not change with shifts in the location of patients, or the age group involved, or the category of disease. It is on the basis of the existence of a central purpose in being that professions are identified and differentiated and by virtue of which they endure over time (Johnson, 1964).

If one accepts that cure is the central purpose of being of medicine, and care is the central purpose of being of nursing, it is easy to recognize that cure and care cannot be mutually exclusive and will result in areas of overlap. Yet the failure to accept this phenomenon of role overlaps is at the heart of professional conflict.

Cure can best be characterized by the functions of diagnosis of pathology and its treatment. Anesthesia, except for a minimal number of diagnostic or therapeutic blocks, is not a primary diagnostic or therapeutic modality, thus does not fit well into the cure model even though at times it gives occasion for diagnosis and treatment. Anesthesia is basically a process through which patients are rendered insensitive to pain with or without unconsciousness and often temporarily paralyzed to facilitate other medical requirements. As a result of the process, the patient is rendered incapable of caring for himself. Thus, the care component becomes critical to the process, mandating vigilance in monitoring aimed at protecting and detecting changes requiring modification of the process to maintain the patient at near optimal status. This is and has been a traditional nursing function (Gunn, 1979).

Certainly there is a role for the medical expert in anesthesia just as there is a very important role for the nurse. The anesthesiologist is the "cure" expert within the field while the nurse is the "care" expert. Their roles inevitably overlap but that does not diminish either in the area of their expertise. This is no different than in medical and nursing roles in obstetrics, pediatrics, psychiatry, or other specialized fields.

While nurses may be principally the care agents, it would be incomprehensible if they were not concerned about effecting that care in such a manner that it has a curative outcome, recognizing that in some instances comfort might be all that is possible. Likewise, while physicians may be the principal cure agents, it would be equally inconsistent if they were unconcerned with care. This interrelationship between cure and care makes role overlap inevitable.

Nurses functioning in expanded roles do share larger role overlaps with physicians than do most other nurses. However, this is also true of nurses functioning in intensive care settings. Role overlaps are not static, but rather shift on the basis of patient or client requirements as well as on the basis of the expertise of the care and cure providers. The question of whether the role shift is toward medicine or toward nursing is totally dependent on patient needs at any given point in time.

Role overlap between physicians and nurses has positive benefits: (1) it provides opportunity for an enhanced continuity of care as well as a more cost-effective basis for care, (2) it affords health clients access to both nursing and medicine, and (3) it sets up an environment in which interdisciplinary cooperation and collaboration can be maximized.

As mentioned in the beginning of this chapter, interprofessional conflict often has as its basis the biological phenomenon of territoriality that finds translation in the human social experiences of individuals, groups, or nations as they strive for status, power, and wealth. While aggressive behavior is characteristic of territorial conflict, survival in our age is seen as being dependent on the development of a society in which conventional competition becomes substituted for territorial warfare, a society in which people learn to cooperate and communicate because the alternative is to destroy themselves.

When legal barriers, as reflected in outdated state practice acts, become perceived as inhibiting a profession's development and growth and denying the public access to needed health services because they have become more protective of the professions which they were designed to regulate than of the society whose safety and general welfare formed the basis of their intent, territorial conflict becomes inevitable. What health care professions, as reflected by medicine and nursing, have yet to learn is that they have more to lose in territorial conflict than they have through cooperation or conventional competition. It is in conventional competition that health care as a private enterprise has its best hope for survival. Competition between medicine and nursing can only exist within the areas of role overlap; professional uniqueness mandates cooperation and collaboration if all the health care needs of society are to be met. It is within the areas of role overlap that professions begin to understand and respect the contributions of each in the achievement of health goals which they hold in common. And indeed, it is in the recognition of those areas outside of role overlap that we come to recognize the extent of our interdependence—society's need for us both and our need for each other.

The question remains as to whether medicine and nursing can rise above instinctual responses to territorial conflict to a degree of maturity at which they are able to work cooperatively and collaboratively, placing society's needs over those of the profession's. Or, are we doomed to repeat the past—over and over again? If the latter, this conflict may be destructive to us both.

Samuel Martin, in addressing the future of allied health education and accreditation, sounded a note of warning that undue restrictiveness is associated with spiraling health care costs. As such, as costs continue to rise and impact industrial production costs in the form of employee benefits, industry may see fit to take over the health care system and, perceiving professional credentialing as a form of trade unionism, substitute a form of institutional credentialing. Martin provides us warning that society might not always be tolerant of those professional territorial conflicts which most often stem from professional protectionism rather than from a true concern for society and its needs (Martin, 1980).

References

Bendixen, H. H. "Debate: Anesthesia Manpower Shortage—Fact or Fiction? Fact," *Clinical Anesthesia* (1967): 16–21.

"Bill to Legalize Administration of Anesthetics by Nurses Causes Difference of Opinion," *Ohio State Medical Journal* 15 (1919):231.

Dripps, R. D. "Decisions for a Specialty," *Bulletin New York Academy of Medicine* 38 (1962):264–270.

Frank et al. v. South et al.: Kentucky Rep. 175:416–428.
Gunn, I. P. "Nurse Anesthetists Should Control The Teaching and Practice of Their Profession." In *Controversy in Anesthesiology*, edited by J. E. Eckenhoff. Philadelphia: W. B. Saunders, 1979, pp. 211–220.
Johnson, D. E. "Directions of Graduate Education for Nursing and Development of Psychiatric-Mental Health Programs," *Report of Work Conference in Graduate Education*. University of Pittsburgh School of Nursing, November 9–13, 1964, p. 51.
"Joint Statement of the American Society of Anesthesiologists and the American Association of Nurse Anesthetists Concerning Qualifications of Individuals Administering Anesthetics," *AANA News Bulletin* 26 (1972):3.
Martin, S. P. "Health Professional Education and Accreditation—A Futuristic View." In *Proceedings of the National Forum on Accreditation in Allied Health Education, April 28–30, 1980*. Washington, D.C.: American Society of Allied Health Professions, pp. 1–32.
Stephen, C. R. "Nurses in Anesthesia," *ASA Manpower Report* (1969), 19.
Storr, A. *Human Aggression*. New York: Bantam Books, 1970, p. 34.
Thatcher, V. S. *History of Anesthesia With Emphasis on the Nurse Specialist*. Philadelphia: J. B. Lippincott, 1953.

Additional Readings

Gunn, I. P. "Preparing Today's Nurse Anesthetists to Meet Contemporary Needs: A Philosophic and Pragmatic Approach," *AANA Journal* 42 (February 1974): 25–38.
Gunn, I. P. "Nurse Anesthetist-Anesthesiologist Relationships: Past, Present and Implications for the Future," *AANA Journal* 43 (April 1975):129–139.
Gunn, I. P. "An Apple Is Not an Orange But Is Good in Its Own Right: A Response to Professional Conflict Between ASA and AANA," *AANA Journal* 45 (December 1977):584–593.

16. Nursing's Pivotal Role in Achieving Competition in Health Care

Claire M. Fagin

Maximizing the Unique Contributions of Nursing to Health Care Delivery System

How do we maximize the potential for nurses' contributions to the health care system at a time of growing concern and action to reduce health care spending? In examining previous proposals with regard to reimbursement for nursing services it is apparent that, for the most part, nursing has recommended *expanding* third-party paid *services* as well as additional categories of practitioners. Specifically, nursing has bemoaned the fact that health promotion and disease preventive services have not been included in benefit packages and that nursing services have not been reimbursed, and has recommended that such other services as home health care be complementary.

During the past 15 years of cost escalation one would have thought such an approach might achieve at least minimal success. It did not. What did achieve some success, however, was the direct reimbursement to some nurses offering services already reimbursed to others, e.g. midwives, nurse psychotherapists, nurse anesthetists, and some nurse practitioners.

A quest for direct reimbursement in ambulatory care, which suggests *substitution* of nurses for other providers on the basis of cost, and both short- and long-term quality, must be explored in relation to the supply of physicians in the United States in the coming decades.

Proposals for direct reimbursement for nurse providers who

From C. M. Fagin, "Nursing's Pivotal Role in Achieving Competition in Health Care." In *From Accommodation to Self-Determination: Nursing's Role in the Development of Health Care Policy.* Copyright © 1982 by the American Nurses' Association. Excerpted with permission of the American Nurses' Association.

substitute for physicians imply head-on competition with physicians for the health care dollar. Since such reimbursement requires changes in legal and regulatory mechanisms, explicit recognition of this problem is essential, and a conscious decision must be made as to whether or not to engage in such competition.

On the ambulatory care scene, regardless of the procompetition strategy eventually agreed upon, the system must be opened to true competition from properly credentialed nurses, home health agencies, and visiting nurse associations, among others. Consumer choice and competition among providers will rest in great part on the removal of restraints to access to appropriate practitioners.[1] In recognition of fiscal restraints, services contemplated are to be substitutive [alternative] rather than supplementary.

Further, nursing should be actively involved in the design of programs of health promotion and disease prevention that will ultimately reduce reliance on higher cost technological interventions.

Reimbursement for Nursing Services in Hospitals and Other Inpatient Settings

Several of the reasons for the limited public awareness of nursing's contributions to health care outcomes are related to the reimbursement system, the organization of nursing services, and the mental associations about nursing that affect nurses as well as lay people. Lack of public access to the data presented here, and reluctance to blow its own horn also contribute to nursing's low profile. An important factor in the equation is the way payment for institutional nursing services is handled in most settings.

In most hospitals, nursing service is an income-producing department in that it is specifically reimbursed by third parties. Nursing service costs, however, as well as certain other service costs, have traditionally been lumped in the multi-purpose category of routine operating costs of institutions. This practice has prevented true cost accounting, hampered the development of a financially responsive health care system, and prevented consumers from evaluating the services received in relation to the cost.

An example of the lack of knowledge the public and nurses themselves possess relating to nursing cost is the confusion about nurses' income as it relates to solutions to the nursing shortage. An argument frequently presented in response to proposals to increase nurses' salaries is the negative effect such increases might have on cost-containment priorities. The public has been in no position to either lend support or denial to such views, and nurses have not come forth with suitable responses. Not only is the public unaware of the percentage of daily rates they are paying for nursing, but also nurses themselves are unaware that salary expenses for nursing personnel have declined as a percentage of hospital expenses since 1968. As the percentage of cost for technology has increased, nursing income has suffered.[2]

The data to support proposals substituting nursing services are available and directly appropriate to the stated goals of pro-competition reform. Indeed, cost control in health delivery stimulated by tax-caps and rebates to the health economical consumer will depend to a great degree on two factors: opening the system to competition and reducing consumer dependence on health care providers. From the standpoint of opening the system, the studies cited earlier have shown that nurses are cost-effective providers of a wide variety of primary care services. Not only are their direct costs lower than those of physician providers, but also the cost of ancillary services is greatly reduced when nurses are the primary carers. These cost benefits must be facilitated by new state and federal legislation. Barriers must be eliminated that prevent direct access to nurses for ambulatory services such as health services for children and teenagers, prenatal and post-natal care, nursing determined home-care, and care of the elderly.

Nursing's use of the certification process to establish credentials for such providers is essential. I would endorse the National League for Nursing recommendation that the appropriate educational credential for these reimbursed providers practicing independently is the master's degree in nursing. For a variety of organized group practices, however, other certification could be considered.

Part of reducing consumer dependence on the health delivery system is the assumption of responsibility and accountability on the part of the consumer. The techniques for accomplishing this basic change are in a state of infancy (if they are out of utero at all). However, various measures (preferably age and cultural group specific) will be required to encourage consumers to make intelligent choices. The question of regulation is intrinsically tied to the level of information available to consumers and the development of their accountability. Accountability can be developed by the quality of the information provided and choices available to use the information, as well as the direct contact with the pocketbook.*

If it reflected the appropriate level and intensity of nursing care for individual patients, the billing of acute care hospitals, nursing homes, and home health agencies would reimburse the institution for nursing care quantified according to the nursing effort involved in patient care. The patient's dependency level and basic, technological, rehabilitative, and supportive care required are the key considerations in classifying the patient for nursing. Such a classification system would also reflect the components of nursing practice affecting nursing care on a uniform basis.

Such billing for nursing care would permit patients, institutions, and providers to understand the cost/benefit of nursing care and allow prospective economic modeling of differing care environments and needs. Most important, it would provide the public with a more accurate understanding of the costs and benefits of specific nursing care.

Consideration must also be given to the substitutability of alternate nursing services for higher cost hospital services. A variety of predominately nursing interventions have been shown to have low cost/high benefit results. Utilization of home care, skilled nursing facility care, nurse aided family care, and rehabilitative care with or without prior hospitalization and *with* nursing judgments should be part of benefit packages available to consumers.

---

*Target approaches in the health area have shown great success in the past 20 years. For example, from 1968 to 1977 death due to heart disease decreased by 22 percent. (Surgeon General's Report. *Healthy People, the Surgeon General's Report on Health, Promotion and Disease Prevention.* Washington, D.C.: Public Health Service, DHEW Publication No. 79-55-81, 1979.) While all of the reasons for this are not totally understood, the prevalence of four risk factors for heart disease also decreased during that time: incidence of cigarette smoking, prevalence of hypertension, amount of cholesterol consumed in the diet, and the frequency of sedentary life styles. Dramatic results have been obtained by the hypertension detection and follow-up program sponsored by the National Heart, Lung, and Blood Institute of the National Institutes of Health. An important health education experiment was conducted by the Stanford Heart Disease Prevention program. Their intensive mass media campaign and face-to-face instruction decreased the incidence of three risk factors for cardiovascular disease among men to a significantly greater extent than with the control group. Other health education programs relating specifically to risk factors for illness have also been moderately successful. Health promotion efforts that are directed towards specific illness, therefore, have been shown to be effective.

Changes in reimbursement policies to encourage such tested models must acknowledge that these services are not, for the most part, medical services.

Conclusions: Summary of Recommendations

A great deal of data suggests the importance of restructuring nursing roles in competitive health plans. To maximize possibilities for the inclusion of nursing in federal legislation fostering competition, I have explicitly recommended third-party reimbursement for nursing services in primary, secondary, and tertiary care; long term care; and alternative care models. In any competitive legislation adopted, nursing services should be included in the minimum benefit package, and nurses must be permitted to compete on an equal basis with other providers. These recommendations acknowledge the constraining role of state laws and regulations in the appropriate utilization and reimbursement of nurses. Nursing should give immediate attention to removal of these constraints, however.

In developing alternatives to high-cost technological care, a clearinghouse for information must be established, and the necessary steps taken to formalize reimbursable substitutes for hospital and institutional care. Utilizing health teaching, family support systems, home visiting, and other predominately nursing interventions under nursing management and design, in consultation with physicians and appropriate others, will bring about short- and long-term cost savings.

In long-term care we will see a variety of demonstrations conducted in the next 5 years. The Robert Wood Johnson Foundation Teaching Home Program, co-sponsored by the American Academy of Nursing, and the national study by the Health Care Financing Administration comparing long-term health care programs in patients' homes with those in nursing homes both offer tremendous opportunity for maximizing nursing's potential. Successful achievements from these and other demonstration projects should be institutionalized in the health care delivery system.

If competition is to be a solution for controlling the major costs of the health care delivery system, hospitals will need to examine all cost and income variables with more discrimination than occurs at present. Specific billing for nursing care will permit patients, institutions, and providers to understand the costs and benefits of nursing care, and will allow prospective economic modeling of different care environments and needs.

Nurses must recognize for what they are, the threats and promises in seeking direct reimbursement for primary care functions. If reimbursement must be substitutive rather than additive, specificity with regard to services and credentialed practitioners is essential. A national network of state leaders should address state laws and regulations with consistent recommendations on this issue. New federal legislation should encourage states to examine and document the state laws and regulations that deny access to the market by credentialed practitioners such as nurse-midwives and certified nurse practitioners.

Use of the term *competition* to describe current proposals will be mere rhetoric unless proposals are altered to include competition among a variety of credentialed providers. The data of the past 20 years speak to the phenomenal contribution of nursing to health care outcomes.

References

1 Dolan. A. K. Anti-Trust Law and Physician Dominance of Other Health Practitioners. *Journal of Health Politics, Policy and Law.* Winter. 1980. 4:4. 675–690.
2 Michela, W. A. Deductions from Revenue, *Hospitals* 52. February 1, 1978, 28.

Bibliography

American Academy of Pediatrics Commmittee on Drugs. Effect of Medication During Labor and Delivery on Infant Outcome. *Pediatrics,* September, 1978, 62:3, 402–403.
Chan, Wan H., R. H. Paul, and J. Toews. Intrapartum Fetal Monitoring: Maternal and Fetal Morbidity and Perinatal Mortality. *Obstetrics and Gynecology,* January, 1978, 40:1. 7–13.
Enthoven, A. C. *Health Plan: The Only Practical Solution to the Soaring Cost of Medical Care,* Reading, Mass.: Addison-Wesley, 1980.
Goodlin, R. C., and H. C. Haesslein. When Is It Fetal Distress? *American Journal of Obstetrics and Gynecology,* June 15, 1977, 128:4, 440–447.
Jacobs, A. Comparison of Critical Incidents About Baccalaureate, Associate Degree, and Diploma Nurses. Chicago: National Council of State Boards of Nursing, Inc., 1981, 104.
Krueter, F. R. *Nursing Outlook,* May, 1956, 5:5, 302–304.
Rooks, J. Testimony to the Subcommittee, December 18, 1980. 153.

Roth, A., *et al.* 1977 National Sample Survey of Registered Nurses: A Report on the Nurse Population and Factors Affecting Their Supply. Springfield, Va.: National Technical Information Service (offset), 1979.

Shenker, L. Clinical Experiences with Fetal Heart Rate Monitoring of One Thousand Patients in Labor. *American Journal of Obstetrics and Gynecology*, April 15, 1973, 115:8, 1111–1116.

IV

Educational Issues

17. Introduction—
Educational Issues: Background Paper

Bonnie Bullough and Vern Bullough

Professional Status and Education:
Historical Background

In the United States, status has traditionally been awarded to those with significant educational accomplishment. The highest status professions, such as medicine, law, and college teaching, are those involving the most education. While wealth is also important for determining status, the most respected persons are those with "old money" who have the sophisticated education to accompany their money. Those occupations with lower educational standards, such as auto mechanic, baker, and police officer, generally are regarded as lower on the social scale no matter what the salary. In fact, one of the distinctions between so-called white collar and blue collar jobs is the nature of education required for the job.

Inevitably also there has been an effort in the United States to use education as a barrier to entrance into the professions. It is not enough for physicians to go to medical school, but we now demand that they complete 4 years of college before beginning medical training. Since this education can be in any field, it serves primarily as a social class barrier rather than to furnish educational prerequisites. Thus professions already within the college or university setting have tended over the course of the twentieth century to increase educational requirements. What once required 4 or 5 years, e.g., medicine, now requires 8 or 9. At the same time occupations not established in the college curriculum have made strong efforts to gain admission, and during the twentieth century such diverse groups as social workers, engineers, physical therapists, nurses, and police (though criminal justice programs) have made great efforts to professionalize themselves through education. This has been easier for some occupations than others.

Nursing has found it difficult for at least two major reasons, first because nurses were overwhelmingly women, and second because the medical world in which they developed was dominated by physicians. These two factors are essential background to the understanding of the educational struggle on which this section focuses. Both the attempt to distinguish between the technical nurse and the professional nurse and the agitation for the 1985 resolution can be understood as efforts to gain professional status. But it also helps explain why nursing in the last two decades has emphasized the social and psychological needs of the patient over the physiological. Quite simply the physicians were believed to be so well versed in the physiological that the only turf which the nurses could carve out for themselves was in the area of the psychosocial support of patients. While the editors of this book do not believe that such a division was either wise or necessary, this is how the nursing leadership perceived it at the time.

Some background is necessary to illustrate the above generalizations. The first question to be dealt with is the fact that nursing was overwhelmingly a woman's profession. This meant that during its early developmental period college education was effectively denied to nurses because until the twentieth century few colleges admitted women at any level. It is true that in the last part of the nineteenth century a number of women's colleges were established but for the most part these steered clear of any vocational or professional training and instead concentrated on the liberal arts. While women's colleges offered intellectual challenges to their students, they also visualized most of their students as potential wives and mothers rather than professionals. Like their male counterparts at Harvard, Yale, and Princeton, the undergraduate degree was in liberal arts. However, the graduates of the men's schools went on to professional schools and became lawyers, ministers, college professors, and physicians while the women were essentially terminal liberal arts students who were well prepared for conversation with their professional husbands.

Though Oberlin College had been fully integrated in 1841, it was not until the rise of the state universities in the last part of the nineteenth century that sexual integration took place on any large scale and even then many of the states established separate colleges for women. Most of the sexually integrated colleges were in the midwest and west while early nursing had developed in the east, which was the most educationally sex-segregated part of the country.

Nursing, however, was attractive to large numbers of women

who were anxious to be economically independent of the men who legally had control over most of a woman's existence. This meant that when the hospital training school model came into the United States from England, large numbers of women flocked to nursing. Florence Nightingale had undoubtedly chosen the hospital model because it was in the hospitals that the English physicians were trained and it seemed natural to train nurses there also. In the United States, however, growing numbers of hospital medical colleges were becoming more firmly affiliated with universities and by the twentieth century this affiliation became almost a necessity. Nursing schools were slow to follow. When nursing schools were first established in the United States, sick care was in a period of transition moving from home to hospital, and the existence of a new professional group—nurses—allowed hospitals to grow and expand at minimal cost. This was because students furnished the basic work force in the hospital, and because they were students they need not be paid. It also allowed medicine to become more specialized as it delegated tasks to nurses. This allowed medicine to deliberately lower its numbers and to raise standards. It also raised physicians' incomes and status by emphasizing longer and longer periods of college education. In fact, it does not seem too strong to state that it was only because nursing education moved into the hospitals that medical education was able to move out.

So effectively did nurses take over menial duties performed either by family members or by physicians that nursing education boomed. From 15 nursing schools in 1890 the number rose to 432 in 1900. Unfortunately, once the hospitals found a source of free labor they were extremely reluctant to do away with it, and nursing has been struggling ever since to overcome its early success. Thus, even though nurses from the first tried to upgrade themselves by getting advanced degrees, they found themselves at a disadvantage because no college or university would recognize their hospital training school experience. If they went to a college, they had to in effect enter as a freshman. Still nurses tried. The beginning of higher education for nurses dates from the time a five-member delegation from the recently organized Superintendents Society (forerunner of the modern National League for Nursing) made an agreement with Dean James Russell of Teacher's College, Columbia University, to offer a course for nurses. He agreed to do so providing they would guarantee an enrollment of 12 persons or pay $1,000 a year. Members of the society screened and admitted students, contributed $1,000 a year, and taught the course, a not very auspicious beginning. Still, in a sense Teacher's College was a natural because it was attempting to upgrade the education of teachers most of whom (at least at the elementary level) lacked college training. In 1905 the Columbia program was lengthened to 2 years, and finally, in 1907, Adelaide Nutting was hired to direct it. Not until 1910, when the program was endowed by Helen Hartley Jenkins, did it become firmly entrenched (Christy, 1969; Cunningham, 1959).

The first basic nursing program in a collegiate institution was started at the University of Minnesota in 1909, although it was not a degree program. Students enrolled in the program were required to meet university standards but in addition to their classwork had to work 56 hours a week on the hospital wards. After 3 years they received a diploma rather than a degree (Gray, 1960). This modest alliance with academia was copied by a few other universities, including Cincinnati, Indiana, Virginia, and Washington (MacDonald, 1965), and finally, in 1916, Cincinnati went further and established a degree option (Roberts, 1961; Stewart, 1945). Other colleges followed but not particularly rapidly for at least two reasons: hospital training schools were unwilling to give up their free labor, and college graduates were not always willing to either work the hours or carry out the menial tasks that nursing programs demanded. For a long time the college-educated nurse was regarded as an elite nurse who ended up teaching or working as a public health or school nurse. However, it was only slowly that diploma nurses themselves moved into the hospital role because there most of the care was given by students.

As the struggle to raise educational standards progressed, nurses and hospital administrators decided that not all nursing tasks required a full 3- or 4-year educational program. The solution was to stratify the role into two levels: registered professional and practical nursing. The first license for practical nurses was established in New York State in 1938 and the idea rapidly gained currency because of the crisis in nursing brought on by World War II (Bullough and Bullough, 1974). By 1960 all of the states and territories had statutes licensing practical nurses (U.S. Dept. of Health, Education and Welfare, 1968). No sooner had this happened than practical nurses repeated the experience of registered nurses and raised their own status by turning many of the lesser tasks over to nurses' aides.

The growing stratification of nursing made it easier to argue that the top strata needed university education. At the same time both medical and nursing care were becoming more complex, so that the need for better backgrounds in the biological and behavioral sciences was more apparent. Gradually more colleges and universities established collegiate programs. It was, however, a slow uphill struggle and it is only now that the collegiate schools are expanding rapidly enough to take over a significant portion of nursing education. Consequently, in the decade of the 1950s another entry into academia opened up through the community colleges. This movement, pioneered by Mildred Montag (Montag and Gotkin, 1959; Montag, 1972), caught on rapidly and associate degree programs are now emerging as the largest source of registered nurse preparation.

The Career Ladder Issue

The associate degree movement is not without controversy. Probably the major issue is whether or not associate degree programs and baccalaureate degree programs should be linked to form a career ladder. In this section a paper by Kramer argues that baccalaureate education is different from other nursing education and it should not be incorporated into a career ladder. Bullough describes a successful career ladder plan used by the Southern California Consortium.

The career ladder issue also has ramifications in the practice setting, in nursing practice law, and in the accreditation process. The issue as it relates to the accreditation body, the National League for Nursing, is discussed by Castiglia, Garvey, and Bullough in this section as a part of their survey of the problems and approaches to educational mobility. Probably one of the more unique models for achieving educational mobility is the New York Regents External Degree Program, which uses testing rather than an educational approach. It is described in this section by Lenberg.

Entry into Practice Issue

The fragmentation of nursing caused by the four types of educational programs (practical, diploma, associate degree, and baccalaureate), all of which at times claim to prepare the basic bedside nurse, has caused considerable confusion in the mind of the public. This is particularly true in light of the controversy outlined above over whether or not these programs should be linked in a clear career ladder or stratification pattern. It is not surprising, then, that the suggestion was made to have one basic baccalaureate educational pattern for all registered nurses and one for practical nurses. The vehicle for enforcing this approach would be the state nurse practice acts. The movement started in New York State in 1974 when the Nurses Association passed a resolution calling for the baccalaureate degree as the minimum preparation for entry into professional practice by 1985. This resolution quickly became the focus of a national discussion and in 1976 the Council of Baccalaureate and Higher Degrees of the National League for Nursing (NLN) passed a similar resolution. The idea gained further momentum when a package of three entry-into-practice resolutions was passed by the American Nurses' Association (ANA) in 1978. Subsequently, various other nursing organizatons have debated the issue and some, including most notably the Association of Operating Room Nurses, have supported the movement. In 1982 the board of directors of the National League for Nursing, representing all of the councils (practical, associate degree, diploma, and baccalaureate), voted to make the baccalaureate preparation the requirement for entry into the practice of professional nursing.

The resolutions are emerging as one of the major issues facing the profession today, although there are differences of opinion as to what the resolutions mean, whether or not they should be implemented, and what their implementation would do for the profession.

The 1978 Entry into Practice Resolutions†

Resolution 56: Identification and Titling of Establishment of Two Categories of Nursing Practice.

WHEREAS, ANA for the past 13 years has upheld the position that the "minimum preparation for beginning professional practice at the present time should be baccalaureate degree education in nursing," and the "minimum preparation for beginning technical nursing practice at the present time should be associate degree education in nursing,"*

THEREFORE BE IT RESOLVED THAT: ANA ensure that two categories of nursing practice be clearly identified and titled by 1980

AND BE IT FURTHER RESOLVED THAT: by 1985

†Reproduced with permission of the American Nurses' Association.
*American Nurses' Association. *Education Preparation for Nurse Practitioners and Assistant to Nurses: A Position Paper.* New York: American Nurses' Association, 1965.

minimum preparation for entry into professional nursing practice is the baccalaureate degree in nursing

AND BE IT FURTHER RESOLVED THAT: ANA, through appropriate structural units, work closely with SNAs and other nursing organizations to identify the two defined categories of nursing practice

AND BE IT FURTHER RESOLVED THAT: national guidelines for implementation be indentified and reported back to ANA membership by 1980.

Resolution 57: Establishing a Mechanism for Deriving Competency Statements for Two Categories of Nursing Practice

WHEREAS, ANA for the past 13 years has upheld the position that the "minimum preparation for beginning professional practice at the present time should be baccalaureate degree education in nursing," and the "minimum preparation for beginning technical nursing practice at the present time should be associate degree education in nursing," and

WHEREAS, Nursing groups throughout the country have developed, or are in the process of developing competency statements of two categories of nursing practice, and

WHEREAS, There is a need for statements to clearly differentiate the competencies for associate and baccalaureate degree prepared nurses

THEREFORE BE IT RESOLVED THAT: ANA established a mechanism for deriving a comprehensive statement of competencies for two categories of nursing practice by 1980.

Resolution 58: Increasing Accessibility of Career Mobility Programs in Nursing

WHEREAS, Since 1965 ANA has supported the position that all nurses obtain educational preparation in colleges and universities, and

WHEREAS, The Commission on Nursing Education has developed standards to ensure quality educational programs, and

WHEREAS, The overwhelming majority of registered nurses currently do not hold a baccalaureate degree in nursing and vocational nurses do not hold an associate degree, and

WHEREAS, Future employment of nurses undoubtedly will be based on academic preparation as well as licensure, and

WHEREAS, There are limited educational opportunities for large numbers of non-degreed nurses in many geographic areas, and

WHEREAS, Flexible and non-traditional programs in nursing education can be developed while ensuring academic integrity,

THEREFORE BE IT RESOLVED THAT: ANA actively

support increased accessibility to high quality career mobility programs which utilize flexible approaches for individuals seeking academic degrees in nursing.

Differing Views of the
Entry into Practice Resolutions

It seems clear that the New York Nurses Association did not have a career ladder in mind when they passed the original resolution. Rather they seemed to have conceptualized the baccalaureate graduate as the registered nurse, while nurses with associate degrees were to be technical or practical nurses. Articulation between the two groups of nurses was not spelled out in the original resolution, although there was considerable sentiment in favor of some type of "grandfather clause" that would allow existing registered nurses the right to retain their current titles. Only new graduates would be required to earn the baccalaureate degree. The resolution passed by the Council of Baccalaureate and Higher Degrees of the NLN used similar wording but members of the council were also ambiguous about a grandfather clause. Possibly more of them knew that a grandfather clause is not a popular concept in the political arena. Legislators tend to argue that the additional education is either needed for patient safety or it is not. They see inequity in allowing present practitioners to hold out with less education than entering candidates are required to have. The other argument against a grandfather clause is that it delays implementation for up to 45 years while the current licensees continue practicing. Thus the humane and politically prudent grandfather clause is not without problems.

The 1978 ANA resolutions were quite different in focus from the original New York proposal. They clearly called for increased accessibility to high-quality career mobility programs using flexible approaches for individuals seeking academic degrees in nursing. Thus, they deal with the problem of the existing work force by advocating continued education rather than the grandfather clause.

The 1982 resolutions by the NLN board of directors was made with career ladder opportunities in mind. This support for educational mobility is a function of time and a growing political sophistication among nurses. Serious attempts to turn the resolutions into laws have taken place only in New York and Ohio. The Ohio Nurses Association has delayed basic reform of the nurse practice act to cover current levels of practice in order to link that reform with a proposal to make the baccalaureate degree a requirement for the registered nurse level. In New York the proposal in the form of a bill has been introduced in every legislative session since 1975. Although it has had the devoted support of several legislators, including most notably Senator Pisani, whose article is included in this section, the bill has never been voted out of committee. Legislators are afraid to support it because they receive a storm of protest whenever it is considered seriously. Eighty percent of the nursing work force in 1975 were diploma or associate degree graduates. They saw the proposal as denigrating their nursing preparation and squeezing them out of the job market. They were particularly angry when the proposal was linked with an anti-career ladder stance.

The New York State Nurses Association has now moved to a pro-career ladder stance but the legislature is cautious about backing any nursing legislation because of the bitter infighting they saw among nurses. It will take a long process of image building to reestablish the Nurses Association credibility. Meanwhile other state associations have watched the New York experience and have reacted with caution.

When the issue is examined on its merits there are arguments to be made both for and against the proposal. Supporters of the idea see it as a means to bring order into a disorderly educational system. They look at the system described above and point out that patients, the public, and colleagues within the health care delivery team would be less confused if we settled on one standard program for the preparation of registered nurses. Advocates look at the growing complexity of patient care and know that nurses need more education in the biological and behavioral sciences as well as in clinical nursing. Moving into the university should improve the knowledge base and enable nurses to give better patient care. University graduation will also "professionalize" the occupation, which will give nurses more status and more power over patient care decisions. These are potent arguments in favor of the resolutions (Christy, 1980; Lynaugh, 1980; Partridge, 1981).

Opponents of the proposal do not perceive the baccalaureate degree as needed for all nursing functions. Some do not even believe that current baccalaureate programs are the best educational preparation for nursing. The American Hospital Association is against the proposal simply because there are not enough existing baccalaureate graduates to staff the nation's hospitals.

With a grandfather clause the existing staffing could continue, but because few legislatures will seriously consider such a clause, the proposal passed into law could cause a crisis in the hospitals. Two articles in this section examine nursing educational preparation from this point of view. One is an official paper prepared by the National Advisory Commission on Vocational Education. The other is a paper written for the Buckeye State Nurses Association, an organization that was born out of the struggle with the Ohio Nurses Association over the resolution.

Clinical Competence

Intertwined with the arguments for and against the baccalaureate program as a requirement for entry into professional practice is a feeling of discontent among some hospital nursing service people about the level of clinical competence exhibited by graduates of generic baccalaureate programs. Three approaches to solving this problem have been proposed. The first is to incorporate more clinical practice into all nursing courses in baccalaureate programs. This would move these programs back in the direction of diploma education with its heavy emphasis on skill training. Many baccalaureate educators are philosophically opposed to such a move. The second proposal is to add a clinical internship to the programs. The chief worry about a required internship is that it might be used to exploit students. The third approach is to leave the programs as they are and let graduates acquire skills in their first year or two on the job in formal or informal internships. The last article in the section by Soukup proposes a short required internship which may serve as a compromise solution to the problem.

Summary

The major issues in education for the 1980s are inherited ones. They are created by a history that produced multiple approaches to basic nursing education. We cannot erase our history; we can only understand it and try to solve the problems related to the multiple entry points. The profession needs to decide whether it wants to continue with many roads to licensure or one, whether it wants to support a stratification system, and whether it wants to foster educational mobility. Those decisions cannot be made in a vacuum. The realities of politics and the need for a viable nursing work force must be considered as these issues are debated.

References

Bullough, B. and Bullough, V. "The Causes and Consequences of the Differentiation of the Nursing Role." In *Varieties of Work Experience: The Social Control of Occupational Groups and Roles,* edited by Phyllis L. Stewart and Muriel G. Cantor. New York: Halsted, 1974, pp. 81–86.

Christy, T. *Cornerstone for Nursing Education.* New York: Teachers College Press, 1969.

Christy, T. "Entry into Practice: A Recurring Issue in Nursing History," *American Journal of Nursing* 80 (March 1980):485–488.

Cunningham, E. V. "Education for Leadership in Nursing, 1899–1959," *Nursing Outlook* 7 (May 1959):263–272.

Gray, J. *Education for Nursing: History of the University of Minnesota School of Nursing.* Minneapolis: University of Minnesota, 1960.

Lynaugh, J. "The Entry into Practice Conflict: How We Got Where We Are and What Will Happen Next," *American Journal of Nursing* 80 (February 1980):266–270.

MacDonald, G. *Development of Standards and Accreditations in Collegiate Nursing Education.* New York: Teachers College Press, 1965.

Montag, M. *Evaluation of Graduates of Associate Degree Nursing Programs.* New York: Teachers College Press, 1972.

Montag, M. and Gotkin, L. G. *Community College Education for Nursing.* New York: McGraw-Hill, 1959.

Partridge, R. "Education for Entry into Professional Nursing Practice: The Planning of Change," *Journal of Nursing Education* 20 (April 1981):40–46.

Roberts, M. M. *American Nursing: History and Interpretation.* New York: Macmillan, 1961.

Stewart, I. M. *The Education of Nurses: Historical Foundations and Modern Trends.* New York: Macmillan, 1945.

U.S. Department of Health, Education and Welfare. State Licensing of Health Occupations. Public Health Service Publication No. 1758. Washington, D.C.: U.S. Government Printing Office, 1968, pp. 9–10.

18. The Nursing Challenge: Eliminating the Two-Step Backward Syndrome

Senator Joseph Pisani

Recently, I had the honor and pleasure of being the guest speaker at graduation ceremonies at one of my local hospitals. It was an unusual graduation because the graduates were all under the age of five years. Each one of them was a severely handicapped child suffering from a developmental disability, an emotional disability or a physical disability or perhaps a combination of them. It was a unique school, multidisciplinary in approach, whose purpose is to try if possible to prepare these very unique children, very special children, to function at some minimal level and be able to enjoy their place in the sun as any normal child would.

As I was visiting with their very special nurses prior to the ceremonies, one of them remarked that I was among [in the presence of] two of my favorite [kinds of] people, namely, children and nurses. And indeed I was. I reflected for a moment as to why I have chosen the problems of children and the problems of nurses as two of my particular legislative concerns. There is a similarity between these two groups. As for children, from time immemorial, they have been deprived of their rights and they have been unable to secure them for the obvious reason that they are unable to speak and act for themselves. *They* need a voice in the legislature. As for nurses, they, too, for too many years have been deprived of their rights and their deserved privileges. They were *not* unable but were too busy serving others to take the time and effort to secure their own rights. They too need a voice in the legislature.

I do not mean, of course, to sail the analogy on to the rocks of chauvinism—either male, legislative or medical. So let me make

Pisani, Senator Joseph. "The Nursing Challenge: Eliminating the Two-Step Backward Syndrome." *Journal of the New York State Nurses Association* (December 1978):26–30. Reprinted with permission of the New York State Nurses Association.

clear that I know that nurses have always had the *capacity* to speak effectively for themselves. And the world, and the medical profession, and hospital administrators have since learned that the nursing profession not only can, but *has,* spoken for itself in New York State and in the nation.

But you were, at one point in time, looking for a friend in the State legislature, and I volunteered.

I have tried to be a voice for nurses ever since that day when I was sitting in my legislative office and a delegation from the nursing profession came in to me and educated me as to what has been going on with respect to your profession, vis-à-vis the other health-related professions. I was convinced then, and I am more convinced now, that you are deserving more in the way of recognition, not for tribute, but recognition in terms of your ability to stand on your own as true professionals and take your rightful place in the spectrum of disciplines and services available to the sick and the needy in our society.

In October, 1970, your Association sponsored a program entitled, "Confrontation with the 70's—Are we to be Spectators or Participants?" I was privileged to speak at that session. In my comments, I told your members that the health care delivery system was literally "up for grabs" and that nursing *must* participate actively in influencing redesign of that system. I urged your members to assist legislators in making informed decisions about the kinds of health care services needed by people—and the role nursing should play in delivering those services.

Following that conference, your Association—largely through you, its members—made a heroic effort to modify the laws of this state to provide for recognition of the independent function of nursing. Most of you will recall that that effort was vigorously opposed by the regulatory bodies, the organized medical profession and organized hospital administration. But nurses stood united in defense of their practice and the public's right to quality nursing care services. Because of that unity the nursing profession and the legislature of this state charted a new course for nursing and health care throughout this country.

As primary Assembly sponsor of the legal definition, I was indeed proud of the leadership demonstrated by nurses in New York. I was proud to be known as organized nursing's advocate in the legislative arena—because it was obvious that organized nursing's objective included a *new* and *better brand* of *health care* for our citizens.

In my view, the 1972 redefinition of nursing was a major step forward. But, I must tell you that I think nursing is now caught in a one-step forward, two-step backward syndrome. Furthermore, I cannot emphasize strongly enough that, unless you resolve this syndrome, you will be completely locked out of any influence or responsibility in the emerging health care delivery system. This is a matter of great concern to me because of my admiration and respect for nursing and nurses—but beyond that, I know that *health care* is *different from* and *greater than* medical care. I believe the nursing profession is the key group in humanizing and integrating health care. I believe YOU MUST assume responsibility and accountability for ensuring that nursing practitioners of the future are bonafide and genuine *colleagues* of physicians, dentists, social workers, physical therapists and other health care providers. Otherwise, health care will remain as inadequate, fragmented and depersonalized as it is today.

The crux of nursing's one-step forward, two-step backward syndrome is your system of education. Like it or not, we live in an academic world—but nursing thus far has not faced up to that reality. You continue to permit—indeeed even defend—a pattern of nursing education which is little more than a dead-end street. Tragically, it is a dead-end street not only for the profession as an entity, but for virtually every individual who enters nursing.

Now let me make one thing manifestly clear. What I am about to say should not and must not be taken as a criticism of the diploma-school nurse. To the contrary I have nothing but respect and admiration for the thousands of nurses who have become members of your profession as a result of diploma-school training. There is no question in my mind that diploma-school nurses have exemplified *all* of the high ideals of the nursing profession and stand second to no one in terms of dedication, ability and knowledge. The fact is, however, that diploma-school training, as good as it may be, has been literally segregated from the main stream of academia, while at the same time our society has become more and more credential-oriented. And that orientation has been geared to those credentials that are granted by the academic community, namely, degree-oriented institutions as opposed to certificate-oriented institutions.

And I'll say another thing: I deeply deplore the fact that there has been little or no articulation between the diploma schools and the academic institutions so that someone with a diploma can move easily sideways into an academic institution and receive full credit for the years spent in a diploma school. The fact is that such is not the case. And the fact is that, for upward mobility, our degree-oriented society looks for degrees as a prerequisite to significant upward mobility. And—try as we might—I cannot foresee in the near future changing the settled prejudice of our modern degree-conscious society.

Let me amplify. As a profession you have enacted a legal definition of nursing practice which *should* permit you to practice as fully autonomous practitioners. But your credentials, the sine-qua-non of professional credibility, are completely inconsistent with those of our autonomous health care providers. As a result, the integrity of the legal definition is subject to constant challenge by those who doubt your qualifications and competence. This poses enormous problems for you as a profession. In practically every year you have been forced to ward off legislative or regulatory efforts to classify vital and legitimate components of your practice as medically delegated and supervised. The resources you have had to expend on these defensive maneuvers have deterred and weakened your ability to take affirmative initiatives in health care. Further, your practitioners are constantly subjected to subtle and not-so-subtle legal and professional challenges. Meanwhile, greater and greater authority and prestige are accorded to physicians' assistants. The bottom line is that patients *still* do not have access to urgently needed professional nursing services. And all the medical care in the world will not compensate for the absence of nursing care.

At other levels, you and your profession are completely knocked out of influence in health care. Because the *value* of your services is underestimated and the competence of your practitioners doubted, you are either not represented at all or are greatly outnumbered in health planning bodies at agency, local, state, and national levels. As a result, the public's *need for and right to* nursing care services is seldom considered or provided for in decisions made by these bodies. A cardinal example is nursing's exclusion from the insurance law which defines health care providers whose services are reimbursable.

Finally, what is the impact of the current pattern of nursing education on those individuals who pursue a nursing career? From my perspective, under present circumstances, too much of nurse training can only be described as a dead-end street. It is sheer folly to expect recognition as a professional nurse *without* a baccalaureate degree. And for those who enter programs outside the mainstream of higher education—i.e., hospital diploma programs, practical nurse programs—academic or career mobility will be virtually non-existent. Let me repeat—we live in an academic world. If nursing is to survive, it *must* change and get into that world.

What I mean to say specifically is that to require a nurse to spend three years in academic and clinical training and receive a diploma and then, after making that great giant step forward, to have to take two steps backward and *lose* years in order to gain entry into the academic community, is what I characterize as nursing's one-step forward, two-step backward syndrome. It is manifestly unfair, it is inequitable and discriminatory to the nurses individually and to the profession as a whole.

I believe the 1985 Proposal is the solution to nursing's one-step forward, two-step backward syndrome. First, it calls for movement of all nursing education into institutions of higher education. For this reason alone, it immediately and automatically enhances and facilitates career mobility. Secondly, it places nursing education on a level more consistent with that of other health care providers. Thus, it increases public confidence in nurses and permits nurses to interact more competently and comfortably with both the public and other health care providers. Third, it emphasizes that there is an intellectual base to nursing practice, thereby refuting the unfortunate perception that nursing care is simply a collection of medically-delegated procedures. Finally, it protects the licenses and practice privileges of practical and registered nurses licensed at the effective date of the law. This provides approximate recognition of those individuals who have met the requirements of existing law and insures that the public will have continued access to their services.

I am fully aware of the objections and challenges to the 1985 Proposal. I know it has been labeled "elitist"—but I believe it is *not* elitist to guarantee to the public that practitioners of nursing will be as competent in their discipline as other practitioners are in theirs. I know questions have been raised about the "expense" of the proposed system—but I believe that qualified nursing care services are essential and, therefore, quality nursing education is as worthy of financial support as quality medical and dental education.

Further, I *know* the present fragmented pattern of nursing education is indefensibly costly to the public and nursing students alike. I know that concern has been expressed that the '85 Proposal may negatively affect minority or disadvantaged individuals who seek a nursing career—but I believe *entrée* to academic credentialing is the greatest possible opportunity for these individuals. I know also that the grandfather provisions are thought by some to be dangerous and confusing to the public—but I believe that individuals licensed under existing law are competent, responsible and fully qualified to continue their practice throughout the transition period. The American public is now very familiar with the steps taken by occupations and professions seeking to insure that their educational systems remain current, and the public understands that imposition of new requirements is not an indictment against those prepared under past requirements.

How can the 1985 Proposal be secured? In exactly the same way the 1972 Definition of Nursing Practice was secured. No external group "gave" nursing that definition—nurses themselves secured it by persuading me and other legislators that it was indeed appropriate.

In my mind's eye I can still see that wave of white hats and white uniforms, men and women alike, all dedicated to the nursing profession, marching up State Street until the entire front of the Capitol was inundated with what history will record to be one of the most impressive, orderly, and magnificent expressions of support for a piece of legislation that has ever been experienced in our State Capital. Yes, against overwhelming odds, in the wake of a Governor's veto, and in spite of the insidious forces then working against us (and still in place, I'm sorry to say), we proved to the legislature that nurses united were deserving of recognition and nurses united can indeed change the course of medical and legislative history.

No external group will "give" nursing the 1985 Proposal. Nurses have persuaded me and some of my legislative colleagues that the 1985 Proposal is necessary. But much remains to be done.

I am sorry to observe that the 1985 Proposal does not mobilize and rally nurses as the 1972 definition did. On the contrary, it has divided and polarized the nursing community. The legislature is not so naive as to expect total unanimity or consensus on any measure. Nor does it fail to perceive that this type of legislation is inevitably threatening to many within the profession. But the legislature does expect support from at least a majority of those who seek legislative support of change.

It is my belief that the majority of nurses agree with and

support the 1985 Proposal. But it has been a silent majority—comprised of some who believe it is so logical it requires no action; comprised of others who believe controversy will be more quickly resolved by avoidance of confrontation; and comprised of many who believe that somebody else will do the necessary work.

I pledge my absolute support of the 1985 Proposal and commit myself to its enactment into law. But I must also tell you I cannot do this alone. *You* must make a commitment to resolve—*this year*—nursing's one-step forward, two-step backward syndrome. You owe it to yourselves and to nurses of the future—and, more importantly—to the public.

Let me, in closing, remind you again of that moving procession up State Street to the State Capitol that took place nearly a decade ago. Not all nurses marched in that parade either in body or in spirit. There were some who had learned to live comfortably most of the time with a definition that said, in effect, that a nurse is a lady who helps doctors by doing their bidding.

But I don't believe that there can be many nurses today who regret the demise of that old definition.

Just so, there are nurses today—good nurses—and I respect them—who oppose our present program. But I sincerely believe that—by 1985 or shortly thereafter—there will be few nurses, indeed, who will regret what we are now about to accomplish.

Therefore, I say to you, let us, with that future day of concord in mind, work together vigorously and effectively now to achieve the 1985 program—to hasten the day when a new and recognized posture of complete professionalism unites the profession of nursing in the vanguard of the health professions.

I pledge to you my efforts toward that proud objective.

19.   The Entry into Practice Issue —
Position Paper

Buckeye State Nurses Association

Introduction

It is with feelings of deep concern that the Buckeye State Nurses Association discusses the issue of educational preparation for entry into nursing practice. In these days of acute nursing shortages, professional burnout, rapid turnover of staffing, employment dissatisfaction, declining enrollments in some programs, and zero growth in others, it would seem that nursing would band together to seek solutions to our common problems. Such, however, is not the case. We are a profession torn apart by ideological differences.

The Buckeye State Nurses Association regards the issue of the educational preparation for entry into nursing practice as a major cause of our professional alienation. We feel that until our ideological differences are worked out, we will not be able to solve our other problems. We would have to agree with Anne Zimmerman who, upon retiring from the presidency of A.N.A. in 1978, remarked that "Until we can make a decision on this issue [entry into practice] and make plans to implement it, progress on all other issues facing this profession will be impaired."[1]

The purpose of our testimony today is to outline three major sources of opposition to the A.N.A. Position on Education for Entry into Practice. And since the original Position Paper of 1965 has remained virtually unchanged except for the 1978 resolution on support for career mobility,[2] it is this initial document which is being addressed.[3]

The two areas to be discussed are 1. the position that all education for those who are licensed to practice nursing should take place in institutions of higher learning and 2. the philosophical division of the two domains of nursing practice into professional and technical.

Reprinted with permission of the Buckeye State Nurses Association, 1981.

Point Number 1:   The position that all education for those who are licensed to practice nursing should take place in institutions of higher learning.

In 1965 a group of eminent educators, motivated by a sincere desire to improve the fragmented and depersonalized care being given by nursing, sought to formulate a plan whereby nursing care could be improved.[4] Influenced by a number of studies on nursing, the latest of which was the 1949 report of Esther Lucille Brown,[5] these educators were convinced that nursing could be advanced if the educational preparation for practice was improved. Their basic premise was that education bore a direct relationship to practice.[6] The group then took the position that in order to improve nursing practice the locus of educational preparation should be transferred from existing diploma programs to institutions within the mainstream of education, i.e., colleges and universities.[7]

Whenever a sociological change of major proportions is considered, it is usually necessary to produce evidence that such a change would benefit society. In order to have arrived at the conclusion that nursing care could be improved by this transfer, it would have been necessary to demonstrate that the clinical performance of graduates of the collegiate programs was superior to that of graduates of the diploma programs. To date, no such evidence has been reported. Early studies done to research this subject did not show consistent findings; and later studies either failed to support earlier ones, or even contradicted them. As late as 1978 it was reported that the systematic study of the differences in the clinical performance of the graduates of the different programs was still extremely limited.[8]

On the contrary, there is evidence to suggest that in the work world graduates of diploma programs (and ADN programs) do as well as or better than baccalaureate-prepared graduates.[9,10] According to a recent survey,[11] 64 percent of diploma nurses were still working either full or part time ten years after graduation. Baccalaureate nurses surveyed at the same point in their careers showed that 59 percent were so employed. Sixty-five percent of diploma nurses were employed in hospitals as compared with 42 percent of BSN nurses. Moreover, diploma nurses were favored for head nurse positions with 24 percent as compared with 13 percent of BSN nurses.

There are currently about 343 diploma programs in the United States. Some of these programs fulfill every requisite for being an institution of higher education.[12] They have excellent faculties, good clinical facilities, ample resources, and well-motivated students. In the state of Ohio which represents the sixth largest state in the union there are 30 NLN accredited diploma programs. These programs fulfill a vital social need. Should the 1965 Position Paper be legislated into law, these 30 programs would cease to have any relevance for nursing education. Presently Ohio has no statewide plan for assuring sufficient numbers of programs to prepare graduates to meet the health needs of the citizens of Ohio. In the absence of such a statewide plan, the collective wisdom of mandating the demise of these programs must be questioned.

And yet the threat of such a mandate has become a reality for Ohio. With the adoption of the "Concepts of Change to the Nurse Practice Act"[13] by the House of Delegates of the Ohio Nurses Association in April 1976, the Association committed itself to the implementation of Concepts Number 5 and 6 which call respectively for the baccalaureate degree as entry into licensed registered nursing and the associate degree for the registered nurse associate. According to A.N.A. it has been only by the resistance from a number of groups such as the ADN nurses, the Ohio Hospital Association, the Ohio State Medical Association and the Buckeye State Nurses Association that attempts at implementation of the concepts have been halted.[14] That these efforts have not been abandoned but merely postponed is evident from the report of the Ohio Nurses Review of September 1980 which states that ". . . both the A.N.A. delegates and the O.N.A. Board of Directors have decided to support a more open-ended approach by not reordering a specific date [for implementation]."[15]

In the absence then of definitive data to demonstrate that graduates of current baccalaureate programs give nursing care which is superior to diploma graduates, and in the absence of responsible statewide planning to insure sufficient numbers of baccalaureate programs to meet the health needs of the citizens of Ohio, the Buckeye State Nurses Association has adopted the position of supporting the current educational system in which graduates of ADN, diploma, and baccalaureate programs become licensed into basic registered nursing. Furthermore, the organization actively supports those programs which emphasize unlimited clinical excellence as well as academic superiority. The organization opposes all efforts which would lead to legislation that would limit licensing for registered nursing exclusively to graduates of baccalaureate programs.[16]

Point Number 2:   The philosophical division of the two domains of nursing practice into professional and technical.

The authors of the Position Paper are to be commended for their insight into the philosophical base for nursing practice. For the authors of the paper, nursing was viewed as encompassing the patient's biophysical health problem, along with its necessary therapeutics, as well as the patient's unique experience of his illness. Thus, the essential elements of nursing practice included both care and cure. In these inter-subjective relationships, the nurse then had a dual concern. She cared for the biophysical needs of the patient but never lost sight of his psychosocial needs. She assisted the patient to find meaning in his illness but was involved simultaneously in his biophysical health problem.

The fundamental philosophical error of the Position Paper was the failure to recognize the radical unity of these two domains of nursing. The authors separated the two inextricably-related domains and assigned them to different categories of practitioners. The major focus of the one was the care aspect; the dominant thrust of the other was the cure aspect. In this system the caring, or professional, nurse would provide ". . . comfort and support in times of anxiety, loneliness and helplessness."[17] She would listen, evaluate and intervene appropriately. She would assist persons in the cure aspect by helping them to understand their health problems and assist them to cope. However, the cure aspect of her practice would be delegated largely to the technician. The technical nurse, on the other hand, would be involved with the physiological reactions of patients and the physics of machines. She would carry out medically delegated tasks as well as tasks assigned to her by the professional nurse.

The authors noted that the role of the technician would assume greater importance in the future. And just as engineering, architecture and medicine had made use of technicians, so too nursing would have a place for this category of worker.[18]

On the basis then of dividing the two aspects of practice into professional and technical, an entire educational system was envisioned. The professional nurse would be prepared in a four year baccalaureate program; the technical nurse would be the product of the two year associate degree program. And in the original document, no provision was made for any articulation between the two programs.

In order to understand how the authors were able to accomplish the separation of the two aspects of nursing into professional and technical, it is necessary to examine the model of man postulated in this division. Conceptualizing nursing as dichotomous presupposes that the patient too can be separated into his component parts; that is, into mind and body. Students of philosophy will recognize this model of man as reminiscent of the mind-body split as described by René Descartes.[19]

During the Renaissance period there was an intense interest in the study of nature and natural phenomena. Science, however, could not progress because it was hindered by theological debate.[20] The question which Descartes addressed was the nature of man. He was able to satisfy both science and religion by advancing the idea that man was composed of two separate substances. Man possessed both a thinking substance, or mind, and a material substance, or body. While the two substances were characterized by intimacy, they were nevertheless distinct. Man's rational soul directed his mechanical body much as a pilot directs his ship. This dualistic philosophy was the dominant thinking about man for a long period of time and it persisted well into the 20th century.

With this model of man as dichotomous, it would be possible for the professional nurse to care for the spirit and the technician to care for the machine-like body. The question must be raised as to whether or not separating the two domains of nursing and practicing them from the perspective of either one or the other is still nursing.[21] Is it truly possible in the real world to be concerned about the patient's unique experience of his illness and not be involved simultaneously in how the person's bodily functions are changed because of the illness? Is it likewise possible in the real world of practice to care almost exclusively for the patient's bodily needs and not be concerned about how the person experiences his world?

Compounding the original philosophical error was the belief that this philosophy enjoyed wide acceptance among professional nurses. The authors of the Position Paper proceeded to assign the titles of professional and technical to even currently practicing nurses as though such titles ". . . were taxonomic terms that truly distinguished observable behavior in the real world."[22] It is small wonder then that nurses were quick to respond with the expression, "a nurse is a nurse is a nurse." Diploma and ADN graduates who were so labeled saw the term *technical* as pejorative rather than descriptive of their actual practice. And, although the label of technician has been modified somewhat over the intervening years, the implications of the original classification of categories of practice have not changed appreciably.

That the professional/technical split enjoyed less than whole-hearted acceptance by the practicing nurses is evident from the 1979 *RN* magazine survey. A significant number of RN's rejected the division. Furthermore, the results of the survey indicated that "... polarization of views on all questions related to the professional/technical proposal is far more pronounced than any difference in background, career status, or affiliation could account for."[23] There has been a similar lack of acceptance of the care/cure dichotomy among nursing educators. In current baccalaureate and associate degree programs there is less than universal differentiation of these two domains of practice in curriculum content. As noted by Verle Waters, "Despite efforts thus far, nursing has not defined and established two separate, identified practitioners and corresponding practice; as a total group, nurses have not had their heart in it because we have yet to develop a plan for implementation which doesn't make large segments of the profession feel discounted."[24]

Is it possible that nurses do not have "their heart in it" because they feel that the underlying philosophy is no longer a viable conceptualization for modern nursing? With the current shift in nursing literature to a more holistic model of man,[25-30] it would appear that differences in the educational preparation for the categories of nursing practice would be based in a philosophical system which more closely reflects current and future practitioners' ideological convictions.[31]

The Buckeye State Nurses Association therefore has adopted the position that in a democratic pluralistic society such as ours there will be variations in the health needs of citizens. In addition, the objectives and career goals of students will differ. Therefore, there is a need for programs of varying length, level of complexity, degree of responsibility, and area of practice (acute care, community nursing, etc.). Programs should be designed to meet the health needs of society as well as career goals of students. However, differentiations in nursing education should rest upon a philosophy that is acceptable to current and future practitioners.[32]

References

1. Zimmerman, Anne. "A.J.N. Interviews the President," *American Journal of Nursing, 78* June 1978, p. 1018.
2. "American Nurses' Association Commission on Nursing Education Report to the 1980 House of Delegates in Response to Resolutions Related to Educational Qualifications for Nurses," Resolution #58, Resolution on Increasing Accessibility of Career Mobility Programs in Nursing, p. 19.
3. "American Nurses' Association First Position Paper on Education for Nursing, " *American Journal of Nursing, 65* December 1965, 106–111.
4. Bullough, Bonnie. "Baccalaureate vs. Associate Degree Nurse: The Care-Cure Dichotomy," *Nursing Outlook, 27* November 1975, p. 692.
5. Brown, Esther Lucille. *Nursing for the Future.* Philadelphia: Wm. F. Fell Co., 1948.
6. Waters, Verle. "Progress of the Nursing Profession in Implementing the ANA 1965 Position Paper." Presented at the ANA National Conference on Entry into Nursing Practice, held February 13–14, 1978, Kansas City, Missouri, p. 6.
7. ANA First Position Paper, *op. cit.* p. 107.
8. Waters, Verle, *op. cit.* p. 5.
9. "Survey of Nursing Service Administrators," Assembly of Hospital Schools of Nursing, American Hospital Association, 1978.
10. Dickerson, Thelma M. "What Differentiates One Nurse from the Next? The Diploma Education." Address presented at the National Conference on Categories of Nursing Practice in Chicago, 1979.
11. "Nursing News," *RN,* June 1979, p. 11.
12. Lysaught, Jerome P. *An Abstract for Action.* New York: McGraw-Hill Book Company, 1970, p. 157.
13. "Concepts of Change to the Nurse Practice Act," *Ohio Nurses Review,* June 1976, pp. 5–7.
14. "Stand on BSN taken by 34 State Associations," *American Journal of Nursing,* April 1980, p. 628.
15. Torres, Gertrude. "Communication with the President," *Ohio Nurses Review,* September 1980, p. 1.
16. "Position Statement on Entry into Practice of the Buckeye State Nurses Association," November 1979.
17. ANA Position Paper, *op. cit.,* p. 107.
18. ANA Position Paper, *op. cit.,* p. 108.
19. Buytendijk, F.J.J. *Prolgeomena to an Anthropological Physiology.* New Jersey: Humanities Press, 1974, p. 14.

204   EDUCATIONAL ISSUES

20. Flynn, Patricia Anne Randolph. *Holistic Health: The Art and Science of Care*. Bowie, Maryland: Robert J. Brady Co., 1980, p. 42.
21. Colaizzi, Janet. "The Proper Object of Nursing Science," *International Journal of Nursing Studies*, 12. Great Britain: Pergamon Press, 1975, p. 199.
22. Lysaught, Jerome. *From Abstract into Action*. New York: McGraw-Hill Book Company, 1973, p. 240.
23. Lee, Anthony, Editor. "Seven out of Ten Nurses Oppose the Professional/Technical Split," *RN*, January 1929, p. 83.
24. Waters, Verle. *op. cit.*, p. 7.
25. Flynn, Patricia A.R. *op. cit.*, p. 17.
26. Colaizzi, Janet. *op. cit.*, p. 199.
27. Cousins, Norman. *Anatomy of an Illness as Perceived by the Patient*. New York: W. W. Norton and Company, 1979.
28. Flynn, Patricia Anne Randolph. *The Healing Continuum: Journeys in the Philosophy of Holistic Health*. New York: W. W. Norton and Company, 1980.
29. Goldway, Elliott, Editor. *Inner Balance: The Power of Holistic Healing*. New Jersey: Prentice-Hall, Inc. 1979.
30. Paterson, Josephine and Zderad, Loretta. "Foundations of Humanistic Nursing in the Healing Continuum," *Journeys in the Philosophy of Holistic Health*. Bowie, Maryland: Robert J. Brady Co., 1980, pp. 95–105.
31. Lambert, Vickie A. and Lambert, Clinton E., Jr. *The Impact of Physical Illness and Related Mental Health Concepts*. New Jersey: Prentice-Hall, Inc., 1979, p. xi.
32. Position Paper, BSNO, *op. cit.*

20. The Education of Nurses: A Rising National Concern— Position Paper

The National Advisory Council on Vocational Education

The National Advisory Council on Vocational Education has been concerned with a proposal of the American Nurses' Association to alter the process of nurse training.

The position paper, "The Education of Nurses: A Rising National Concern," is the Council's official response to that proposal.

The American Nurses' Association (ANA) has proposed a change in the process by which our nation prepares its nurses for practice. This proposal calls for reducing a four-level system to two levels of nursing: the professional nurse, who would be required to have a bachelor of science degree in nursing, and an assistant technical nurse, who would have an associate degree in nursing, and work under the supervision of the professional nurse. Implementation date for this proposal is targeted by the ANA as 1985.

The four ways in which nurses may prepare at present are: registered nurses, who may receive their education through a four-year program leading to a baccalaureate degree, required for certain administrative, managerial, and some community health positions; a two-year associate degree program, offered by two- and four-year colleges and universities; a three-year diploma program combining on-the-job training administered by hospitals with liberal arts courses taught at colleges and universities. All of these registered nurses shall have taken an examination administered by a state board of nursing in order to receive licenses. Of the 1.2 million R.N.'s licensed, 13 percent have the bachelor of science, 20 percent an associate degree, and 67 percent are di-

National Advisory Council on Vocational Education. "The Education of Nurses: A Rising National Concern—Position Paper." Issue Paper No. 2, May 1980.

ploma nurses. A fourth category, licensed practical nurses, are trained in various educational settings, including high schools, vocational schools, colleges, and hospitals over periods of nine to eighteen months. They also must pass an examination, different from the registered nurses', for licensing. Approximately 650,000 L.P.N.'s are presently licensed.

The changes called for in the ANA proposal are drastic. The diploma nurse and the licensed practical nurse, the two largest categories, are eliminated outright; and the status of the associate degree nurse becomes that of technical assistant instead of full-fledged nurse. Eighty-seven (87) percent of all nurse training programs would be altered or eliminated. Only the bachelor of science program would remain intact.

It is important at the outset to understand the nature of the American Nurses' Association. The ANA is a professional, registered nurses' organization, and is a union with a membership of somewhat fewer than 180,000, approximately *15 percent* of the total number of R.N.'s in the country. They do *not* represent the licensed practical nurses, nor do they represent over one million R.N.'s who are not members. They appear to be disproportionately influential because the 85 percent of the nation's R.N.'s who are not members of ANA are either unaffiliated or belong to small, independent nurses' associations with little influence. [These independent nursing organizations have recently joined together to oppose ANA with a coalition known as the Federation of Independent Nursing Organizations (FINO)]. Essentially, ANA strength and power emanate from their well-financed, well-organized, tri-level structure at the national, state, and district levels. With a payroll annually of over two million dollars, they are able to support state and national lobbyists who articulate their position.[1] The opposing nurses and the general public have no such united strength.

The American Nurses' Association asserts its proposal would bring a change for the better. The rationale is that a bachelor's degree for all practitioners would improve the quality of nursing care, and would therefore be in the public interest. Their position rests on the premise that nurses with baccalaureate degrees are better nurses.

The National Advisory Council on Vocational Education wrote to the American Nurses' Association, asking if they had any

1. *Labor Organization Annual Report*—Form LM-2; File no. 000-233

definitive proof of the superiority of baccalaureate degree nurses. Despite the fact that their case rests on this premise, they replied that further study is needed.

It was reported in the proceedings of the 1978 ANA Convention that one speaker stated the following:

> There has been, since 1965, a great deal of interest in differences in the nursing practice of graduates of associate and baccalaureate degree programs, but systematic study of differences in clinical performance of graduates has been extremely limited. . . . What one study shows in differences in technical or communication skills, another fails to support, or contradicts. For each claim of distinction, other claims oppose that point of view. We are left with only individual differences as the differences in performance of graduates in work settings. That may not be the whole story, but the rest of it, for the moment is not clear.

An analysis of over 50 studies prepared by the Department of Health, Education and Welfare's Division of Nursing supported this conclusion, for the most part. In addition, the Council examined several other studies which raised doubts that the ANA position was tenable.[2]

In the face of lack of evidence that the proposed change would improve the quality of nursing care, the National Advisory Council was concerned about possible adverse effects of such change. It was reasonable to assume that this change could drive the cost of health care services upward; that it could shut down large numbers of the nation's nurse preparation programs; that it could result in the loss of jobs for some nurses; and that it would reduce available options and eliminate opportunities for many of our nation's aspiring young nurses, many from minority groups.

A consideration of costs led to the conclusion that longer training periods would increase expenses for provision of health care services. One analyst estimates that, if all nurse candidates must attend four-year schools, in order to achieve the same number of nurses we now have, training costs could rise by 39.5 per-

---

2. *Prediction of Successful Nursing Performance,* Parts I & II. P.M. Schwirian, Ph.D. DHEW Publication no. HRA 77-27, pp. 163–164
American Journal of Nursing, Feburary, 1979, pp. 305–308. "How do Graduates of Different Types of Programs Perform on State Boards?"
R.N. Magazine—March, 1980, pp. 28–78. "Is the BSN Better?"
"Effects of Education on Nursing Performance," Lyman C. Dennis, II, Ph.D. and Janice K. Janken, R.N., M.S.N., September 22, 1978, Medicus Systems Corporation, Washington, D.C.

cent, in terms of the current dollar alone. Figures projected for 1985 revealed that training costs could rise by more than 57 percent.[3]

Sharp cost increases are corroborated in U.S. News and World Report, April 21, 1980, p. 78–79. The article, "Biggest Boosts Yet in College Fees," states:

> $10,000 for a year of college? It's coming next fall as one school after another falls behind in the race against inflation. Boosts in college costs in prospect for next fall are going to shock even the most inflation-wary students and their families. Increases in the double-digit range will be typical for most institutions, with some schools raising tuition and living costs by nearly 20 percent.

It's obvious what deleterious effect this will have on BSN training costs. Projected further, the increases will be reflected in higher costs of maintaining government hospitals and government military services, medicare costs, and private sector health costs, if the BSN should become mandatory.

It also is possible that the proposed change might result in a shortage of nurses. Recent ANA news releases indicate that the nationwide nursing shortage is approximately 100,000. The proposal conceivably could result in a further shortage, for, if all nurses were required to embark on a four-year training period, educational institutions would not be able to produce graduates at the present rate. Thus, the number of nurse candidates would be reduced. Such an additional shortage would prove costly, both in terms of dollars and decreased health services.

The National Advisory Council on Vocational Education has concluded that adoption of the ANA proposal would certainly affect nursing programs. According to 1977 data, there are 2,711 programs preparing nurses in this country. Of this number, only 349 are baccalaureate programs. All others—associate degree, diploma, and licensed practical nurse programs—either would be eliminated or drastically transformed. Over 87 percent of all the nurse preparatory programs in the United States would be affected (National League of Nursing).

The Council also is concerned about the effect on currently practicing nurses who do not have the baccalaureate degree. The ANA proposal calls for "grandfathering" them into the system—

3. Andrew K. Dolan, "The New York State Nurses' Association, 1985 Proposal: Who Needs It?" *Journal of Health Politics, Policy and Law,* Winter, 1978, pp. 508–536

allowing them to retain their licenses. However, the question is whether or not these nurses would be able to hold their jobs, or have job mobility, after establishment of the baccalaureate degree as a required credential. "Grandfathering," however, would then apply to registered nurses *only*. The ANA represents registered nurses exclusively, and allows no room in its proposal for the licensed practical nurse. Therefore, any LPN planning to continue a career in nursing would be forced to seek additional training, obtaining the associate degree as a minimum.

The National Council believes that adoption of this proposal would reduce career options. It seems reasonable enough to require, as the present system does, that certain administrative positions be assigned to nurses with baccalaureate degrees. However, should the nurse not aspire to such a position, the need for the bachelor's degree is less apparent. Associate degree programs already have proved that all the required health care courses can be accomplished in the space of two years, and the two-year program, as offered by community colleges, provides a low-cost, locally accessible option for students who otherwise would not have the opportunity to pursue a registered nurse career. In this group are members of disadvantaged populations—racial minorities, displaced homemakers, and persons who may not have immediate geographic access to universities. In these cases, the curtailment of career opportunities is particularly regrettable.

Although licensed practical nurses possess less technical knowledge than registered nurses, they nevertheless constitute the backbone of direct patient care in this country. The LPN course of instruction lasts only nine to eighteen months, and in some cases is available in secondary schools, thus providing a career option which is even more accessible than that provided by the associate degree program. The ANA proposal would appear to eliminate this option.

Finally, there is the diploma nurse, graduate of an intensive three-year, in-hospital course of instruction, which provides more on-the-job training than any other nurse-preparation program. An excellent statement of the value of this type of training and its desirability as a career option was carried in the March, 1979 issue of RN Magazine. A graduate of a diploma program, then studying for her baccalaureate degree, was quoted as follows:

> My diploma school training was so difficult and demanding that it weeded out those who didn't have tremendous dedication to

bedside nursing. At the time I didn't know what kept me going, but now, some twelve years later, I do know—interest in people and a tremendous satisfaction in caring for them.

In my experience, the BSN programs have eliminated the struggle and sacrifice and supplanted them with a traditional academic schedule—semester breaks, vacations, no night work, and no long hours facing crisis after crisis. That to me is the test of nursing mettle. I've met excellent AD and BSN nurses, but initially their patient care approach is different. Only after going through reality shock and adjusting to the demands of nursing—sometimes grudgingly—do they learn the great feeling one obtains from caring for others. Diploma students learn that from the beginning, or they drop out or are dropped.

It is within the prerogative of most state legislatures to change licensing laws pertaining to nurses. To date, no state legislatures have adopted changes as recommended by the ANA. The New York State Legislature, for the past three years, has considered the ANA program, and has declined to accept ANA recommendations.

Nevertheless, enactment of ANA's position has become fact in many of our health-care institutions. Promotions are being denied on the basis of merit, experience, and ability, in favor of arbitrary new job descriptions requiring a bachelor of science degree of head nurses, supervisors, coordinators, and such. Information suggesting the likelihood of enactment already has resulted in declining enrollment in diploma, associate degree, and licensed practical nurse schools. The diploma schools are rushing to link up with universities and are abandoning their diploma status, causing students and institutions to face dramatic tuition increases, longer training periods, and resulting in the denial of initial entry to many prospective students because of these factors. An attempted change in testing and credentialing to differentiate among the R.N. levels is looked upon by many as a first step in implementation of the 1985 ANA position. These elements apparently affect the very high attrition rate, i.e., the dropping out of nurses due to a sense of hopelessness and uncertainty. The injection of these career-threatening factors is demoralizing, and has created a general sense of fear and confusion which pervades the profession. If this trend is permitted to continue, and if a strong counter move is not initiated, the result will be a grave loss to the public of vitally needed health care personnel and the vocational institutions which train nurses. The ANA policy will become a *de facto* law—it actually will be in place without so much as approval by a single state legislature. When all major avenues of entry into the profession are closed due to lack of support, the proposal already will be implemented. The ANA illusion is slowly becoming a reality.

In the interest of the public good, this cannot be permitted to continue. The present proven system of four routes to a nursing career must not be traded for a system whose potential for success is based on mere conjecture. In the face, then, of all these considerations—cost in terms of dollars, reduced options, loss of valuable members of the health care profession, and reduction of opportunities for special and disadvantaged populations—the National Advisory Council of Vocational Education has concluded that implementation of the ANA proposal would not be in the national interest. The investigation of the issue gathered opinions and information from various health care and educational organizations. Most of them also are in opposition to the proposal. A summary of the rationale of eight different organizations on this subject is presented in the Appendix to this paper.

On March 19, 1979, the National Advisory Council on Vocational Education moved to disseminate its findings concerning the issue of entry-level nursing, and adopted a resolution opposing the position of the American Nurses' Association. The resolution, unanimously reaffirmed at the Council meeting of November 2, 1979, is as follows:

WHEREAS: The American Nurses' Association has taken the position that minimum preparation for beginning professional nursing practice should be baccalaureate degree education in nursing and that all associate degree nurses should serve as professional nurses' assistants; and

WHEREAS: There is no conclusive evidence that this proposal will result in improved health care services; and

WHEREAS: Implementation of the position would eliminate the diploma nurse and the licensed practical nurse; and

WHEREAS: Diploma nurse training programs, licensed practical nurse training programs and associate degree programs currently offer viable options to persons desiring a career as a nurse; and

WHEREAS: All four types of nurse training programs produce valuable members of the health care delivery system; and

WHEREAS: Implementation of the American Nurses' Association's position would increase the cost of health care services; and

*WHEREAS: Implementation of the proposal would result in disenfranchisement of career opportunities for and discrimination against several disadvantaged and special populations including (1) racial minorities, (2) displaced homemakers, and (3) those who do not geographically have access to universities;

THEREFORE, BE IT RESOLVED: That the National Advisory Council on Vocational Education oppose the position of the American Nurses' Association and support the continuance of all four routes to a career in nursing: baccalaureate degree, associate degree, diploma, and licensure of practical nurses.

The National Council thus reached its conclusion that it is not in the national interest to alter the manner in which nurses are prepared, and recommends that the ANA proposal not be adopted.

Appendix: Positions of Health and Relevant Educational Associations with Respect to the ANA Proposal

Pro

National Student Nurses' Association

Rationale: Nursing as a profession lags far behind other health professions in the length and breadth of its education for beginning practice. In fact, nursing lags behind teaching, library science, engineering, and a host of other fields. NSNA believes it is time that nursing share an education that is at least similar to those of other professions. In addition, and perhaps more important, the knowledge needed for the practice of nursing has increased exponentially and continues to do so. A nurse without a broad education in the arts and sciences simply is not able to adjust to the changing world of health care. As professional nurses expand their practices, assistants to nurses, by whatever name, must be prepared to step into the breach with sufficient education to carry the responsibilities many of them now are assuming. The NSNA does not believe that costs should rise except

*This clause was added at the November 2, 1979 meeting.

as costs generally rise. The cost of educating nurses would be borne more equitably by the people as a whole. If national health insurance comes into being, costs of nurses' services would be a part of that cost. Actual nursing service costs today are not accurately known. NSNA recommends that NACVE accept ANA's position as inevitable and work with community colleges to help them plan programs that will meet the needs of students who plan a career in nursing short of professional nursing.

Con

American Association of Community and Junior Colleges
Rationale: To increase the entry level degree requirement would reduce the number of persons qualifying for registered nurse practice. The persons most likely to be unable to meet the requirement would be those community colleges which have been most successful in drawing into such programs persons with low income, from traditionally non-college-attending families, and older women with responsibilities at home. Locally accessible, low-cost community college ADN programs have opened up nursing careers to these and other persons who would be shut out if attendance at four-year colleges became a requirement.
American Health Care Association (formerly the American Nursing Home Association)
Rationale: Nursing homes and other long-term care facilities provide unique clinical settings. Most facilities are relatively small, give significant decision-making responsibilities to licensed nurses, and often are located in non-urban areas. AHCA's greatest concerns are that the 1965 position, if implemented, would adversely affect the clinical competence of new nursing graduates, diminish the nurse manpower pool, and prevent facilities from meeting staffing requirements.
National Federation of Licensed Practical Nurses
Rationale: There are no acceptable bases or demonstrated needs from which alteration of the requirements for the licensure of practical nurses can be effected in the present. The present licensing credential for practical/vocational nursing is sound and should be allowed to continue.
National Association for Practical Nurse Education and Service, Inc.
Rationale: Existing practical/vocational nursing programs have demonstrated that they can prepare knowledgeable, skilled and

dedicated health care providers. Practical nursing programs have provided rewarding career opportunities to literally thousands of highly committed, competent persons because of their shorter period of training, lower tuition and vocational focus. These characteristics make practical nursing accessible and acceptable to many persons interested in and adapted to caring for the sick, who otherwise would be lost to the nursing profession due to lack of finances and the need to enter the employment market as rapidly as possible. The critical issue of ever-increasing costs in health care must be borne in mind in any consideration of extending the length of time for the education of health providers. The expense of education is a serious concern and, in response, we believe that nurses should be prepared in as short a time as is consistent with high quality graduates.

American Vocational Association

Rationale: No conclusive evidence has been presented to support the contention that these changes will improve the quality of health care, or better meet the basic health needs of society, or provide better educational opportunity to those who desire entry into practice in the health field; the changes are being proposed without adequate input and cooperative planning with all representative worker, employee, consumer and educational groups; and implementing the changes would lead to rapidly escalating costs of preservice education and subsequent manpower shortages in the health field. (From AVA resolution passed at the December 1978 convention.)

*National League for Nursing**

Rationale: Support for the four types of nursing programs—associate degree, baccalaureate and higher degree, diploma, and practical nursing—represents the League's belief in a value system that reflects the health care needs of a pluralistic democratic society as well as the needs of a profession in the process of growth and change. The impetus for the right of access to health care, and the economic, social and political factors affecting society at large will continue to influence the development of health care. Thus, the League believes that in the interest of the nation's health, individuals who wish to enter nursing should be free to choose from a number of alternatives, each of which legitimately fulfills the purpose of the profession's uppermost goal: to meet the health care needs of the nation.

*The position of the NLN was changed in 1982 to one of support for the ANA proposal.

Abstaining

American Medical Association
Although the American Medical Association is not officially commenting on the position of the ANA, in their "Statement on Medicine and Nursing in the 1970's," they state that they support all levels of nurse education—diploma, baccalaureate, associate degree, and practical nursing.

American Hospital Association
A poll of the State Hospital Associations produced the following results: There were 44 responses out of 51. Twenty-three have adopted a formal position against ANA's, 19 are opposed to ANA but have not taken a formal position, and 2 have said they could adapt to the ANA position but not by 1985.

Division of Nursing, Department of Health, Education and Welfare (now Department of Health and Human Services).
No comment provided.

21. Philosophical Foundations of Baccalaureate Nursing Education

Marlene Kramer

Despite its scary, high-sounding quality, the title seems destined to evoke a "ho-hum, here we go again" reaction. In the hope of avoiding this, I'll move quickly to the questions to which I intend to provide straight answers: What is baccalaureate education in nursing? Specifically, what constitutes the upper division nursing major? Finally, how do baccalaureate and technical nursing education articulate? As these questions are addressed, the philosophical foundations of baccalaureate nursing education will perhaps emerge.

Kramer, M. "Philosophical Foundations of Baccalaureate Nursing Education." *Nursing Outlook* 29(4) (April 1981):224–228. Copyright © 1981 by the American Journal of Nursing Company. Reprinted with permission of the American Journal of Nursing Company and the author.

Since it is imperative that hospital administrators, the lay public, physicians, and fellow nurses understand the answer to the first question—what is baccalaureate nursing—I shall avoid jargon and instead use the terms and analogies that I think are most meaningful and useful in interpreting the current mixed-up situation in nursing education. By way of comparison and contrast, I shall discuss technical education, since doing so may help to clarify the concept of baccalaureate education.

Differences in Functions

Stated in practical terms, the goal of baccalaureate nursing education is to prepare a liberally educated person to function as a professional nurse in a variety of nurse roles and health care settings. Roles are made up of a constellation of functions. Most baccalaureate programs prepare their graduates for the functions inherent in five specific roles or positions: the caregiver function, which is the mainstay of the staff nurse position in both hospitals and community health agencies; the beginning managerial-leadership function, which is inherent in such roles as team leader, assistant head nurse, or head nurse in centralized settings; the health promotion and health supervision function, which predominates in positions in community health nursing, school nursing, and mental health clinics, and is needed in the hospital staff nurse position; the teaching or counseling function, which is or should be an integral part of almost every nursing position; and the health and illness screening function, which predominates in primary care, but is also increasingly demanded in hospital staff nurse positions (at least the illness-screening part). In contrast, the purpose of ADN programs is to prepare technical nurses to function in the caregiver role of the hospital staff nurse.

Both kinds of educational programs must accomplish their respective goals with the greatest possible amount of efficiency and economy of resources. Any educational program could do an absolutely superb job if it had all the time and resources its leaders wanted and felt were needed, but educators must accomplish a far harder task: to do what is required in the available time and with the available resources. It stands to reason that the primary and most immediate consumers of the product of educational programs—that is, hospital nursing service administrators— may not be as satisfied with the new baccalaureate graduate as with the products of technical nursing programs, particularly diploma programs. After all, one cannot possibly commit as much time or as many resources to the preparation of a person for five functions as one can when preparing someone for one predominant function. As a general rule of thumb, it can be estimated that approximately 60 percent of baccalaureate nursing education is devoted to preparation for the caregiver function, in contrast to 90 to 100 percent of education in diploma and ADN programs. A technical nursing program in which all or most of the time can be spent preparing for the singular caregiver function that predominates in the hospital staff nurse position should produce a better, immediately marketable hospital staff nurse.

Educators and service personnel alike must look beyond the immediate situation, however; the baccalaureate nurse graduate is prepared for a greater variety of functions, which will come to the fore after the initial adjustment period.

It is imperative that nursing service administrators decide upon the particular mix of role functions that are needed for a particular position. Job descriptions should then be written accordingly and the kind of nurse who possesses those functions hired for the position. For example, if a particular position requires the occupant to function as a caregiver for patients who have common, recurring problems, then the appropriate employee is one with technical education. If on the other hand, the position requires the occupant to spend about half the working day in assessing patient's knowledge and understanding of surgical procedures and postoperative activity, and planning and providing teaching, then the appropriate nurse for the position is one who has knowledge and skill in the assessment and teaching function (that is, a baccalaureate graduate).

Liberal Education

If we move to the second question, what is the upper division baccalaureate nursing major?—or, to put it another way, how do we accomplish the purpose of baccalaureate nursing education?—we may find it useful to examine that purpose segment by segment. If indeed the purpose of baccalaureate education in nursing is to prepare a liberally educated person, we may find it helpful to consider what this means. Liberal education and a liberally educated person have been described in various ways. Among the descriptions are these: self-actualized, broad development of one's interests and talents, knowledge for joy, not connected or concerned with immediate use; and knowledge acquisition as a consummatory event. However it is described, the common element of a liberal education is the idea of enrichment of the self, through a study of the liberal arts, humanities, and sciences—a kind of learning and development that permits and stimulates constant and continuous growth as a person. A liberal education ensures that later on in life, through good and bad times, one will never become bored with oneself and that when one knocks on the doors of the self, someone will answer. This last effect has been highlighted by research into the effects of long imprisonment and isolation on the human spirit, which has shown that the chances of mental survival and growth without deleterious effects is markedly improved in direct proportion to the extent to which the prisoner was liberally educated.[1]

Aside from its effects on the person, a liberal education also provides the base for professional study and practice, usually within the first two years of the nursing program. This is probably one of the least understood concepts in the development of a professional nurse. Perhaps an analogy to the planting of a garden would be of help in explaining this concept. When one is going to prepare a plot of soil for a garden, it is customary to spade the soil and prepare it by using a broad-spectrum fertilizer, which would be useful to any kind of plant. A liberal education is analogous to this general preparation and cultivation of the soil, into which the seeds—the preparation for various nurse role functions—of professional nursing are planted. In the process of growing and developing, the plants (the various role functions of nursing) use up some of the nutrients from the soil, but the soil is never left bereft. The goal in preparation is to feed and nurture all of the plants that grow in the soil.

In the preparation of a technical nurse, the analogy goes like this: one area of the garden is well fertilized, well cultivated, and liberally supplied with exactly those nutrients needed for a specific kind of seed, rather than a variety of seeds; as a result of this special care, the plant flourishes. So also with technical nursing education, wherein the goal is to provide those specific arts and science courses directly needed to nourish the seed of technical nursing. It is quite possible that a plant in the technical garden might be stronger and healthier than the various plants in the baccalaureate garden, but it cannot replace them; all are needed. Both kinds of products are excellent in their own way. As Gardiner admonishes, we must strive for and honor excellence everywhere.[2] Nursing needs both excellent technical and excellent professional nurses.

Further Differentiation between the Two

How do the professional and technical nurse differ with respect to function? As Montag reminds us, there are two basic premises from which technical nursing was developed that have never been retracted: first, that the function of nursing can and should be differentiated, and second, that these functions lie along a continuum, with professional at one end and technical at the other.[3] There are some functions of nursing that are common to both the technical and professional nurse.

Specifically, the major focus of technical nursing programs is the preparation of nurses to give care to patients and clients with common, recurring problems. This function includes routine teaching—for example, teaching diabetic patients how to test urine for sugar and acetone—and predictable nursing interventions for common and recurring problems. The management-leadership function is minimal for the technical nurse and is focused mainly on the management of care for her own group of patients. A technical nursing program includes only minimal practice in either health screening and assessment or in health promotion and supervision, but it usually includes opportunity to develop skill in illness screening and monitoring. The predominant focus of technical nursing programs is on and should be on cure.

Recently some research has been reported, however, showing that technical nurses in a particular articulated consortium program in California have moved from a reportedly dominant cure orientation six years ago to a more care and health promotion orientation now.[4] This really doesn't say anything except that many technical nursing programs simply are not teaching and focusing on what they are intended and supposed to—namely, the preparation of skilled, excellent nurses for the caregiver function. These research results simply support what many nurse leaders have been saying. In dedication and devotion to the cause of articulation, many ADN programs have tried to be or become all things to all people; they have included leadership, public health nursing content, and other content irrelevant to technical nursing in an effort to become mini-baccalaureate programs. In so doing, they have lost sight of their primary mission and goal—to prepare warm, sensitive, caring nurse technicians who are skilled and competent in the caregiver function.

Professional Functioning

Continuing on with the next part of the definition—to function as a professional nurse—what exactly does that mean? I could use all of the usual clichés about the criteria for judging a profession—a scientific body of knowledge, a code of ethics, and so on—but I think the essential ingredient of the practice of the professional nurse is the fact that she consistently and constantly sees and nurses the individual and family as a whole entity. This total, comprehensive view of the individual is first, foremost, and paramount. From this flow all the other characteristics of professional nursing—such as humanistic and individualized care. It is the holistic view and the constant concern to return the individual to an even higher state of wellness that marks the professional nurse. To achieve this goal, the professional nurse must exercise all of the functions described earlier in this paper—the caretaker, teaching/counseling, managerial, and health supervision, and screening functions. This is what constitutes professionalism and identifies the professional nurse.

The technical nurse, on the other hand, is a competent nurse, an expert, in one function—the caretaker nurse role function. As in any other discipline, a technician is a person who through repeated performance of a singular function acquires tremendous skill and competence. This nurse should reach a high order of excellence, comparable in many ways to the skill of the surgeon, who approaches the zenith of his technical competence during a surgical procedure. I think it needs to be said loudly and clearly: a technical nurse is not an unkind, unfeeling nurse who is only concerned about manual-technical skills, equipment, and their application and use on the patient. Such a statement denies any comprehension or understanding of the *care*giver function. Care is the essence, the end goal, the product of a technical nurse's performance; skills are the means by which this end can be achieved.

How is the liberally educated person prepared to function as a professional nurse in a variety of nurse roles and settings? In the preparation of the baccalaureate nurse, this is done by utilizing and building upon the liberal arts base in the development of the five major role functions described earlier and providing the opportunity for practicing these role functions in a variety of settings. Some settings provide more opportunity for some role development than others. In an acute care hospital, for example, the dominant orientation and function is the cure and care of sick people. This is not a particularly suitable place to develop health supervision or health/illness screening functions. This is the major reason why clinical practica in baccalaureate programs take place in many different settings—in clinics, communities, homes, industry, and schools, as well as in hospitals. Although it is true that at present, 80 percent of the nurse work force are employed in hospitals that care for only 20 percent of the ill population, and correspondingly 20 percent of the nurse work force care for 80 percent of the population in the community, this will not always be true. Although there will always be sick people to care for in both hospital and home, and relatively healthy people who need help to maintain or improve their status of health, we will need both professional and technical nurses working in hospitals, as well as increasing numbers of professional nurses to function in the other areas of health care.

Another result of baccalaureate education is that the caregiver function of the hospital staff nurse role as conceptualized and practiced by the professional nurse is not exactly the same as that of the technical nurse. This difference can be illustrated by using the generally agreed upon steps in the nursing process: assessment, planning, interventions, and evaluation. Although both professional and technical educational programs prepare their graduates to carry out all components of the nursing process, there is relatively more emphasis on assessment and evaluation in professional programs and on planning and intervention in technical programs. And this is as it should be; but it also means that the technical nurse will be the most immediately marketable and useful to the employer, because it is planning and doing that is most immediately needed in the cure-dominated hospital marketplace. It will still be a while before nurses shift from dependence on and acceptance of the physician's assessment and evaluation of the patient to carrying out these aspects of care for themselves and planning and executing nursing care accordingly.

Repeat Learning or New Learning?

In summary then, the purpose of upper division baccalaureate nursing is to utilize the liberal arts and science base to develop the five principal role functions of professional nursing to be exercised in all areas of the nursing process, but particularly in assessment and evaluation. In light of this, I'd like to pose, answer, and explain the question that RNs so often ask when returning to school for their baccalaureate: "Why do I have to have more clinical practice? I've been through all that; why do I have to learn it all over again?" The answer is that they don't have to learn it all over again; the "it" that one is learning after one has acquired a liberal education is different from the "it" that one learned before.

Taking a blood pressure, for instance, is a very common procedure that is learned early in virtually all nursing programs. Does an RN returning for a baccalaureate have to take blood pressures in the clinical area? The answer is clearly yes. There is no doubt that technical nursing programs do a quite adequate job in teaching their students the mechanical procedure of taking blood pressures and the general interpretation of systolic and diastolic sounds. Such learning is built upon that physiological base that nurse educators have determined as adequate. What a nurse hears in a blood pressure, the interpretation of the various Korotkoff's sounds, what they mean, their relationship to nursing interventions is quite different, however, when she has a broad base of physiology and chemistry than when she does not.

The RN student who has acquired her liberal arts base *after* learning a nursing skill or procedure needs some reexposure to previously learned skills, procedures, and interventions. It does not have to be great and certainly the focus is not and should not be on the skill and manipulation of the equipment per se, but rather on the interpretation and assessment of underlying health and illness states. It is educationally predictable that with some learning of this type, transfer to other areas will probably occur. But there does need to be opportunity to learn and to practice nursing assessment, interventions, and evaluations after acquisition of the liberal arts base.

In assessing the diploma school or ADN nurse for entry into upper division baccalaureate nursing following the acquistion of the liberal arts base, both her knowledge and experience in all five functional areas need to be assessed. This is crucial and is not in any way satisfied by passing grades in the NLN achievement exams or state boards. The assessment depends upon the structure, meaning, and interpretation that the faculty of the particular baccalaureate program has given to the five role functions. If the RN student has been working, it is highly likely that she will have little or no difficulty in demonstrating competence in the caretaker function for patients with common and recurring problems, but what still remains to be assessed is the extent of her accomplishment in the other four functions, as well as her understanding of the differences in the caretaker role for the professional nurse described earlier. The RN student has a right to show whether she has competence in the areas of the five role functions and if so, to what extent. The baccalaureate educator is responsible for devising fair methods for assessment and evaluation of these abilities and competencies.

Whither Articulation?

How do baccalaureate and technical education articulate? This question is easy to answer, but my answer will not be popular. In two words: It doesn't. It was never intended to; it should not; it does not need to; it is a bastardization of both technical and professional nursing to force technical education to be the first two years of a professional education. To say that the two must, can, or do articulate is to deny the essential purpose and philosophy of both. For reasons I've already described, one of the major characteristics of professional nursing is that it builds on a broad liberal arts base. The road to professional nursing is no more through technical nursing than the road to being a dentist is through a dental hygienist program, the road to being a surgeon through the barber's shop, or to being an agricultural engineer through first being a farmer.

I want to make it clear that I am not saying that there cannot be career mobility in nursing. On the contrary; there can and should be, but career mobility is not the same as articulation. Technical education programs were designed to be and are terminal, in the sense of "complete." Although some nurse educators have now declared they are no longer terminal or complete, rooftop declarations do not alter the facts.

The tremendous fixation on articulation and the resulting development of programs that aim first and foremost for such articulation, have led to the corruption and bastardization of both technical and professional nursing programs. Technical programs that try to be all things to all people, try to be mini-baccalaureate programs and do not do well the job that they are supposed to do. Baccalaureate programs that lose sight of their own goals and purposes offer nothing more than both an inferior technical and professional education. They simply exist to grant a union card.

Excellence versus Union Card

I do not believe that the RN who wants career mobility wants an inferior education. Baccalaureate programs that are primarily focused on articulation and the granting of a union card, rather than on the development of a liberally educated professional nurse, are a disservice not only to the public and to the profession. But most of all, they are a disservice and an insult to the RN who wants a good education that is relevant and meaningful, at reasonable cost and convenience.

It is not a matter of finding fault and fixing blame. We are all in this educational morass together. I sincerely hope that by getting together and clearly interpreting our goals and purposes to one another and to the RNs in the community, we will be able to work together. Our goal must be not to articulate something that mixes about as well as water and oil, but to develop excellence in both technical and professional nursing programs, and to ensure the humane, kind, caring treatment of RN students desiring career mobility.

References

1. Schein, E. H. The Chinese indoctrination program for prisoners of war; a study of attempted brainwashing. *Psychiatry* 19:149–172, May 1956.
2. Gardner, J. W. *Excellence.* New York, Harper & Row, 1962 (Paperback, 1971).
3. Montag, Mildred. Looking back: associate degree education in perspective. *Nurs.Outlook* 28:248–250, Apr. 1980.
4. Bullough, Bonnie, and Sparks, Colleen. Baccalaureate vs associate degree nurses: the care-cure dichotomy. *Nurs.Outlook* 23:668–692, Nov. 1975.
5. Bullough, Bonnie. Associate degree: beginning or end? *Nurs.Outlook* 27:324–328, May 1979.

22. The Associate Degree: Beginning or End?

Bonnie Bullough

Although there is a certain amount of positive and negative opinion in nursing about the career ladder at any level, probably the most controversial line is the one between the associate degree programs and the baccalaureate programs. This link has been made even more of an issue by resolutions passed in 1976 by the Council of Baccalaureate and Higher Degree Programs of the National League for Nursing, and in 1978 by the American Nurses' Association.

Each of these bodies accepted a movement which originated with a resolution by the New York Nurses Association to make the baccalaureate degree the level at which nurses enter professional practice; the operational date for this change was to be 1985.[1] However, this resolution does not have the same meaning for everyone. Some educators conceptualized the terms "baccalaureate" and "professional" as applying only to graduates of generic baccalaureate programs. Others, including the A.N.A. House of Delegates, look upon alternative pathways as legitimate. A resolution also passed in 1978 by the A.N.A. urged nurses to actively support high quality career mobility programs that use flexible approaches to assist individuals seeking academic degrees in nursing.[2-4]

Some of the controversy about upward mobility for graduates of associate degree programs stems from the original philosophy of the community college movement in nursing. Although two levels of nurses were suggested by Brown in *Nursing for the Future* and support for the concept was given by the American Association of Junior Colleges and the National League for Nursing during the period following World War II, the idea was brought to

Bullough, B. "The Associate Degree: Beginning or End?" *Nursing Outlook* 27(5) (May 1979):324–328. Copyright © 1979 by the American Journal of Nursing Company. Reprinted with permission of the American Journal of Nursing Company and the author.

fruition in a cooperative research project started in 1952 by Montag.[5,6] She carried out a five-year demonstration project involving eight community colleges and effectively demonstrated that students could acquire the necessary knowledge and skill both to pass state board examinations and to function as bedside nurses in two years.[7-9]

However, Montag firmly believed that associate degree and baccalaureate programs could not and should not be articulated. She argued that the objectives, content, and teaching methods of the two types of programs were so different that the "ladder concept of curriculum development was indefensible" and that the two year programs should be terminal.[10]

Her philosophy was supported by most of the leading educators of that era and was amplified in the 1965 American Nurses' Association position paper on nursing education, which differentiated the "technical" from the "professional" nurse by assigning them different functions. The technical nurse was to be responsible for medically delegated tasks that would assist the patient in moving toward recovery, while the professional nurse's practice was more theory-based and emphasized the social-psychological aspects of care. The philosophy of the paper precluded easy mobility for nurses with associate degrees, because the baccalaureate was conceptualized as building upon a liberal arts education rather than upon a lower division nursing degree.[11] In previous research, this dichotomy in orientation has been characterized as a focus toward "care" or "cure," with the position paper and other nursing authorities arguing that the associate degree focus should be cure, while the baccalaureate focus should be care of the patient.[12]

In spite of this clear-cut division, a review of the contemporary nursing literature suggests that the original conceptualization of the associate degree as both technical and terminal has to all intents and purposes been abandoned.[13] In 1971, Kohnke interviewed a group of deans and directors of both baccalaureate and associate degree programs. She found that at least half of them did not accept the dichotomy of focus of the two levels and that the two types of programs were quite similar.[14] Moreover, there seemed to be little differentiation between the functions of associate degree and baccalaureate level nurses in the hospital setting.[15] In reality, it seems the associate degree nurse has emerged as the basic hospital nurse.

The entry level competencies of the AD nurses were recently

outlined by the Council of Associate Degree Programs of the National League for Nursing. As outlined in this document, the role of this basic registered nurse seems much broader than the one presented in the 1965 A.N.A. position paper, and it is certainly well beyond the scope of the technician pictured in the writings of Montag. The current expectations include knowledge and skill related to the assessment, planning, implementation, and evaluation of nursing problems in both the social-psychological and physiological realms. Moreover, the paper concludes with a statement that associate degree nurses are members of the nursing profession; in no place in the document is the term, "technical," seen as pejorative by many, used.[16]

While these developments may be a disappointment to some nursing educators, they are not surprising in light of American values and the political realities of the world in which we live. Graduates of associate degree programs constitute a major portion of the nursing work force. After its cautious experimental phase, the community college concept spread rapidly. In 1960 there were 57 programs in operation, and by 1977 there were 656 associate degree programs (as compared to 367 diploma and 349 baccalaureate programs).[17,18]

The trend to emphasize the associate degree level for the preparation of the basic registered nurse is even more marked in California, where there are 60 community college, 4 diploma, and 19 baccalaureate programs. These data suggest that associate degree preparation is the major model for the education of basic registered nurses. The political realities of the situation suggest that graduates of the largest program need not accept terminal or technical status unless they want it. The question therefore arises: Do they?

To find out what students in the Orange County/Long Beach nursing consortium thought about upward mobility and whether they exhibited the care-cure dichotomy in their orientation to nursing, the research described in this article was planned. The Orange County/Long Beach consortium of schools was formed in 1971 to improve the articulation between the various levels of nursing education in that part of Southern California. In order to furnish opportunities for nursing personnel to move up the educational ladder, five community colleges and two universities formed a multiple entry, multiple exit consortium. These seven schools prepare licensed vocational (practical) nurses, registered nurses at the associate degree and baccalaureate levels, and nurses at the master's level. At the associate degree and baccalaureate levels there are both generic and career ladder programs. Although the aide level is not formally included, the licensed vocational nurse programs are set up so that students can, if necessary, terminate at the end of the first semester to work as aides.

It is interesting to note that while there was no conscious effort to follow the model outlined by Wood in the UCLA Allied Health Professions Project, the levels of education available in the consortium schools correspond remarkably well to those she arrived at by analyzing the functions of nurses and searching for reasonable lines of demarcation.[19] The development of the consortium has been described in more detail in a previous publication.[20] This article will focus on the views of consortium students as they relate to current issues in the structuring of nursing education.

Some qualification is necessary. These students might not represent the total population of nursing students in the country. First of all, they are from California, where community colleges are of long standing and many graduates move on to baccalaureate schools; secondly, because they are members of the consortium, they exemplify students nurtured in an environment where expectations for continued growth through further education is the norm, rather than exemplifying students whose education has involved no such consistent expectation.

In the spring of 1977, a teacher in each of the seven consortium schools served as a sponsor of the research on her campus. She contacted students during or after class and asked them to fill out questionnaires. This process yielded a sample of 132 vocational nursing students, 130 vocational nurses who were working on their associate degree, 643 generic associate degree students, 227 registered nurses working toward a baccalaureate, 168 generic baccalaureate students, and 49 master's degree nurse practitioner students.

Student Aspirations

The fact that 26 percent (357) of the students in the seven schools were in career ladder programs suggests the popularity of the concept. Nonetheless, we still wanted to see how many of the current students planned to continue their education after they finished their current program. As can be seen in Table 22–1 the responses show that students at every level either are sure they want further education or are still entertaining such a possibility.

Table 22–2 furnishes more information about the desire for

Table 22–1   Percentage of students at each level planning to continue education definitely, possibly, or not at all.

Current Program	Yes	Perhaps	No
Vocational nurse	59	33	8
Career ladder associate degree	52	35	13
Generic associate degree	54	38	8
Career ladder baccalaureate	50	40	10
Generic baccalaureate	35	52	13
Master's degree	20	44	35

further education. It shows the level of aspiration of students in each type of program. As can be noted by looking at the totals at the bottom of the table, the baccalaureate degree seems to be the major goal among the total student sample. Until that degree is reached, most students are unwilling to look upon themselves as having finished their education. Only 27 percent of the career ladder associate degree students and 24 percent of the generic AD students see their education as terminal.

The finding that more career ladder baccalaureate students than generic students were planning to seek the master's degree is interesting. In talking to the two groups of students this difference seems related to the fact that the career ladder students are somewhat older; their median age is 31 while the median age of the generic students is 22. Many of the career ladder students returned to school for the express purpose of achieving the master's level nurse practitioner preparation. More of the young generic students want to work as a nurse for a while before making a decision about further education, although even among this group, half are planning to continue with schooling.

The Care-Cure Dichotomy

What about the other aspect of the original philosophy of the associate degree education, which is said to be focused on the technical, cure-oriented aspects of nursing as opposed to baccalaureate care-oriented elements of nursing? This study afforded an opportunity to look at the orientation of nurses at all four levels and to compare the orientation of career ladder and generic students.

Table 22–2   Percentage of students in each educational program aspiring to reach each educational level.

	Level Aspired to					
Current Program	LVN	AD	BS	MS	DR	OTHER*
Vocational nurse	23	23	35	13	2	3
Career ladder associate degree		27	43	24	4	2
Generic associate degree		24	51	21	2	2
Career ladder baccalaureate			34	59	4	3
Generic baccalaureate			46	47	4	3
Master's degree				75	14	10
Total group	2	16	43	32	3	3

*Most students who indicated some other goal specified nurse practitioner.

This aspect of the research represents a partial replication of a study conducted in 1974, when the care-cure scale was developed. In that study, the orientation of nursing students from associate degree and baccalaureate programs from a random sample of Southern California schools was studied. Seventy percent of the baccalaureate students and 42 percent of the associate degree students scored on the care side of the scale, while 30 percent of the baccalaureate and 58 percent of the associate degree students were on the cure side of the scale. While these differences were statistically significant they did not represent a dichotomous situation; they could hardly be used to specify two discrete sets of functions. Differences in orientation were found to relate to the students' perception of the faculty and curriculum orientation.[21]

Following the completion of that study, further analysis of the scale items was done and an alternative form of the scale was constructed for use with licensed vocational nurses.* Most questions are the same on both scales; a few are different. Each of the questions called for the nurse responding to make a choice between two different work roles or between two tasks within a role. One question on the registered nurse scale, for example, asked: If the choices of work were as triage nurse in an emergency room or as a patient teacher in a diabetic clinic, which would you choose? An example of the choices given to LVNs included a role drawing

*This version of the scale was authored by Jean Dunworth.

blood at a blood bank or giving care through a visiting nurse agency. The current reliability coefficient of the registered nurse scale is alpha=.62 while the alpha score of the LVN scale is .59.

Findings Related to Orientation

Table 22–3 compares the orientations of the consortium sub-samples. Most of the groups are split at the middle of the scale suggesting some sort of balance between extremes. The exceptions to this middle ground are the career ladder baccalaureate students and the master's level nurse practitioner students, both of whom score high on the care side of the scale.

In order to find out the students' view of their course of study, the students were asked whether the *curriculum* in their schools was oriented more toward physiology and pathology—so that they could help the patient get well, or toward psychosocial skills—so that they could help the patient cope with his illness. Table 22–4 shows the responses to this question. The curriculum focus seems more dichotomized than the students' own orientation. It seems that the students have found some sort of balance for themselves; some are opting for roles that emphasize treatment, while others look to giving emotional support. This will probably help them fill a variety of roles in a growing health care delivery system. Most of the students scored towards the median on the scale; they want to fill a variety of functions and, apparently, to give holistic health care.

Table 22–3   Percentage of students in each educational level with care and cure orientations.

	Orientation	
Current Program	Cure	Care
Vocational nurse	49	51
Career ladder associate degree	49	51
Generic associate degree	51	49
Career ladder baccalaureate	44	56
Generic baccalaureate	50	50
Master's degree	22	78

Chi square 17.7, 5df; p=<.01

Table 22–4   Percentage of students at each level describing their program as emphasizing physiology and pathology or psychosocial skills.

Current Program	Physiology and Pathology	Psychosocial Skills
Vocational nurse	63	37
Career ladder associate degree	23	77
Generic associate degree	39	61
Career ladder baccalaureate	2	98
Generic baccalaureate	16	84
Master's degree	29	71

Chi square 164.51, 5 df; p=<.0001

Given the fact that most students perceived their curriculum as focused heavily on psychosocial aspects and that 98 percent of the faculty in the career ladder programs were described as oriented toward "counseling and giving emotional support to patients," one might question the concept of a "bridge year." Both Fullerton and Long Beach have established this with a view to resocializing the "cure" oriented registered nurse students, perhaps because they erroneously assume that associate degree programs do not include a psychosocial focus.

While curriculum might be thought to create some of these students' orientation, it cannot explain the orientation of the master's level nurse practitioner students. The students seemed more care-oriented than their curriculum. This finding came as a surprise in light of criticism of the practitioner movement which has held that as nurse practitioners gained medical skills, they would lose their focus on nursing's roots in caring. These data suggest that this has not happened. These findings are supported by a longitudinal study done by Linn in 1972 with two small groups of practitioner students. He found no significant difference in the care orientation of beginning and graduating family nurse practitioners.[22]

The data related to an orientation toward care versus cure suggests that while the differences in orientation between levels of students are statistically significant, they do not represent a dichotomy in focus. The definitions of the scope of function of these two levels of nurses outlined in the 1965 A.N.A. position paper use this dichotomy. These data suggest that those definitions need to be reexamined and updated if they are to be used for educational planning or as a basis for legislative proposals.

Implications

To the extent that the California experience applies to other states, this research has some far-reaching implications. It seems apparent that the associate degree in nursing is not and should not be thought of as a terminal degree. Any state or group of nurses that is considering setting up such a program should be aware of this reality. The norms of the community college movement are against such a conceptualization; community college teachers and administrators believe in and plan for upward mobility for a significant portion of their students. While students who lack the ability to continue their education beyond this level are certainly weeded out, this does not mean that teachers in community colleges support those outside planners or nurse educators at other levels who assert that the associate degree is terminal.

Given a supportive atmosphere such as that found in the territory of the Orange County/Long Beach Nursing Consortium, most students will at least entertain the possibility of further education. Given a less supportive atmosphere, a cycle of frustration and aggression seems likely. This sort of atmosphere undoubtedly creates divisiveness in the ranks of the profession.

Planners who are eagerly looking toward an all-baccalaureate registered nursing work force by 1985 need to deal with a growing associate degree population as well as the traditional diploma graduates. Since the diploma schools are gradually being converted to degree programs at either the associate degree or baccalaureate level, they pose no problem if one takes a long enough view of the statistics. The associate degree movement, however, is growing rather than declining, and the needs of this largest group of students cannot be overlooked if any long-range plan for nurse education is to be viable.

References

1. New York State Nurses Association. *Resolution on Entry into Professional Practice.* Albany, The Association, 1974.
2. American Nurses' Association Convention '78. *Am. J. Nurs.* 78:1230–1246, July 1978.
3. ANA convention: 1978. *Nurs.Outlook* 26:500–507, Aug. 1978.

4. Styles, M.A., and Wilson, H.S. The third resolution. *Nurs.Outlook* 27:44–47, Jan. 1979.
5. Brown, E. L. *Nursing for the Future; A Report Prepared for the National Nursing Council.* New York, Russell Sage Foundation, 1948.
6. Rines, A.R. Associate degree education: history, development, and rationale. *Nurs.Outlook* 25:496–501, Aug. 1977.
7. Montag, M. L., and Gotkin, L. G. *Community College Education for Nursing.* New York, Blakiston Division, McGraw-Hill Book Co., 1959.
8. Montag, M. L. *Evaluation of Graduates of Associate Degree Programs.* New York, Teachers College Press, 1972.
9. Anderson, B. E. *Nursing Education in Community Junior Colleges.* Philadelphia, J.B. Lippincott Co., 1959.
10. Montag and Gotkin, *op.cit.*, p. 25.
11. American Nurses' Association. *Educational Preparation for Nurse Practitioners and Assistants to Nurses; A Position Paper.* New York, The Association, 1965.
12. Bullough, Bonnie, and Sparks, Colleen. Baccalaureate vs. associate degree nurses: the care-cure dichotomy. *Nurs.Outlook* 23:688–692, Nov. 1975.
13. Bensman, P.A. Have we lost sight of the AD philosophy? *Nurs. Outlook* 25:511–513, Aug. 1977.
14. Kohnke, M. F. Do nursing educators practice what is preached. *Am.J.Nurs.* 73–1571–1573, 1575, Sept.1973.
15. Sheahan, Sister Dorothy. The game of the name: nursing professional and nursing technician. *Nurs.Outlook* 20:440–444, July 1972.
16. National League for Nursing, Associate Degree Programs. Competencies of the associate degree nurse on entry into practice. *Nurs. Outlook* 26:457–458, July 1978.
17. American Nurses' Association. *Facts About Nursing.* New York, The Association, 1961, p. 98.
18. Johnson, W. L. Educational preparation for nursing—1977. *Nurs. Outlook* 26:568–573, Sept. 1978.
19. Wood, Lucile. Proposal: a career plan for nursing. *Am.J.Nurs.* 73:832–835, May 1973.
20. Cobin, Joan, and others. A five level articulated program. *Nurs.Outlook* 24:309–313, May 1976.
21. Bullough and Sparks, *op.cit.*
22. Linn, L.S. Care vs cure: how the nurse practitioner views the patient. *Nurs.Outlook* 22:641–644, Oct. 1974.

23. Expanding the Options through the External Degree and Regional Performance Assessment Centers

Carrie B. Lenburg

The change in perspective about the need for and types of educational mobility options has been marked, if not dramatic, since the mid-1970s. Very few leaders in nursing or in education now dispute the need for additional educational opportunities for those already in the field of nursing; to the contrary, most are interested in exploring nontraditional modalities which are both educationally and economically sound. Much has been written about the "open curriculum," career (educational) mobility, and nontraditional education patterns in nursing (Lenburg, 1975; NLN, 1977). Most of the approaches used in these programs, however, have rested on the basis of the conventional instructional campus-based model. The external degree model, epitomized by the New York Regents External Degree Program (NYREDP), provides a radical departure from this traditional approach in that it focuses entirely on the objective *assessment* of academic achievement which is prescribed by the program's faculty. By using assessment rather than conventional instruction and supervision of learning, it is a true alternative,* a totally different philosophic and educational approach.

During the decade of the 1970s, the Regents External Degree Nursing Programs (REDNP) were developed, implemented, studied, and accredited. After years of controversy, the REDNP is viewed now by many as an alternative which embodies a creative solution to one of the most difficult problems facing the profession: assisting thousands of nurses to upgrade their knowledge and competence while earning recognized academic credentials commensurate with their professional responsibilities.

---

*Alternative is defined as that providing or necessitating a choice between two entities.

Foundation for the Alternative

REDNP is an alternative model which creatively blends the central elements of three important educational movements: adult education, competency-based education, and objective comprehensive assessment. From the adult education movement it takes the philosophy that deliberate diversity, flexibility, individualization, learner responsibility, and experiential learning are academically acceptable and appropriate for adult learners. From the competency-based education movement it takes the philosophy that abstract objectives and degree requirements should be made explicit, stated in measurable terms, and given to the student to guide the course of learning. From the assessment movement it takes the philosophy that essential learning can be documented through objective written and performance examinations or other academically sound assessment procedures, and that learning so documented is equivalent to that gained through conventional instructional methods.

This blending of philosophies has resulted in a nursing program in which adults experienced in some aspects of nursing (or related health disciplines) may combine past and present learning, may use any resources and facilities available to them, and may establish their own time schedule and pace for completing degree requirements. But they *must document* attainment of required knowledge and clinical competence using rigorous objective theory and performance examinations in nursing. The external assessment model epitomizes a shared educational responsibility: the nursing faculty is responsible for determining what shall be learned and for creating the instruments for objecive assessment, and the students are responsible for learning and for demonstrating achievement of the required competencies. The *process* of learning is totally individualized.

The external degree is considered a true alternative because it is concerned only with assessment of learning rather than with the teaching process. This assessment approach allows maximum flexibility for all aspects of learning but it prescribes specific and objective methods for documenting achievement of predetermined objectives and competencies. In contrast, conventional instruction-oriented programs are designed so that the learning process is directed and controlled by the faculty, with less time devoted to comprehensive objective assessment of specified competencies.

When a program evolves from the philosophy that the center of education is learning and that learning can be documented objectively and comprehensively, then the roles of students, faculty, and administration are altered drastically. And so are the academic traditions, tools, and procedures. Academic programs can be envisioned on a continuum, with the instructional model at one extreme and the assessment model at the other. Many conventional instructional programs move toward the center of the line when they offer opportunities for assessment of prior learning acquired outside their classrooms, i.e., advanced placement. The number of credits that potentially can be awarded for such learning varies from one institution to another and is controlled by the administration and/or faculty. Credit by examination, special assessment, and portfolio review are three procedures commonly used in combination with required classroom instruction. Usually, they are options within the instructional model, placing the program somewhere toward center on the continuum (Keeton et al., 1976; Lenburg, 1981; Meyer, 1975).

In contrast, a total assessment program establishes the degree requirements and offers examinations and other assessment procedures to meet those requirements *without providing instruction* (Nolan, 1975). Students are encouraged to seek and to use all learning opportunities available to them, structured or nonstructured, on campus or at work, individual or group, past or present. Transfer credits are accepted from accredited institutions, and when the student has studied and feels ready, he takes written and performance examinations to document achievement. The faculty designs the program, develops and implements the examinations; it does not provide instruction, except in the form of program objectives and the study guides that outline content, objectives, and suggested learning activities for each nursing examination. Students determine their own time schedules, sequence of study, pace of meeting degree requirements, resources for learning, and even their own role models and facilitators or mentors. In every respect the learning process is flexible and self-directed and the learner is fully responsible for achieving the stated competencies and for documenting them through successful completion of the assessment procedures developed by the faculty (Lenburg, 1979 a and b).

Such an external academic model has obvious and major implications for faculty and administration, for budgets, schedules, and facilities. As inflation and budgetary restrictions become more and more oppressive, the external assessment model in nursing provides an alternative worth exploring because it puts minimum strain on faculty time and on institutional resources and facilities while accommodating an almost unlimited number of adult learners. During the 1970s it received growing recognition in general higher education; perhaps the time for its expansion in nursing is now at hand.

Historical Perspective

In the early 1970s the Commission on Nontraditional Study was created to study ways of increasing flexibility and individualization in higher education. *Diversity by Design* describes the 3-year effort of the commission and its resulting recommendations (Commission, 1973). Another important book to come from that study was Houle's *The External Degree,* which traces the philosophic and historical emergence of the external degree as an educational entity (Houle, 1973). The work initiated by the commission continued through national surveys and conferences for both the undergraduate and graduate degree levels. In 1976, a survey conducted by the Bureau of Social Science Research at the request of the National Institute of Education revealed that some 134 different colleges and universities offered 244 external degree programs. More than 54,000 students were enrolled. Only two of these programs existed just 10 years earlier, in 1965. This national survey also provides important information about the programs and the students participating in them (Sosdian and Sharp, 1978). Based on 10 years of progress and study, the external degree model no longer can be considered rare or experimental; it is part of the spectrum in higher education and will become even more important in the 1980s than it was in the past decade.

REDP in Review

The New York Regents External Degree Program (NYREDP) is one form of external degree and is unlike most others. Its focus is entirely on assessment and it requires no classroom attendance or instruction; however, students who choose to take college courses may do so and transfer the credits from any accredited institution. The program is free of time and space restrictions and allows students to learn however, wherever, and whenever it suits their needs. It is, in fact, *a national examining university,* in which students enroll regardless of place of residence, employment, age, background, or any other characteristic (Nolan, 1975). They are fully responsible for their own learning and then for document- ing their ability to meet the faculty-prescribed knowledge and skills embodied within the degree requirements. The number of transfer credits is unrestricted, and such credits may be used along with approved proficiency examinations, special assessment, and specifically designed performance examinations to meet de- gree requirements. By requiring the use of rigorous objective and comprehensive assessment procedures, the learning process can be as individualized and flexible as the student's circumstances dictate, while assuring academic quality and integrity.

Since 1970, when the New York Regents External Degree Pro- gram was launched by Ewald Nyquist, then commissioner of educa- tion, it has fired the imagination and interest of thousands of adult learners and many educators. Currently, the University of the State of New York, governed by the Board of Regents, offers eight ex- ternal degree programs including those in nursing, business, and the arts and sciences. More than 25,000 candidates are enrolled and approximately 15,000 degrees have been awarded since the first commencement was held in Steptember 1972.

Of particular importance, both associate (ADN) and bache- lors (BSN) degrees in nursing are available, with approximately 3,500 ADN candidates and over 6,000 BSN candidates enrolled actively. By June 1982, more than 1,200 associate degree nursing candidates had completed the program and more than 350 others had met requirements for the bachelor of science (nursing) de- gree program. Candidates in the nursing programs (like all of the other REDPs) meet degree requirements while they live and work in any of the 50 states, the District of Columbia, the territories, or more than a dozen countries abroad. Follow-up studies for the past 6 years have documented that employers have a high regard for REDNP graduates. Moreover, approximately 80 percent of all accredited masters programs in nursing accept BSN graduates of the REDNP. Candidates and graduates are enthusiastic about the program and consider it as the only way they could have obtained the degree while working. Most of them think of the REDNP as more than just another nontraditional program; it is the *only viable alternative* to the instructional, campus-binding programs which had put education outside their reach (Lenburg, 1976).

During the past decade of development and implementation of the REDNP, nurse educators and leaders in the profession cautiously watched, some with concern and others with fascination. Skepticism initially characterized even those who became the faculty for the nursing programs, and understandably so, as nothing like this had ever been done before in nursing or in other applied disciplines. Some nurses spoke out against the idea from the outset and, sadly, never changed their minds. Others were willing to wait and see, and others had the courage to become involved and to develop the idea to its full potential, determined to meet academic and professional standards of excellence.

Now that both the associate and bachelors nursing programs have been completed and accredited, many of these same leaders in nursing education and service have accepted the external degree route as a highly desirable alternative for capable and motivated nurses. That which once was viewed as an extreme and dangerous departure from conventional practice is slowly being accepted as a distinctive method by which the spectrum of academic possibilities can be broadened—even in nursing. The assessment model is now more attractive, for adoption and for adaption, by other systems and institutions.

The Integration of Adult Education, Competency-Based Education, and Assessment Philosophies

Cross (1978), Houle (1973), Keeton et al. (1976), Knowles (1975), and Valley (1975) are among the leaders in the field of higher education, who have written extensively about the educational needs of adults as well as the changes needed in the higher education system to accommodate them. Primarily, adults need academic opportunities that are realistic and sensible and that take into account prior learning that is comparable to that expected of more conventional degree seekers. They need flexibility in meeting degree requirements and in time schedules to prevent unnecessary disruption in meeting work and family responsibilities. They also need recognition for previous learning.

Adults also need diversity in teaching-learning strategies even more than younger, less experienced students. Learning methods that promote flexibility include the following: contract learning, personalized self-instruction, preceptorships, correspondence study, self-paced modular learning, flexible-progress approach, and other versions of independent study (Cole, 1978).

The competency-based education movement emanates from the need for more accountability in education, the escalating cost of education, and the concern with declining performance abilities of graduates. American pragmatism dictates that education should be cost-effective and that it should prepare graduates for their responsibilities in the world of work. The competency-based philosophy requires that the goals for learning be made explicit and that the broad objectives be broken down into measurable units, focusing on the students' performance of specific skills. A recent book by Grant and associates, *On Competency* (1979), provides a good general discussion of competency-based education.

In addition to specifying what shall be learned in terms of measurable skills, a competency-based system requires that the faculty develop and use procedures that facilitate comparable and consistent evaluation of the students' achievement. This is illustrated, for example, at Alverno College, which is well known as a pioneer in the development of a competency-based liberal arts program (Alverno College, 1979). The college also has taken the leadership in developing a competency-based nursing program which is fully accredited by the National League for Nursing. Students in this college know in advance the educational outcomes they are expected to meet; they also know the methods by which their achievements will be measured. Once the outcomes of learning have been specified and measures to evaluate them have been developed, students are held accountable for achieving the designated level of competence.

Even with this quick review, it is readily evident that the beliefs and practices associated with adult education and competency-based education are essential in the REDNP assessment model. The knowledge and competencies required to practice nursing (technical and professional) have been identified and explicitly written by the faculty, and have been made available to students through study guides and other program materials. Students may use any learning approaches they choose, any time schedule that suits their needs, and any resources at their disposal. However, when they declare themselves to be ready, they must take high level theory and performance examinations that assess their achievement of the competencies identified by the faculty as mandatory for the degree. The program values prior learning, maximum flexibility, and learner responsibility. Moreover, the program functions as a total assessment alternative because the expected competencies are explicit and public, learning is the responsibility of the learner, and the objective examinations are tailor-made to document all essential outcome behaviors (Lenburg, 1979b).

The integration of these three educational philosophies forms the basis for the kind of assessment-oriented degree completion programs needed by thousands of nurses who are motivated, capable, and experienced but who lack academic credentials. While campus-based instructional programs must continue to serve the needs of novice generic students, as well as many experienced nurses, the alternative provided by the assessment model could be adopted and adapted by individual institutions and statewide educational systems to meet the academic needs of a large number of nurses seeking college degrees.

Internal and External Pressures for Change

Many internal and external forces are forging the need for change in both nursing education and service. Fagan, McClure and Nelson, Cleland, and others provide an excellent background for understanding the dimensions of the problem currently confronting the nursing profession in a reference edited by Linda Aiken for the American Academy of Nursing (Aiken, 1982). It is well recognized that many components of the problem relate to the initial and subsequent educational preparation of nurses. As long as 80 percent of practicing nurses do not hold the minimum of a baccalaureate degree, the profession will be limited in its ability to reach its potential for providing quality health care. Educational mobility, therefore, is one of the major points for consideration in rectifying the problem. However, conventional methods alone are grossly inadequate to meet the continued educational needs of a profession the size of nursing. A rational and viable alternative is needed in the spectrum of options. That alternative provides for marked increase in external learning and objective academic assessment.

An assessment-oriented nursing degree program can meet the needs of the profession as well as those nurses seeking academic credentials who can practice according to the specified competencies. Because its focus is on *assessment of learning*, there are few, if any, restrictions on the numbers of students that can be enrolled in a particular program. The influence on faculty-student ratio, clinical resources and facilities, and budget are markedly minimized, while the opportunities for learners are maximized. Even when educational advisement and some instruction are provided, the benefits of an assessment program for experienced adult learners make it a plausible and desirable alternative for thousands of nurses who want a career as "professional" nurses and for the institutions seeking to assist them (Lenburg, 1980).

Probably the most significant social-political forces which mandate increased educational mobility opportunities for nurses include the ailing national economy, demographic shifts in the population, advances in technology, and recognition of the need for lifelong learning. These and other external pressures are motivating many nurses to seek BSN degrees and others to enter nursing for the first time. For working adult students, however, the problem of paying for costly campus study is compounded by their inability to take time from work and family responsibilities to attend conventional courses. Other problems relate to the psychological distress associated with required repetition of prior learning and the loss of autonomy in making decisions about how to best spend their money, time, and effort.

Within this context, some exciting possibilities are emerging that have the potential for changing the options available in higher education, even nursing education, particularly for adult learners. For example, significant advances have been made in video and computer technologies which make extra-institutional learning more accessible to adults. A recent issue of *Curent Issues in Higher Education* explores the impact of educational technologies in detail (American Association for Higher Education, 1981b). Perhaps an even more profound change is the increasing opportunities for education in business and industry and their partnership with academic institutions (American Association for Higher Education, 1981a). Nursing education is not immune to these changes.

During the 1980s, such advances will exert a positive influence on the further development of external degrees and the use of extra-institutional learning and assessment procedures. The availability of home video playback units and home computers already is assisting many adult learners at home. The technology is available, and, in time, nursing faculties will develop study modules for video and computer units that can be used at home and at work as well as in the classroom. In the future, many innovative nursing programs will use these technologies, in combination with academic advisement and rigorous assessment procedures, as part of their educational programs in order to make it economically and educationally possible for self-directed, motivated nurses to obtain external degrees.

Regional Performance Assessment Centers

The assessment-oriented external degree in nursing is an alternative which complements the conventional instructional model. It is not a replacement for other types of educational programs, nor is it for adult learners, but it is an alternative tailor-made for the times. Currently, the REDNP is the only existing assessment degree program with a major in nursing; however, other institutions have expressed an interest in pursuing the use of its examinations for their own students. These nursing examinations are used to convert prior learning into academic currency at the associate and bachelors degree levels. Credit by examination already is a widely used concept and in some instances more than 50 percent of nursing credits may be earned this way.

While many nursing programs want to offer more assessment options or even an entire external degree, they have been frustrated primarily by one crucial factor—the difficulty of objectively documenting clinical competencies in nursing. Nursing is an applied discipline and the *performance of nursing* in actual or simulated situations is an essential component of the students' ability to be measured. The lack of objective performance examinations in nursing was an overriding obstacle in the past. However, through funding from the W. K. Kellogg Foundation, the NYREDP was able to secure the time and expertise needed to develop several objective performance examinations in nursing. These performance examinations are required along with the theory examinations for the nursing external degree programs; they also may be used by others.

While it is now possible for students to take the written nursing examinations at one of the 200 locations in the network established by the American College Testing Program,* the performance examinations are available only at designated assessment centers. Five performance test sites are located in New York State. The first performance assessment center established outside the

*The American College Testing Program is under contract to administer the written examinations developed by the New York College Proficiency Examination Program and the Regents External Degree Program in their Proficiency Examination Program (ACT-PEP).

State of New York is in Long Beach, California, through a contract between REDNP and the California State University Consortium. The second regional performance assessment center was established in Atlanta, Georgia in cooperation with the Georgia State Nurses Association and a coalition of other nursing and health care groups. The Rocky Mountain Performance Assessment Center is being developed in cooperation with Metropolitan State College in Denver and is expected to be functioning by the autumn of 1982. These and two other centers are being established through a 4-year grant from the W. K. Kellogg Foundation (see Figure 23–1).

The concept of the regional performance assessment center (RPAC) serves the dual purpose of testing REDNP candidates, as well as students from other programs, who choose to use the performance examinations in nursing. It opens the way for increased assessment options for programs designed to assist experienced students. The regional assessment center is the connecting link, the previously missing concept in the educational mobility chain, which can enable nursing programs to offer clinical assessment alternatives to capable nurses in their geographic area. The idea of regionally located assessment centers initially emerged from the desire to assist thousands of REDNP candidates who had to travel to New York to take the mandatory performance examinations in nursing regardless of where they lived (Lenburg, 1981). However, the obvious needs of other educational mobility programs and thousands of degree-seeking nurses made it mandatory that the envisioned assessment centers be developed to serve the purposes of other programs as well as REDNP. At the same time this proposal was funded, Patricia Cross called for the development of "regional centers" for adult learners in higher education in a publication entitled *The Missing Link* (Cross, 1978). Obviously, the need for the economical and efficient use of resources is essential in higher education as well as in nursing.

The existence of dual-purpose, regional performance assessment centers for nursing makes it possible for nursing programs to design and implement high-quality educational mobility programs that incorporate totally or in part the external degree assessment model. Existing standardized written examinations in nursing as well as criterion-referenced performance examinations in nursing could be adopted by programs of single academic institutions or by statewide academic systems. The examinations could be used in their current form or be adapted to meet specific

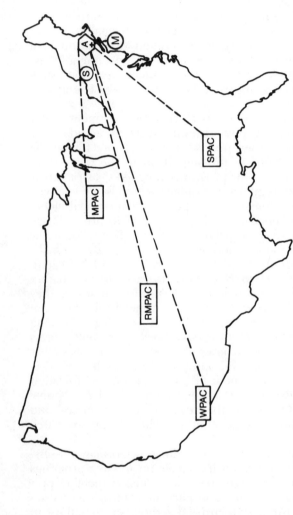

Figure 23–1 New York Regents External Degree Nursing Program, Dual-Purpose Regional Performance Assessment Center Network.

Performance Assessment Centers:

In New York: Albany, Mineola (Long Island) and Syracuse
WPAC: Western Performance Assessment Center, Long Beach, California
SPAC: Southern Performance Assessment Center, Atlanta, Georgia
RMPAC: Rocky Mountain Performance Assessment Center, Denver, Colorado
MPAC: Midwest Performance Assessment Center, (in process)
(The location for the fifth center is undetermined at this time.)

populations and specific needs. They could be used as the base for a total assessment external degree program (similar to the NYREDNP) or to provide a variety of flexible opportunities along the continuum between the total instruction model and the total assessment model as suggested earlier (Lenburg, 1981).

The Regional Performance Assessment Center (RPAC) is envisioned as a freestanding autonomous entity established for the purpose of administering the REDNP performance examinations. It is *not* a branch, extension, or satellite of the REDNP. It is a testing center. The examinations and all related protocols remain the property of the REDNP but the center has full authority for scheduling, administering, and marketing the examinations in the region. After the initial year of training and development, each center is expected to be self-sufficient based on examination fees. The REDNP faculty and staff provide the training program and maintain the examinations and study guides; the center invites local nurse educators who meet the criteria and complete the intensive orientation course to become clinical evaluators. Evaluators are paid by the center on a per diem basis (see Figure 23–2).

The center, in cooperation with the REDNP, also invites local clinical facilities that meet the criteria to enter into a contractual agreement to allow the administration of the clinical examinations. Therefore, the center itself is an administrative entity, where scheduling, advising, and processing occur. The examinations are administered in settings appropriate to their content: adult and pediatric patient care units in general hospitals and ambulatory clinics, or classroom and laboratory for simulated examinations.

Quality control, academic and clinical integrity are assured through careful selection and orientation of personnel and through contractual agreements. The RPAC provides the administrative testing service using local clinical resources; the faculty and staff of the REDNP retain sole responsibility for the content and protocols of the examinations. Qualified local nurse educators administer the examinations only after completing the orientation course required by the REDNP. Therefore, whether the students who take the examinations are enrolled in the REDNP or in other programs, they and their program can be assured that the specified nursing competencies are being documented consistently and objectively.

In another effort to assist educational mobility programs,

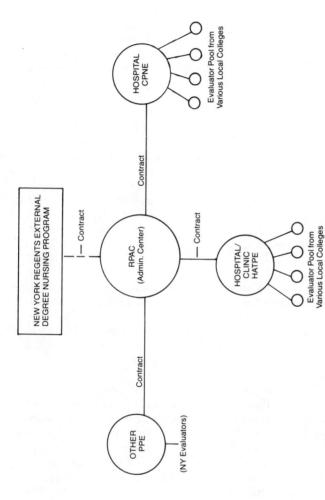

Figure 23-2 Regional Performance Assessment Center.
CPNE: Clinical Performance in Nursing Examination (adult and child patients in hospital)
HATPE: Health Assessment and Teaching Performance Examination (ambulatory clinic)
PPE: Professional Performance Examination (videotape simulations)
RPAC: Regional Performance Assessment Center (administrative headquarters)

the REDNP currently is undertaking a project to make available modified versions of the nursing examinations. Currently, the existing theory examinations are available through the American College Testing Program and the performance examinations are essentially available through the RPACs. However, both types of examinations will be made available by 1983–1984 also in modular components that will increase the options and thus promote the possibility of a better fit between the program's curriculum needs and the available tests. In addition, some examinations will be consolidated into more comprehensive tests, which require less time but yield more information. These new developments will expand the number and variety of both written and performance examinations available to nursing programs throughout the country. This project is funded by a grant from the Kellogg Foundation and will greatly enhance the educational mobility opportunities in nursing. Creative options, therefore, are ready to be designed and implemented using the concepts embodied in the assessment external degree approach and the newly developed RPACs.

Moreover, in the future the REDNP staff and faculty plan to work with statewide educational systems or individual institutions to establish additional performance assessment units, modeled after the initial five regional centers. The development of these additional centers will be dependent on sufficient local funding, clinical facilities, clinical evaluators, and a commitment to the dual-purpose concept. Both comprehensive and modified versions of the performance examinations will be made available at the assessment centers.

Some Problem Areas to Consider

While external degree programs offer a viable educational alternative, they are not without problems. *Change* magazine has published several articles over the past few years which present the problems and deficiencies of external and other nontraditional programs as perceived by a number of leaders in higher education. Basically, the problems for faculty relate to limited academic preparation in the spheres of adult education, competency-based education, and objective assessment. Graduate programs and continuing education for nurse educators will have to correct these deficiencies in the near future if nontraditional programs are to be successful. Current teachers and would-be teachers of nursing will have to learn and implement the philosophies and procedures required by these three educational movements. Lenburg has described in detail the problems associated with implementing objective clinical assessment (Lenburg, 1979b). Some teachers fear they will have no role in an assessment program, but in fact their role is critical—yet different. Some of the major problems result from the difficulty teachers have in completing the necessary role transition.

Students also experience problems in external-type programs, primarily related to the following areas: individual accountability for learning; limited instruction and guided clinical experience; required documentation of both theory and performance using objective examinations; responsibility for planning, for finding resources, and for self-regulation to accomplish the goal. Athough external degree programs provide flexibility and independence, these very assets often present stumbling blocks for students. Many students need instruction and guided learning and are ill suited for self-directed external programs. One of the biggest problems students face is understanding the significance of having a choice and the consequences of their behavior in relation to the choices they make.

Institutions are concerned with problems that relate to a range of topics, such as the differences in administration of external programs, budgets, assisting students, using regional assessment centers, and program accreditation. These problems are discussed in many of the previous references but the entire April 1979 issue of the *Peabody Journal of Education* is devoted to assessment and also deals with these problems (Lenburg, 1979b).

Accreditation of nontraditional programs, especially external degree types, has been (and probably will continue to be) a problem in higher education and particularly in nursing education. However, accrediting bodies, such as the National League for Nursing and the Council on Postsecondary Accreditation (COPA), are beginning to realize that educational changes are required and that the approval process must be modified accordingly (COPA, 1978). Recently, the NLN has made significant changes in the process of accreditation. The accreditation of the REDNP in 1981, after a long and complex process, established a precedent and therefore was a major accomplishment. Other external assessment programs are sure to follow suit, although each will be reviewed with care to assure quality.

Summary

As illustrated by the NYREDNP model, the external degree assessment alternative is now possible and is being accepted widely by academic institutions. By combining the best of adult education, competency-based education, and objective assessment philosophies, an external degree allows maximum flexibility and individualized learning while ensuring academic quality and integrity. It does so by using rigid standards of assessment to document achievement of competencies prescribed as essential for the degree. By incorporating educational technologies, existing high-quality theory and performance examinations, and instructional and advisory services, external degree programs can be developed to serve a major need of the nursing profession. During this time of transition related to education preparation for practice, external degree assessment programs can be used to help the profession reach its goals.

The development of regionally located performance assessment centers will make it possible for many nursing programs to design nontraditional and flexible curricula around the availability of proficiency and performance examinations. The notion of purchasing high-quality written and performance examinations developed by others is becoming more and more attractive as educational budgets are cut and generalized inflation increases. While some dangers exist in such programs, they probably are no greater than the problems experienced by instructional programs—only different.

The development of regional assessment centers requires the intensive training of a large cadre of capable and reliable clinical evaluators (credentialed nurse educators). In time, with the growth in numbers of centers and numbers of students seeking to take these examinations, the position of clinical evaluator could become a full-time entity, requiring specialized educational preparation and perhaps even required continued education and certification.

Variations of the external degree assessment model provide the alternative approach needed by adult learners, by institutions, and by the profession. Academic caution and common sense must be used in developing, implementing, and monitoring external programs to avoid their abuse and prostitution. However, potential problems should not deter a full exploration of their use in professional education, particularly in the continued academic preparation of those who are committed to a career in professional nursing. The alternative is ready to be adopted and, ultimately, to be adapted to help the profession meet its obligations to its members and society.

References

Aiken, L. H., Ed. *Nursing in the 1980's Crises, Opportunities Challenges.* Philadelphia: J. B. Lippincott, 1982.

Alverno College Faculty. *Assessment at Alverno College.* Milwaukee: Alverno Productions, 1979.

American Association for Higher Education. *Current Issues in Higher Education: New Technologies for Higher Education,* Vol. 5. Washington, D.C., 1981a.

American Association for Higher Education. *Current Issues in Higher Education: Partnerships with Business and The Professions,* Vol. 3. Washington, D.C., 1981b.

Cole, C. C. *To Improve Instruction.* ERIC Research Report No. 2. Washington, D.C.: ERIC Clearinghouse on Higher Education, American Association for Higher Education, 1978.

Commission on Nontraditional Study. *Diversity by Design.* San Francisco: Jossey-Bass, 1973.

Cross, K. P. *The Missing Link: Connecting Adult Learners to Learning Resources.* New York: College Entrance Examination Board, 1978.

Council on Postsecondary Accreditation, *Assessing Nontraditional Education.* Summary Report of The Project to Develop Evaluative Criteria and Procedures for The Accreditation of Nontraditional Education. Washington, D.C.: Vol. 1, 1978, p. 128.

Grant, G. and Associates. *On Competency.* San Francisco: Jossey-Bass, 1979.

Houle, C. O. *The External Degree.* San Francisco: Jossey-Bass, 1973.

Keeton, M. T. and Associates. *Experiential Learning Rationale, Characteristics, and Assessment.* San Francisco: Jossey-Bass, 1976.

Knowles, M. S. *Self Directed Learning.* New York: Associated Press, 1975.

Lenburg, C. B. *The Clinical Performance, Examination: Development and Implementation.* New York: Appleton-Century-Crofts, 1979a.

Lenburg, C. B. "Emphasis on Evaluating Outcomes: The New York Regents External Degree Program," *Peabody Journal of Education* 56 (3). Nashville: George Peabody College for Teachers, 1979b.

Lenburg, C. B. "The External Degree: An Alternative Ready for Adoption." In *Current Issues in Nursing,* edited by J. McClosky and H. Grace. Boston: Blackwell Scientific, 1981, pp. 177–196.

Lenburg, C. B. *Open Learning and Career Mobility in Nursing.* St. Louis: C. V. Mosby, 1975.

Lenburg, C. B. "The Promise Fulfilled: The New York Regents External Degree Program in Nursing," *Nursing Outlook* (July 1976).

Lenburg, C. B. "In Search of The BSN: How to Decide Which Program Does you Justice," *RN* 43(3) (1980):60–63.

Meyer, P. *Awarding College Credit for Non-College Learning.* San Francisco: Jossey-Bass, 1975.

National League for Nursing. *Selected Readings from the Open Curriculum Literature: An Annotated Bibliography,* 2nd Ed. New York, 1977.

Nolan, D. J. "Toward an Examining University: The New York Regents External Degree." In *Formulating Policy in Post Secondary Education—The Search for Alternatives.* Washington, D.C.: American Council on Education, 1975.

Sosdian, C. and Sharp, L. *The External Degree as A Credential: Graduates' Experiences in Employment and Further Study.* Washington, D.C.: National Institute of Education, USDHEW, 1978.

Valley, J. "The External Degree: Does It Hold Promise For Nursing Education?" In *Open Learning and Career Mobility in Nursing,* edited by C. B. Lenburg. St. Louis: C. V. Mosby, 1975, pp. 353–361.

24. Models for the Baccalaureate Education of Registered Nurses

Jane Garvey, Patricia Castiglia,
and Bonnie Bullough

The approximately 1 million registered nurses in the United States are graduates of three types of basic nursing programs: diploma, associate degree, and baccalaureate. Table 24–1 shows the distribution of the graduates and indicates that the nursing educational system is in transition with a growing emphasis on baccalaureate education. Moreover, a significant portion of the graduates of diploma and associate degree programs are entering baccalaureate programs. The desire of registered nurses for more education stems from two sources. First, the technology of health care has become more complex, and nurses have taken on expanded roles in acute, primary, and long-term care. These expanded roles require education to at least the baccalaureate level and often to the masters level. A second motivating factor comes from the profession itself, which has been pushing its members to achieve more education through the sponsorship of the series of resolutions calling for the baccalaureate degree as the basic educational level for licensure as a registered nurse (New York State Nurses' Association, 1974; ANA, July 1978, August 1978).

While no state legislature has yet passed such a law, the resolutions have created a motivational backdrop which causes registered nurses who are denied entrance into baccalaureate programs to feel frustrated.

Baccalaureate Education

When West and Hawkins surveyed nursing education in the middle of the twentieth century, there were 201 baccalaureate programs. Of the 201, 61 (30 percent) were generic baccalaureate programs. While a handful of these baccalaureate programs had adopted the university norm of 4 years, most were still using the

Table 24–1   Graduations of registered nurse students from initial professional programs in the United States.

Year	Number	Percent Diploma	Percent Associate Degree	Percent Baccalaureate
1950	21,379	93	—	7
1955–56	30,236	89	1	10
1959–60	30,113	84	3	14
1964–65	34,686	77	7	16
1969–70	43,639	52	27	21
1974–75	74,536	29	44	27
1978–79	76,415	19	48	33
1980–81	74,890	17	50	33

Sources: Margaret West and Christy Hawkins, *Nursing Schools at Mid Century,* New York: National Committee for Improvement of Nursing Service, 1950, p. 72; American Nurses' Association, *Facts About Nursing,* New York: ANA 1959 Edition, p. 71; 1967 Edition, p. 96; National League for Nursing, *NLN Nursing Data Book,* 1979, p. 2; National League for Nursing, *State Approved Schools of Nursing RN 1981,* pp. 59–77; Personal communication, National League for Nursing—Research Department.

5-year pattern, which was essentially a 3-year diploma nursing program plus a 2-year liberal arts component, with or without advanced nursing content in public health or nursing education. The other 70 percent of the schools had both diploma and baccalaureate options or were simply hospital schools with college affiliations that allowed students to go on for a degree (West and Hawkins, 1950). The colleges granted 20–60 units of blanket credit to cover the hospital training.

Probably the major defect in the 5-year plan was its lack of integration; the link between the nursing program and the collegiate component was not always clear. Consequently, a movement grew up among nursing educators to develop a more integrated baccalaureate model. Cincinnati was the first program to move in this direction, claiming a 1945 date for its integrated baccalaureate program. It was quickly joined by several other programs across the country. The time was right for educational innovation in the period following World War II.

This was the era in which the associate degree programs described in Chapter 22 were developed. As indicated, Mildred Montag, the founder of the associate degree nursing programs, believed that the philosophy and objectives of associate degree and baccalaureate nursing programs were completely different, so that no mechanism for articulation was included in the early planning. Thus when the profession did try to move toward improving articulation, it was not only faced with a large contingent of diploma graduates, but also groups of practical and associate degree nurses. The reorganization of the National League for Nursing Education into the National League for Nursing in 1952 did nothing to solve the problem because eventually each level was established as a separate council and communication between the councils dwindled.

The height of the separatist movement came in 1963 when a statement was issued by the Council of Baccalaureate and Higher Degree Programs of the National League for Nursing. It called for a single pattern for baccalaureate education with a genuine upper division collegiate major in nursing (Lenburg, 1975). As this position was adopted and made a criterion for accreditation, the blanket credit mechanism was dropped, so that graduates of diploma programs were effectively cut off from higher education unless they were willing to repeat their education. Associate degree and practical nurses with college credits in nursing were also blocked because their credits were lower division and could not be transferred to fill the upper division nursing requirements.

This decision to move to the single-track baccalaureate seems to have been made in a serious effort to raise the educational standards and to professionalize the occupation. This was also the goal of the 1965 American Nurses' Association position paper, which clearly reiterated the separatist ideology, positing a technical and professional nursing role with no mobility between the two (ANA, 1965).

This move toward higher standards and professionalization ran into difficulty from the rank and file of nurses. The large cadre of nurses that was cut off from upward mobility through the educational system became frustrated and bitter. They made their discontent known to legislators and college officials. In the decade of the 1970s the California legislature passed a whole series of career ladder laws mandating that transfer credits be accepted, that practical nurses be required to take no more than 30 nursing units to complete registered nurse requirements, and that all students be allowed to sit for licensure after 36 months in the nursing program (Cobin et al., 1976). The need for better articulation between nursing programs was identified as a crucial goal for the profession in the 1970 report of the National Commission for the Study of Nursing and Nursing Education. (1970).

Finally in 1970 the Council of Baccalaureate and Higher Degrees also recognized the problem and issued a statement in support of an open curriculum (Lenburg, 1975, p. 28). This was followed by an open-curriculum project that included two surveys of schools and a conference. The conference was held in 1973 and featured 32 open-curriculum projects from 51 schools that reported their experiences.

The first survey of the schools done in 1972 resulted in the publication of the *Directory of Career Mobility Opportunities in Nursing*. The state-approved nursing schools of both the registered and practical level were surveyed, yielding a total of 2,687; out of this group, 1,500 programs met minimum criteria of acceptance of transfer credit for advanced placement (Lenburg, Johnson, and Vahey, 1973; Notter, 1973). By the 1974 revision of the directory 65 percent of the group allowed some advanced placement. From that survey four types of open-curriculum patterns were identified:

1. Programs accepting only licensed personnel, including licensed practical nurses or registered nurses.
2. Programs providing advanced placement opportunities through testing procedures or other exams.
3. Multiple-exit programs in which students can exit and re-enter at two or more levels.
4. Programs awarding a degree on the basis of an examination or transfer of credit without requiring attendance at the program (Notter, 1976).

Models for Baccalaureate Programs for Registered Nurses

Gradually more nursing schools opened their doors to registered nurse students. In 1979 the National League for Nursing reported that 306 of the 353 basic baccalaureate programs were admitting some registered nurses. In addition, there were 93 baccalaureate programs that admitted only registered nurses (NLN, 1980). In 1981 there were 106 registered nurse programs (NLN, 1981). The four categories outlined by the National League for Nursing project can be collapsed into three major models for registered nurse education. All use generic terminal objectives but vary in the process by which these objectives are obtained. The three models are as follows:

1.   The generic baccalaureate pattern, which uses the 4-year baccalaureate program as the model for curriculum planning.
2.   Direct articulation model, which uses the career ladder pattern in planning curriculum. Candidates cycle through nursing knowledge and skills more than once.
3.   The assessment model, which uses testing rather than course work as its basis for granting credentials.

These three patterns are described in more detail below.

The Generic Model

The generic model is the most common approach. The basic tenet of the model is that professional education for nursing must be designed within the baccalaureate framework. Historically, this position was articulated in the 1965 American Nurses' Association position statement. For almost 20 years this position, stating that all nursing courses must be upper division courses, has had a major impact on nursing curricula. Accreditation by the National League for Nursing has served to enforce this position statement and thereby to promulgate the generic model. Therefore, most schools that have tried to "open" or "individualize" instructions for learners with differing entering backgrounds have related their attempt to the established generic program.

The mechanism for making input adjustments to the learning situation include advanced placement by the acceptance of transfer credit, by examination(s), and/or by crediting life experiences. Placement in the learning situation is determined by performance currently evaluated or accepted documentation of past performance.

Most programs admitting registered nurse students today utilize advanced placement concepts by assessing past learning in relation to the objectives identified for the generic student. The most common form of assessment is the challenge or proficiency examination (Lenburg, 1975, p. 201). A challenge examination tests essential content. If the examination is passed, college credit is awarded. Most challenge examinations are designed to test knowledge. There are, in addition, a few schools that test clinical competence. Challenge examinations may be designed by faculty in a particular school or they may be standardized tests such as the College Proficiency Examination (CPE) or tests developed by the College Level Examination Program (CLEP), the American College Testing Program (ACT), the National League for Nursing achievement tests, and, most recently, the New York Regents External Degree associate and baccalaureate level examinations. College proficiency examinations have offered both a solution and a problem. They have offered a solution by providing a route to college credit by examination, thereby eliminating the necessity for registered nurses to attend courses which to some degree are repetitious of those learnings included in their basic nursing programs. Problems encountered in the use of these examinations arise when attempts are made to exempt students from specific courses. The examinations are oriented to the medical model curriculum, including medical/surgical, maternal/child, and psychiatric nursing, at a time when the integrated-curriculum model has gained momentum. It is difficult, if not impossible, to match the examinations to specific courses. In response to these problems, teacher-made tests and clinical performance evaluations have gained popularity in recent years. The use of CPEs, the more recently popular teacher-made challenges, and clinical performance examinations propose a comprehensive testing of nursing knowledge.

The valuation of the clinical performance of applicants is the area most difficult to assess in terms of both time and financial cost. Sometimes the rationale for not testing clinical ability is the stance that passing a cognitive challenge examinations at a lower level places the student in an upper division nursing course where satisfactory clinical performance verifies lower level clinical ability.

The issue in crediting relates to the goal of challenge examinations. The goal is embedded in one of two beliefs. The first of these beliefs acknowledges the problem in transfer of credit and seeks to provide a mechanism whereby registered nurses from diploma schools may legitimately accrue credits toward the baccalaureate degree. The second belief is that thorough testing of all nursing knowledge and validation that applicants do indeed possess the knowledge and skills commensurate with the license is necessary. The second position, then, regards with suspicion both the quality of the diploma programs, even though they have been approved by the state and the National League for Nursing, and the power of the state to grant licensure.

Which belief is supported (accrual of credit or validation of learning) makes considerable difference in the approach to challenge. In the situation where accrual of credit is the goal, the use of the examination will be predicated on granting credit without concern for comprehensive generalist types of knowledge. When validation of learning is sought, then it becomes necessary to test each area of nursing comprehensively. Whichever the goal and subsequent choice, the CPEs in themselves are inadequate means by which to determine placement of registered nurses within degree programs.

Transfer of credit for advanced standing is applicable for associate degree graduates and for students from other baccalaureate programs. Transfer credits in these cases generally present few problems. Considerations include the number of credits which can be transferred into the program at that institution and the number of credits transferable in the major area of concentration, i.e., nursing. Generally, diploma schools do not generate transferable credit. The exception occurs when the diploma program is affiliated with a college or university where students take some of their course work. In this situation the college credits may be considered for transfer; however, the nursing courses required in diploma schools do not qualify for college credits.

Credit for life experiences is another approach that is possible within the generic model. This method may be evidenced by the requirement of a license to practice nursing and/or work experience as the basis for admission. State board examinations are viewed as testing a level of knowledge and practice. This method credits the identification of common knowledge and skill levels, thereby enabling the identification and development of a curriculum built on this base.

The most significant point concerning the generic pattern is that an established generic program provides the framework within which individualization is recognized and implemented. All graduates of the generic program show how they have traversed a similar learning process and met the same terminal objectives as baccalaureate students. The chief advantage of this pattern is the mingling of registered nurse and generic students, which theoretically aids the socialization into the role of the baccalaureate nurse by incorporating the philosophy and values associated with the role. The disadvantages include the cost, the substantial time commitment required, and perhaps the inappropriate assignment of learning experiences.

Direct Articulation

The basic assumption of a career ladder pattern is that it is reasonable to cycle students through nursing content more than once. Certainly basic learning theory would support this assumption. We know people learn by reiteration. Yet the idea was unpopular in nursing for a while in the 1960s and 1970s. Some nurse educators argued that the only sound educational pattern was one that started with complete focus on the liberal arts and ended with a total focus on nursing. Because of this rather hostile climate of opinion the career ladder model has emerged haltingly.

The State College of Arkansas seems to be one of the first multiple-entry and multiple-exit programs at the baccalaureate level. It was set up as a formal funded project called Career Options in Nursing Education with the acronym CONE. The CONE project conceptualized the curriculum in an upward spiral. The first cycle was a 1-year practical nurse program, the second time around terminated with an associate degree registered nurse, and the third cycle, a 2-year cycle, produced a registered nurse with a baccalaureate degree (Garner, 1975).

The Orange County Long Beach Consortium started from two focal points. In 1967 the Long Beach City College started experimenting with an articulation pattern between nurses' aides and vocational nurses. By 1971 a formal core curriculum with three exit points and two entry points was set up (Drage, 1971; Venner, 1978). At the same time a consortium of schools started to meet informally in nearby Orange County. The focus of the consortium was to encourage articulation between schools. Kellogg funded the project and the Long Beach schools joined the effort. At the completion of the funded project in 1979, the career ladder included five levels of nursing personnel (aides, practical or vocational nurses, associate degree registered nurses, baccalaureate level nurses, and clinical specialists or nurse practitioners with masters degrees (Lysaught, 1979).

There is an important difference between the articulation which can occur with prior planning in one school as in the Arkansas example, and the articulation within the consortium model. Articulation between schools has to be accomplished by negotiation rather than purposeful planning, and that is a different sort of challenge. Nevertheless, it is important because that is how most articulation is now occurring.

The problem in the negotiated articulation is that both partners in the articulation plan have their past lives and past philosophies to deal with. Often each group of educators feel that theirs is the best of all approaches. For example, many diploma educators consider their programs best because of their heavy clinical orientation. Associate of arts educators tend to look upon their programs as the most solidly planned, and baccalaureate educators tend to feel that the 4-year generic model with the sciences first and the nursing content later is the only appropriate way to educate nurses. Consequently, negotiations between any two of these groups will take time. Both parties need to be persuaded to actually look at the other programs to see their strengths and to assess the gaps which need filling with further education. Only then can rational planning take place.

The most common type of articulation now emerging is the freestanding registered nurse program. The National League for Nursing reported in 1979 that there were 93 such programs in existence. These programs usually articulate with local associate degree and diploma programs but try to make requirements general enough to fit most other lower division nursing programs. The key to planning an upper division articulated program is a thorough analysis of not just the single registered nurse (as is the case with the generic model) but the total class of registered nurses so that the program can be designed to fit this learner population.

A well-known example of an upper two program is the one at Sonoma State which was established in 1972. It admitted only registered nurses and tried to include only new learning in the program. Sonoma even experimented with a highly successful family nurse practitioner program as one element in its baccalaureate program. Other students wrote their own objectives for a senior specialty that involved them in a variety of roles as infection control nurses, critical care specialists, and rural public health nurses (Searight, 1976).

An articulated program that addresses the abilities and needs of the registered nurse student has been designed and implemented at the State University of New York at Buffalo. It differs from the Sonoma model in that it stands beside and uses courses from the generic program. The plan is based on identification of the competencies of registered nurse students and subsequent modifications of the existing generic program. Content and objectives of courses were examined and resulted in the development of 2 nursing courses for registered nurse students which would complement the 6 nursing courses taken by generic students. These 2 nursing courses as well as an additional 8 courses taken by both generic and registered nurse students constitute the 38 nursing credits required for registered nurse students compared to 53 credits for generic students. Of the 8 courses, 2 contain modified clinical components (Garvey, in press).

Assessment Model

The basic assumption of the assessment model is that learning occurs in a variety of ways and in many instances outside any formal instructional setting. The goal of assessment programs is to ensure that learning has occurred and no attempt is made to identify the how or where. The New York Regents External Degree (NYRED), more fully described in Chapter 23, is the most well-known example of the assessment models. This program grew out of the College Proficiency Examinations. Begun in 1963, the College Proficiency Examinations provide opportunities to accrue credit by examination. They are widely recognized in colleges and universities as an acceptable credit mechanism. These examinations offer isolated credit by examination but not a degree program. The NYRED, on the other hand, does offer complete degree programs. Established in 1971, it is a network of programs offered under the aegis of the University of the State of New York. These programs are unique in that they grant credit through assessment rather than instruction. Traditionally credit has been granted through colleges and universities where students have enrolled in courses with prescribed objectives, defined content, and regular sessions in which instruction is given and regular attendance expected within the limits of a semester. Following testing which purports to assure that learning has occurred, a prescribed number of credits is awarded. Many courses taken in similar fashion constitute the degree program (Lenburg, 1979).

The NYRED removes the instructional component, the attendance requirement, and the limitations of time. Courses are designed which constitute the degree framework. Objectives and content are developed for each course and students prepare independently for the assessment examinations assisted by study guides. Following successful achievement credit is awarded, and through similar preparation and testing the total credits within a specific degree program are completed and the degree awarded.

There are three different nursing degree programs available through NYRED: two associate degree and one baccalaureate degree. All three of these programs are fully accredited by the National League for Nursing.

The NYRED program provides an alternative education program for highly motivated, self-directed individuals. It is not intended to replace traditional educational programs but to augment them. It serves the purpose of validating learning. Some universities are now using selected NYRED examinations to validate portions of a traditional degree program.

Summary and Conclusions

The process for facilitating the movement of diploma graduates into and through the baccalaureate in nursing degree programs has become increasingly problematic. Three models of facilitation have emerged: the generic model, the career ladder model, and the assessment model. Each model proposes a different process whereby registered nurse graduates of diploma and associate degree programs may complete baccalaureate degree requirements selecting the model most appropriate for that particular setting.

These models and variations of these models are becoming increasingly available in nursing education. No one model is likely to provide the solution. Suitable selection or adaptation of a model depends on local needs and resources.

There is a maldistribution of universities in the United States. Certain states and urban centers abound with universities that offer a wide variety of programs. Other areas have few universities and limited programs and some large areas have no university available. The decision, then, as to what model to adopt requires consideration of these basic resources.

In areas where there are no universities, an assessment model could be considered. The New York Regents External Degree is available nationwide and offers access to the baccalaureate degree in nursing to those areas with no available university. In areas where universities are available but do not offer a baccalaureate degree in nursing, selection of the career ladder model appears most appropriate. In areas where universities offering the baccalaureate in nursing degree are available, the generic model might be the easiest to institute, although an articulated upper two program might be more satisfying to the registered nurse population.

Further consideration of the characteristics of the learners within each area with respect to educational background, years of nursing practice, life style, and cognitive mapping will assist in selection of a program which will address the needs within a given area.

In reviewing the evolution of nursing education, it becomes apparent that changes in programs and the development of new programs have been in response to a need for nursing education at a particular time. At this time nursing education must first recognize the need to increase the access of registered nurses to baccalaureate nursing degree programs; second, analyze existing resources; and third, select the appropriate model to facilitate the accomplishment of this goal.

References

"American Nurses' Association Convention '78," *American Journal of Nursing* 78 (July 1978):1230–1246.

"A.N.A. Convention," *Nursing Outlook* 26 (August 1978):500–507.

American Nurses' Association. *Educational Preparation for Nurse Practitioners and Assistants to Nurses.* 1965.

Cobin, J., Traber, W., and Bullough, B. "A Five Level Articulated Program," *Nursing Outlook* 24 (May 1976):309–313.

Drage, M. "Core Courses and a Career Ladder," *American Journal of Nursing* 71 (July 1971):1356–1358.

Garner, J. "Career Options in Nursing Education at State College of Arkansas." In *Open Learning and Career Mobility in Nursing,* edited by C. B. Lenburg. St. Louis: C. V. Mosby, 1975, pp. 313–327.

Garvey, J. "An Alternative Baccalaureate Curriculum Plan for RNs," *Journal of Nursing Education* in press.

Lenburg, C. B. (Ed.). *Open Learning and Career Mobility in Nursing.* St. Louis: C. V. Mosby, 1975, pp. 20–29.

Lenburg, C. B. "Emphasis on Evaluating Outcomes: The New York Regents External Degree Program," *Peabody Journal of Education* (April 1979):212–221.

Lenburg, C. B., Johnson, W. L., and Vahey, J. A. T. *Directory of Career Mobility Opportunities in Nursing.* New York: National League for Nursing, 1973.

Lysaught, J. P. *You Can Get There From Here: The Orange County/Long Beach Experiment in Improved Patterns of Nursing Education.* Battle Creek, Mich: W. K. Kellogg Foundation, 1979.

National Commission for the Study of Nursing and Nursing Education,

Jerome P. Lysaught, Director. *An Abstract for Action.* New York: Blakiston, 1970, pp. 114–117.

National League for Nursing. *NLN Data Book, 1979.* New York: 1980, p. 3.

National League for Nursing. *State Approved Schools of Nursing RN 1981,* 39th Edition. New York: NLN Pub. No. 19-1853, 1981.

New York State Nurses Association. *Resolution on Entry Into Professional Practice.* Albany, N.Y., 1974.

Notter, L. (Ed.). *Proceedings: Open Curriculum Conference I.* New York: National League for Nursing, 1973.

Notter, L. E. "The NLN Open Curriculum Project." In *Accountability and the Open Curriculum in Baccalaureate Education.* New York: National League for Nursing, 1976, pp. 21–30.

Searight, M. W. *The Second Step: Baccalaureate Education for Registered Nurses.* Philadelphia: F. A. Davis, 1976.

Venner, M. F. *An Evaluative Study of an Open Curriculum/Career Ladder Nursing Program.* New York: National League for Nursing, 1978.

West, M. and Hawkins, C. *Nursing Schools at Mid-Century.* New York: National Committee for the Improvement of Nursing Service, 1950, pp. 10–14.

25. Reality Shock Alleviation: Student Experience in a Preceptored Advanced Clinical Nursing Practicum

Mary Claire Soukup

Reality Shock

The concept of reality shock as identified by Kramer (1974) is one of the most devastating experiences the new graduate of nursing will have to undergo. Numerous writers have provided suggestions to assist the student in this transition. Alhadeff (1979) speaks directly of her initial experiences and cites the importance of orientation programs, as well as strong efforts to foster the realization that one cannot know everything at once.

Utilization of internship, externship, and preceptor programs are explored in articles by May (1980), Huchstadt (1981),

Bushong and Simms (1979), and Walters (1981). All these articles speak to alleviating reality shock. One of the earliest users of the preceptorship program in the undergraduate setting was Boston University, which initiated a credit-granting course in March 1974. This program is described by Scipien and Pasternack (1977).

As a diploma graduate, I myself cannot recall any particular instance of reality shock because I was exposed gradually to the real world of nursing with each day's progression in my initial program. Yet during the last 20 years of my teaching of nursing in two baccalaureate programs, whenever the topic of insecurity came up, the faculty blissfully assured students that this was a process all new graduates had to work through. Our colleagues in nursing service frequently expressed the opinion that additional and more refined clinical skills should be taught in the basic program. However, we as baccalaureate educators recognized the need for a broad educational program which included not only a substantial body of biological and behavioral science but nursing theory as well. We wanted graduates who could thoroughly understand the concepts of humanistic patient care. Such a program necessarily demanded many classroom hours, so that it limited the time available for clinical experience. Consequently, graduates of a program such as ours were caught in conflicting sets of expectations. On one hand, the nursing faculty wanted them to understand all of the humanistic concepts of client care. On the other hand, the prospective employers in nursing service wanted them to be experts in the skills of nursing care.

A New Course

In 1978 the faculty at the State University of New York at Buffalo admitted that these conflicting expectations were basic to the reality shock experienced by new graduates and they designed a course to deal with the problem. The course, titled Advanced Clinical Nursing, is conceptualized as a 4-week culminating experience. Its primary purpose is to aid students in their transition from the student role to that of graduate nurse. Focus of the course is a 5-day-a-week experience in close association with a clinical preceptor. It furnishes an opportunity for students to provide for continuity of patient care, to refine their nursing skills, and to obtain a more realistic view of the real nursing work world. Four objectives of our school philosophy are particularly emphasized: the nursing process, communication, health teaching, and collaboration with other health professionals.

Since the spring of 1979, over 400 students have taken this culminating course either in the fall or spring semester immediately prior to the completion of their studies. Students choose their own setting and compile their own proposals, which must include their rationale for selection of the type of setting, behavioral objectives, and a built-in means of evaluation. These proposals are then read by selected faculty reviewers who aid in proposal refinement. Students may request out-of-town placement if they have a grade point average of 3.0 (B). Most generic students elect an adult medical or surgical experience. Psychiatry receives the least number of requests.

The registered nurse students choose a wider variety of placements. While some seek to update skills in basic nursing areas, the majority select specialty areas including trauma, ICUs, coronary care, in-service education, discharge planning, infection control, hospice, and occupational health nursing. Since these registered nurse students have previously been exposed to the consecutive 5-day weekly experience, we allow them to complete their 20-day experience 2 days a week throughout a semester. This freedom enables them to take over the same time period other courses required for graduation.

After review, the proposals are sent to the course coordinator and placements are sought. About two-thirds of the students are placed locally, while the remainder choose out-of-town locations. To date placements have been made in 15 other states as well as Canada. The students are expected to assume responsibility for arrangements and expenses relative to transportation, housing, food, and communication with the faculty advisor.

Local hospitals or agencies are asked to provide the course coordinator with the name of a liaison person. The proposals are sent to the agencies and the liaison person suggests a suitable nurse to act as the student's preceptor and role model. As defined in the course syllabus, a clinical preceptor is a registered nurse employed by the health care facility selected for student placement. This individual is selected by a joint collaborative effort between the agency liaison and the coordinator. If the placement is a distant one, the agency assumes responsibility for determining and identifying the preceptor. The selection of a preceptor should be based on that individual's clinical expertise, familiarity with the agency, and interest in working with baccalaureate nursing students. The preceptor must be available to the student in order to provide direct supervision when needed. Many preceptors treat the student as a beginning practitioner, newly placed on the unit. The students are able to progress to varying degrees of independence, based on their adeptness, knowledge, and adaptability.

A faculty advisor is assigned to students on a ratio of 12 to 1. This advisor reads the student's proposal, suggests revisions if they are needed, reviews experience logs, and encourages students in the attainment of their personalized objectives. The advisor maintains close contact with the preceptor and can be reached easily should any difficulty arise. It is the policy of the School of Nursing not to usurp the preceptor's role. Visits by the advisor are kept to a minimum in order to make the experience more realistic for the student. In those few instances where difficulties arise, preceptors generally want to work the situation out directly with the student rather than bring in the faculty advisor to mediate. For the first time in the student's educational experience the solution or intervention came from a representative of Nursing Service. Also, the preceptors feel free to independently intervene and are accepting of and reponsive to this responsibility.

The faculty advisor can discern from reading the weekly logs required of all students that a gradual growth in ability, independence, and increased confidence has been achieved by the students. They had been encouraged to solve problems and frequently arrived at very creative solutions. The students were able to view a more complete picture of patient care because they were able to follow the preceptor's time schedule. Also, many students found themselves assigned to shifts other than the day shift and had opportunities for weekend work experiences. This reflected a truer picture of work hours. Students experience reality shock while in this course but, with aid from the preceptor and the faculty advisor, they are better able to cope with it. Although most students start working immediately with the preceptor, some institutions have an orientation program. For example, one local hospital offers a 2-day orientation before the students enter the units for direct patient care.

When the agency approves of a student placement, two signed copies of our contract are forwarded, with the request to sign one and return it to our institution. The other copy is retained in their files. A separate malpractice insurance rider is also sent to the institution, as all of our students are covered by malpractice insurance. A course syllabus and our program philosophy are also sent to each institution and each preceptor.

The students, on completion of the experience, write a self-evaluation including a recommended letter grade as based on their objective attainment and overall performance. Preceptors are also requested to write summary statements of students' progress, which includes letter grades. Faculty advisors then arrange interviews with each student. Based on these three sources, a final grade is given to the student.

Informal Evaluation of the New Course

Student comments about the experience speak of nursing "in the real world." Some were surprised to see how physically tired they became on a realistic work schedule. All students experienced a variety of refinement of nursing skills which increased their confidence in their ability. Many relied heavily on this opportunity to strengthen these skills prior to graduation. Most important of all, students were afforded the opportunity to follow through on nursing plans because of the continuity of the experience. In previous clinical experiences, plans were often made with a minimal possibility of follow-through because of the necessary brevity of the clinical exposure.

The comments from preceptors reflect an interest in aiding the student in objective attainment. Most felt that they themselves personally profited from this experience of exposure to a student because it offered them an opportunity to hone their teaching skills. Some students have also provided a stimulus for the preceptor to initiate further educational studies.

The agencies have been cordial and helpful in accepting the students and in choosing preceptors who would function as true role models. These agencies also profit by being able to have immediate feedback from the preceptors. They can then, if they so desire, offer the student a position based on an on-the-job evaluation of the student's performance. The offer of a position, which happens frequently, certainly bolsters the student's sense of worth. Moreover, the young graduate who has become more familiar with shift and weekend assignments at this facility is better prepared to evaluate this job offer with a realistic view toward future functioning.

All preceptors receive a certificate of merit from our university as well as an official thank you letter. All in all, we feel we have been successful with this course offering. We have now arrived at the point where several of our preceptors were once themselves preceptored students.

Written Evaluation of the Course

In addition to these informal evaluations of the course, data were also gathered by means of questionnaires from students and preceptors. Selected findings from these two sources are reported here. The student response rate was 95 percent. Table 25–1 shows the students' evaluations of their experience. As can be noted, student opinion was highly favorable with 98 percent indicating they were able to achieve the objectives they had outlined for themselves and a majority responding favorably on the other parameters of the questionnaire.

In order to identify the characteristics of a good clinical placement site, the students who felt their placement was a good one were asked to give the reasons they favored it. Table 25–2 shows these responses. Two major thoughts seem to emerge from this table. First, students valued a setting in which they felt

Table 25–1 Student responses to simple yes/no questions.

Item	Total in Agreement ($n = 92$)	Percent Agree
Opportunity was given for continuity of patient care	86	93
The student felt she or he had achieved the behavioral objectives	90	98
The agency did permit flexibility in the implementation of the student's objectives	80	87
The preceptor was viewed as a good role model	81	88
The student would recommend future placements here for other students	81	88

Table 25–2   Recommended future placement (reasons most frequently given by students in recommending placement of future students in the same location they utilized).

Reason for Placement*	Number of Times Given	Percent of Times Given
A helpful, accepting, friendly, open hospital staff	57	62
An excellent learning situation	29	32
Wide variety of patient conditions	16	17
Excellent preceptor available	8	9
Exposure to new and challenging experiences	8	9
This experience gave the student confidence	7	8

*Generally, students gave more than one reason in response to this question.

welcome, where the staff was accepting and helpful. Second, they valued sites in which they felt they were able to learn, including those with a variety of patient problems, a good preceptor, and new and challenging experiences.

Responses to the preceptors' questionnaire were also highly favorable. Ninety percent indicated that they would choose to participate again and 94 percent felt that the experience of being a preceptor had facilitated their own professional growth. Preceptors did, however, have some suggestions for improving the course. Table 25–3 shows these responses. While 76 percent indicated that no change was necessary, there were a few people who felt the need for a bit more structure. They also wanted closer contact with the advisor and an opportunity to meet the student ahead of time.

It may be possible to provide these individual preceptors with the structure they need on an individual basis and leave the majority of the placements as they are by individualizing the relationship with the preceptors and giving a bit more structure to those who want it.

An unanticipated benefit of the course has been the influence of the experience on preceptors. Table 25–4 shows the educa-

Table 25–3 Preceptors' suggestions for course improvement as it relates to the preceptor's role.

Suggestion*	Number of Times Advanced	Percent of Times Suggested
No change necessary	68	76
Closer contact with faculty advisor	6	7
Opportunity to meet with student previous to assignment to unit	5	6
Greater knowledge of student's previous clinical experience	4	4
Availability of a more structured preceptor evaluation tool	4	4
Opportunity for evaluation of the preceptor by either the faculty advisor or the student	3	3

*Some preceptors included more than one suggestion.

Table 25–4 Education background of the preceptor.

Education Level	Number ($n =90$)	Percent
AAS	16	18
AAS and studying for BS	2	2
Diploma	26	30
Diploma and studying for BS	6	7
BS	31	34
BS and studying for MS	4	4
MS	5	6

Table 25–5   Reasons advanced for desire for future participation as a preceptor.

Reason*	Number of Times Given	Percent of Times Given
Enjoyed working with and helping student achieve objectives and combat reality shock	26	29
An excellent course leading to student growth	22	24
Impressed by professionalism of the student	17	19
Student was subsequently offered a position in the agency	16	18
Student became an integral part of the staff	9	10
The student was of direct assistance to the preceptor	4	4
Desire to have had a similar experience as part of my own initial program	3	3

*Some preceptors indicated more than one reason for desiring future participation.

tional level of the preceptors. Table 25–5 reveals the reasons the preceptors answered positively when asked if they would be interested in future participation in this course.

Summary and Conclusion

Thus, it appears that the course entitled Advanced Clinical Nursing offers a successful model for the alleviation of reality shock. Student success, agency satisfaction, and faculty approval attest to the usefulness and validity of this clinical nursing practicum in assisting the final semester senior student to acquire a greater refinement in nursing care skills.

As we look forward to the future placement of senior students in a preceptored practicum, experience has taught us to carefully monitor the following aspects of the course:

1. The *student proposals* should contain objectives which are realistically geared to the 4-week time frame and are within the allowable limits of the agency.

2. *Preceptors* who are good role models should be selected. They should be fully informed of the student's objectives and should provide adequate information on hospital philosophy and policy.

3. *Agencies* chosen should be accepting of students and should be able to provide the student with opportunities for continuity of care, multiple experiences, the flexibility required for goal attainment.

4. The *students* themselves should prepare for this experience by reviewing nursing procedures to which they have already been exposed. If they are assigned to a specialty unit, i.e., orthopedics, they should prepare themselves in this specialty area.

5. The *faculty advisor* might be alert to the need on the part of some preceptors for a greater knowledge of the student's previous clinical experience, for a closer contact with the faculty advisor, and for an opportunity for a previsit interview with the student.

References

Alhadeff, G. "Anxiety in a New Graduate," *American Journal of Nursing* (April 1979):687–688.

Bushong, N. V. K. and Simms, S. "Externship: A Way to Bridge the Gap," *Supervisor Nurse* (June 1979):14–17, 22–23.

Huchstadt, A. "Work/Study: A Bridge to Practice," *American Journal of Nursing* (April 1981):726–727.

Kramer, M. *Reality Shock: Why Nurses Leave Nursing.* St. Louis: C. V. Mosby, 1974.

May, L. "Clinical Preceptors for New Nurses," *American Journal of Nursing* (October 1980):1824–1826.

Scipien, G. and Pasternack, S. "Creating More Confident Baccalaureate Graduates," *American Journal of Nursing* (May 1977):818–820.

Walters, C. R. "Using Staff Preceptors in a Senior Experience," *Nursing Outlook* (April 1981):245–247.

V

Nursing Law and Politics

26. Introduction—
Nursing Practice Law

Bonnie Bullough

The laws governing nursing practice are derived from two major sources: written statutes and decisions made by courts. This chapter will focus on the nurse practice acts, which are bodies of law written by state legislatures to regulate nursing. The next chapter will cover the issue of malpractice as it is shaped by court decisions. Other selections in this section will highlight the legislative process and legislative issues.

While the regulation of occupations is a function of the central government in most countries, the United States uses a federation model and occupational licensure is one of the responsibilities retained by the states. Legal precedents for occupational licensure were established by physicians. With the organization of the American Medical Association (A.M.A.) in 1847, doctors started lobbying for such legislation. In 1873 they succeeded in getting a licensure act through the Texas State Legislature (V. L. Bullough, 1980, pp. 14–20). In 1881, a similar statute passed in West Virginia, but it was challenged in the courts. The case reached the U.S. Supreme Court in 1888 and the court ruled that occupational licensure was a valid exercise of the political powers of the states. After that date medical licensure spread rapidly throughout all of the states (Derbyshire, 1969).

The fact that medical licensure came first has implications for other health occupations since their licenses in effect became amendments to the medical practice acts.

The History of the State
Nurse Practice Acts

The history of American nurse practice acts has been conceptualized by Bonnie Bullough as falling into three phases: (1) 1903–1938, the early nurse registration acts, (2) 1938, the era in which the scope of nursing function was defined, and (3) 1971 to the present, the era of expanding functions for registered nurses (B. Bullough, 1976, 1980, 1982).

The organization which did the most to lobby for registration of nurses was the Nurses' Associated Alumnae of United States and Canada, the precursor to the American Nurses' Association (ANA). It was founded in 1896 to seek recognition for trained nurses, to lessen competition from untrained nurses, and to upgrade the educational standards for nurses.

To facilitate the registration campaign in the states, constituent state nursing organizations were established to do the necessary work with the legislatures. This was not an easy task in an era when women did not have the vote, but by force of enthusiasm and numbers they were able to convince legislators. North Carolina in 1903 became the first state to pass a registration act, followed by New York, New Jersey, and Virginia in the same year. One by one other states followed suit until by 1923 all of the states then in the union had a nurse registration act. These first phase acts are properly called registration acts rather than practice acts because none of them included a statement outlining a scope of practice. The term *registered nurse* was defined as someone of good character who had completed an acceptable nursing program and passed a board examination (B. Bullough, 1980).

The second phase in the development of nursing licensure started in 1938 when the first mandatory practice act was passed in New York. This law established two levels of nurses, registered professional and practical, and restricted nursing functions to members of these two groups (editorial, 1939; Jacobson, 1940). This event marked the beginning of a new focus for the efforts of nurse activists, whose primary goal became the achievement of mandatory licensure.

While mandatory licensure can be thought of as a long-range aspiration from the beginning of the century when abortive attempts were made to restrict the title "nurse," the goal did not seem realistic until the New York nurses broke the barrier. Their efforts, and those of nurses in several states which followed their precedent, were facilitated by the development of licensure for practical nurses, the group which had previously opposed restricting the title of nurse. Employment patterns for nurses were changing in this period from private duty to hospital nursing, and hospital administrators argued with some justification that all nursing functions did not require the standard 3-year training period which by then was the norm. The development of the practical nurse as the basic bedside practitioner helped all nurses argue more successfully for licensure for all practitioners.

Besides being linked with the stratification of the nursing role, mandatory licensure included another interesting side effect. In order to pass a mandatory act of any kind, it was necessary to spell out the scope of function of the occupation which was being protected against encroachment. The older nursing laws merely made it illegal for an unauthorized person to use the title "registered nurse," but it was not illegal for such a person to practice nursing. If the new mandatory laws were to make it illegal for an unauthorized person to practice nursing, a definition of the scope of practice had to be written into the law so that violations of the mandatory provisions could be identified. Eventually a scope of function statement came to be thought of as a goal in and of itself (Lesnick and Anderson, 1947).

The American Nurses' Association in 1955 joined the effort to write scope of function statements with the adoption of a model definition of nursing. Professional practice was defined as

> the performance, for compensation, of any acts in the observation, care and counsel of the ill, injured or infirm or in the maintenance of health or prevention of illness of others, or in the supervision and teaching of other personnel or the administration of medications and treatments as prescribed by a licensed physician or a licensed dentist; requiring substantial specialized judgment and skill and based on knowledge and application of principles of biological, physical and social science. The foregoing shall not be deemed to include any acts of diagnosis or prescription of therapeutic or corrective measures (ANA, 1955).

By 1967, 15 states had incorporated the language of this model into their state laws and another 6 states had used the model with only slight modifications (Fogotson et al., 1967). A regrettable feature of this model act, as well as the other similar definitions of nursing practice, was the disclaimer, which clearly spelled out the fact that nursing did not include any acts of diagnosis or the prescription of therapeutic measures. Since prior to the era of mandatory licensure nurse registration acts did not define nursing, there was no disclaimer. The disclaimer created problems for the profession at a later date.

Actually, by 1955 when the model act was issued by the ANA, nurses were observing patients, collecting data about their conditions, and acting on such data to deliver nursing care. They were in fact making diagnostic decisions and treating people on the basis of those decisions. The disclaimers in the scope of practice statements were out of date at the time they were written. The behavior on the part of nurses seems like a manifestation of a minority group withdrawal. It is a type of alienation or anticipatory self-discrimination. Rather than risk a rebuff or a possible boundary dispute with medicine, nurses almost unconsciously decided to deny their role in the patient care decision-making process. Similar patterns of anticipatory withdrawal are a fairly common phenomenon among other minority groups; the ghetto walls are often as well policed from the inside as the outside. Feelings of alienation, powerlessness, and fear prevent people from challenging discriminatory practices (B. Bullough, 1967).

The Third Phase in Nursing Licensure: Factors Influencing the Development of a Specialty Level in Nursing

The third phase in the history of nursing licensure can be dated from 1971, when Idaho revised its practice act by inserting the following clause after the prohibition against diagnosis and treatment:

> except as may be authorized by rules and regulations jointly promulgated by the Idaho State Board of Medicine and the Idaho Board of Nursing which shall be implemented by the Idaho Board of Nursing (Idaho Code, 1971).

Following the passage of this amendment, the combined boards met and adopted regulations which called for agencies employing nurse practitioners to draw up policies and procedures to guide the practice of nurse practitioners. Thus, the Idaho legislature and boards established the precedent of defining the scope of function of nurse practitioners as different from that of registered nurses and utilized the power of the boards to define the details of that difference. Thirty-seven states have adopted this approach. In most of these states a legislative mandate was given to the board of nursing or the boards of nursing and medicine to devise a mechanism for dealing with the expanding functions of nursing. However, in Wisconsin, Delaware, and Tennessee the boards of nursing were able to take on this responsibility without new statutory law.

The other major approach to the accommodation of the nurse practitioner role was to expand the basic definition of the registered professional nurse by omitting or limiting the disclaimer against diagnosis and treatment by nurses, or by rewriting the definition of the registered nurse using broader language. New York in 1972 was the first state to use this approach; 35 states have now followed that precedent. From these numbers it is obvious that there is significant overlap with some states both expanding the role of all registered nurses and assigning the details of specialty nursing roles to the boards to write.

One of the reasons for the double-barreled approach is that the simple mechanism of expanding the definition of all registered nurses has not proven completely effective for nurse practitioners. This is, however, partly due to an unfortunate choice of words in the 1972 New York act which was copied in 19 other states. The attempt was made to differentiate between a nursing and a medical diagnosis using the following language:

> Diagnosing in the context of nursing practice means that identification of and discrimination between physical and psychosocial signs and symptoms essential to the effective execution and management of a nursing regime. Such diagnostic privilege is distinct from a medical diagnosis (New York State Education Law).

This language suggests that the act of diagnosis is somehow different when performed by a nurse than a physician, but it does not actually operationalize the difference. The phrase "nursing diagnosis" also focuses diagnosis on the health professional rather than the patient, which further confuses the issue.

Probably the only operational definition of a nursing diagnosis and a nursing regime that would hold up over time and empirical study would be a diagnosis and therapeutic plan done by a nurse as opposed to one carried out by a physician. This was in fact the approach used by some nurse practitioners for a time. They claimed that the work role of the practitioner fell under the general rubric of the terms "nursing diagnosis" and "nursing regime." However, more recently a backlash movement by at least one conservative New Jersey board of medicine member has pointed up the problematic aspect of this conceptualization of the scope of nursing functions. The New Jersey physician claimed that the state nurse practice act which invoked this language did not cover the nurse practitioner role (News, 1978; Regional Review, 1978; Adler, 1979).

Similarly, the attorney for the New York Board of Regents (which carries the ultimate regulatory power over occupations in the state) has ruled that the language is too vague to cover nurse practitioners. Thus, it is clear that the "nursing diagnosis" language is flawed. Yet some expansion of the definition of the scope of functions is needed. All nurses engage in acts of diagnosis and they should be allowed to do this without fear of legal action. States, such as California, which have expanded the definition without invoking the term "nursing diagnosis" seem to be on firmer legal grounds (California, 1974).

Probably the ideal nurse practice act would include an expanded scope of function for all nurses as well as special provisions for specialists including nurse practitioners, nurse midwives, nurse anesthetists, and clinical specialists. The differentiated scope of function for these specialists means that the nursing role is being restratified with the development of a specialty level and that specialty level is now being certified by the states.

The certification movement dates from about 1975 when regulations covering nurse practitioners started appearing. Then the states began collecting together existing laws and regulations for nurse midwives and anesthetists to cluster them with the practitioner provisions. In some states new laws covering anesthetists and midwives were written. Recently in a few states clinical specialists have been added to the list of certified nurses. Table 26–1 shows the current pattern of certification in the states.

The major objection to state certification comes from nurses who believe that the profession should certify advanced practice rather than the states. This is the model used by medicine. However, even that argument is defused by the fact that many of the states are using national certifying organizations as the testing bodies for state certification.

Since the American College of Nurse Midwives and the American Association of Nurse Anesthetists are the oldest accrediting bodies, states started by recognizing national certification by these groups as a criterion for state certification. However, more recently (since 1977) states have started recognizing certification of nurse practitioners by the American Nurses' Association (ANA), the National Board of Pediatric Nurse Practitioners and Associates (NAPNAP), or the Nurses' Association of the American College of Obstetricians and Gynecologists (NAACOG). In some states this certification by a national certifying body is an alternative to graduation from a state-accredited program; in others, certification by the national body is an additional requirement for state certification. The double requirement of an accredited program and national certification is the usual pattern for nurse anesthetists and nurse midwives; it is a beginning trend for nurse practitioners and clinical specialists.

Implications of the Certification Movement

The position paper promulgated by the American Nurses' Association in 1965 suggested that the two levels of registered nursing practice should be at the associate (technical) level and the baccalaureate (professional) level (ANA, 1965). That proposed dichotomy was never institutionalized in law and only occasionally in the practice setting. A careful examination of current practice acts and regulations suggests that it is time to lay that paper aside and look at what has actually developed. The current trend to certify specialists suggests that the advanced level of nursing practice is the specialty level rather than the baccalaureate degree. While many of today's nurse practitioners are graduates of short-term continuing education programs, the trend is in the direction of masters degree education for nurse practitioners as well as other specialists. Thus in terms of educational preparation the pattern which is emerging starts at 1 year for the practical nurse, includes a minimum of 2 years for the registered nurse, and moves on to the specialty level at 6 years. It would appear that from the point of view of the law the baccalaureate level is a way station on the path toward a nursing specialty rather than a major endpoint in and of itself.

Disciplinary Actions by Boards of Nursing

In spite of the pressure for change to accommodate an expanded scope of nursing practice, it is only occasionally that a state board of nursing will move to discipline a nurse who has violated the written scope of practice by allegedly stepping over into medicine's territory. Usually complaints about nurses exceeding their legal limits are handled with warnings rather than actual suspension or revocation of the nurse's license. The outstanding exception to this generalization occurred in the 1977 action against an Idaho nurse, Jolene Tuma.

Tuma was a clinical instructor in a nursing school. She supervised students in the clinical setting. One morning in 1976 she and the student under her supervision were assigned the task of caring for a patient with chronic myelogenous leukemia. The pa-

Table 26–1 State certification of nursing specialties.[a]

	Nurse Practitioners		Midwives		Anesthetists		Clinical Specialists	
	State Cert.	National Cert.	State Cert.	National Cert.	State Cert.	National Cert.	State Cert.	National Cert.
Alabama	X		X	Mand.	X	Mand.		
Alaska	X	Recog.						
Arizona	X		X	Recog.				
Arkansas	X	Recog.						
California	X	Recog.	X	Recog.[b]	X	Mand.		
Colorado	X	Recog.	X	Mand.				
Delaware	X	Recog.	X	Mand.				
Florida	X	Recog.	X	Recog.	X	Recog.	X	Recog.
Georgia	X	Mand.	X	Mand.	X	Mand.		
Hawaii	X	Recog.	X	Mand.	X	Mand.	X	Recog.
Idaho	X		X	Mand.	X	Mand.	X	
Iowa	X	[c]		[c]		[c]	X	[c]
Kansas[d]	X	Recog.	X	Mand.				
Kentucky	X	Mand.	X	Mand.	X	Mand.		
Louisiana	X	Recog.	X	Mand.	X	Mand.	X	
Maine	X		X		X			
Maryland	X		X	Mand.				
Massachusetts	X	Mand.	X	Mand.	X	Mand.	X	Mand.
Michigan	X	Mand.	X	Mand.	X	Mand.		
Mississippi	X	Mand.	X	Mand.	X	Mand.		
Montana			X	Mand.				
Nebraska	X	[c]			X	Recog.	X	
Nevada	X	Mand.[e]						

New Hampshire		X	Mand.		
New Mexico		X	Mand.		Mand.
North Carolina	Mand.	X	Mand.		
North Dakota	Mand.	X	Mand.	X	Mand.
Oklahoma	Mand.	X	Mand.	X	
Oregon		X	b		
Pennsylvania		X	Mand.	X	
South Carolina		X	Mand.		
South Dakota		X	d		
Texas	Mand.	X	Mand.	X	Mand.
Utah	Recog.	X	Mand.	X	
Virginia	Mand.	X	Mand.	X	
Washington	Mand.	X	Mand.		Mand.
West Virginia	Recog.	X	Recog.	X	Mand.
Wisconsin		X	c		
District of Columbia		X			
Virgin Islands		X			

[a] The following states and territories are omitted from the table because they do not certify any advanced level of nursing practice: Connecticut, Illinois, Indiana, Minnesota, Missouri, New Jersey, New York, Ohio, Rhode Island, Tennessee, Vermont, Wyoming, Guam, and Puerto Rico.

[b] State gives its own midwifery exam.

[c] Regulations not yet available.

[d] The certification law in Kansas has been declared unconstitutional so it is not operative.

[e] Recognizes only the ANA examination.

"Mand." indicates that national certification is mandated for state certification. "Recog." indicates that national certification is recognized as one option for demonstrating competence in the field. An educational program of a given length or a continuing education requirement is the usual other option. Where the certification column is blank there is no requirement for or recognition of national certification.

tient had been informed the night before that her prognosis was very grave and that she would need to go through a course of chemotherapy. Her physician had also warned her about the serious side effects of the drugs, including hair loss, infections, and ulcers of the mucous membranes.

During the morning care process the patient expressed her distress and indicated doubts about having given consent for the chemotherapy. Tuma listened to her, answered questions, and encouraged the patient to tell about past coping mechanisms including religion and dietary regimes. Tuma supported her interest in alternatives to the chemotherapy and the two discussed a plan of action. The patient was so pleased that she asked Tuma to return that evening to discuss the nontraditional alternatives with the patient's family.

Obviously Tuma had some doubts about her actions because she confided in the student that what she was doing was illegal and she did not notify the physician of her intended action. The family did, however, notify the doctor. He took no steps to stop Tuma but told them to get her name. He discontinued the intravenous chemotherapy at 8:00 P.M. because of the patient's wishes to explore other alternatives. The conversation took place. It included a discussion of laetrile and even the possibility of the patient's signing herself out of the hospital. However, after all of these possibilities were discussed in depth the patient and her family decided she would go ahead with the chemotherapy. It was therefore restarted at 9:30 P.M. so the delay was negligible. The patient did indeed develop the severe side effects she had feared, including ulcers in her mouth, but by that time she was moribund. She died 2 weeks after the incident.

The hospital reported Tuma to the Idaho Board of Nursing. She was charged with unprofessional conduct on the grounds that she had interfered with the doctor-patient relationship. Her license was suspended by a hearing officer who was acting for the board. When the case was appealed through the judicial process the courts reversed the decision because the Idaho State Nurse Practice Act does not spell out interfering with a physician-patient relationship as unprofessional conduct. The court also held that the hearing officer had exceeded his power (Tuma, Hearings and Briefs, 1976, 1977).

The case is a complex one. Tuma can certainly be faulted for not communicating her plans to the physician and most readers will question her support for laetrile, yet her actions alternatively can be conceptualized as support of the patient's wishes rather than for laetrile. There is no clear right and wrong in this case. It is also interesting that the courts were less willing to punish her for her independent actions than the Board of Nursing.

Other Implications of Violations of Scope of Function Statements

Violation of the provisions of the nurse practice acts can on occasion be contributory factors in a civil law suit. This was demonstrated by the Washington case of *Barber* v *Reiking* (1966). This case focused on a practical nurse who was employed in a physician's office. She was giving an injection to a child when a needle broke off in his buttock. Surgical removal was difficult and was not accomplished for 9 months. The family sued both the physician and the nurse and after a lengthy court battle both were found negligent because the mandatory nurse practice act of the State of Washington at that time reserved injections to registered nurses (Creighton, 1975).

Other Disciplinary Functions of Boards

While scope-of-function problems are interesting, they are not a major problem for boards of nursing. Most licenses are suspended or revoked for other reasons. Each state lists the grounds for disciplinary action. In some states the grounds are specific to nursing, while in others they are more general and apply to all professions. Iowa uses this general format and indicates that the license to practice a profession shall be revoked or suspended when the licensee is found guilty of any of the following offenses:

1. Fraud in procuring a license.
2. Professional incompetency.
3. Knowingly making misleading, deceptive, untrue, or fraudulent representations in the practice of a profession or engaging in unethical conduct or practice harmful or detrimental to the public. Proof of actual injury need not be established.
4. Habitual intoxication or addiction to the use of drugs.
5. Conviction of a felony related to the profession or occupation of the licensee or the conviction of any felony that would affect his or her ability to practice within a profession. A copy of the record of conviction or plea of guilty shall be conclusive evidence.

6.   Fraud in representations as to skill or ability.
7.   Use of untruthful or improbable statements in advertisements.
8.   Willful or repeated violations of the provisions of this act (Law of Iowa, 1980).

The Iowa list is of fairly recent vintage and is therefore more specific than some of the earlier lists that included such phrases as "unprofessional conduct." It also includes professional incompetence as a grounds for revocation. Unfortunately, however, incompetence is difficult to prove so licenses are seldom threatened for this reason. The most common ground for discipline is narcotic addiction or alcoholism, and when the two are compared narcotic abuse is the more common ground for revocation. This is probably because narcotics are so readily available to nurses, yet the crime is easily detected because it usually involves falsifying the narcotic records and so the state can clearly prove its cases against nurse addicts. Alcoholic nurses buy their drinks outside the hospital, so that their problem is less easily documented. While addiction and alcoholism would be victimless crimes under ordinary circumstances, in nurses they clearly impair the ability to give safe care and so have been ruled valid reasons for suspending or revoking licenses.

This emphasis means that incompetence, negligence, and/or other types of substandard nursing care usually go unpunished by the state. This situation has caused consumer discontent and that discontent is reflected in the increased number of malpractice suits. Certainly the consumer concern is more marked relative to medicine than nursing, but the trend to include nurses in malpractice suits is growing. This problem will be discussed in detail in the next chapter, which focuses on the relationship of nursing to the courts.

References

Adler, J. "You are charged with. . . " (Guest Editorial), *Nurse Practitioner* 4 (January/February 1979):6–7.
American Nurses' Association. *Educational Preparation for Nurse Practitioners and Assistants to Nurses.* 1955.
"A.N.A. Board Approves a Definition of Nursing Practice," *American Journal of Nursing* 55 (1965):1474.
Barber v. *Reiking,* Washing P 2d 861, 1966.

Bullough, B. "Alienation in the Ghetto." *American Journal of Sociology* 72 (March 1967):469–478.

Bullough, B. "The Law and the Expanding Nursing Role," *American Journal of Public Health* 66 (March 1976):249–252.

Bullough, B. (Ed.). *The Law and the Expanding Nursing Role,* 2nd Ed. New York: Appleton-Century-Crofts, 1980.

Bullough, B. "The Relationship of Nurse Practice Acts to the Professionalization of Nursing." In *The Nursing Profession: A Time to Speak,* edited by N. Chaska. Hightstown, N.J.: McGraw-Hill, 1982.

Bullough, V. L. "Licensure and the Medical Monopoly." In *The Law and the Expanding Nursing Role,* 2nd Ed., edited by B. Bullough. New York: Appleton-Century-Crofts, 1980, pp. 14–22.

California Business and Professions Code, Chap. 6, 1939, amended 1974.

Creighton, H. *Law Every Nurse Should Know,* 3rd Ed. Philadelphia: W. B. Saunders, 1975, p. 19.

Derbyshire, R. C. *Medical Licensure and Discipline in the United States.* Baltimore: Johns Hopkins University Press, 1969.

Editorial: "All Those Who Nurse for Hire!" *American Journal of Nursing* 39 (1939):275–277.

Fogotson, E. H., Roemer, R., Newman, R. W., and Cook, J. L. "Licensure of Other Medical Personnel," *Report of the National Advisory Commission on Health Manpower,* Vol. II. Washington, D.C.: U.S. Government Printing Office, 1967, pp. 407–492.

Idaho Code, Section 54-1413(e), 1971 revision.

Jacobson, M. "Nursing Laws and What Every Nurse Should Know About Them," *American Journal of Nursing* 40 (1940):1221–1226.

Law of Iowa 1980, Chap. 147.55.

Lesnick, M. J. and Anderson, B. E. *Legal Aspects of Nursing.* Philadelphia: J. B. Lippincott, 1947, p. 47.

New York State Education Law. Op Title 8, Article 130, Section 6901.

News: "Nurse Practitioners Fight Moves to Restrict Their Practice," *American Journal of Nursing* 78 (August 1978):1285, 1308, 1310.

Regional Review. *Nurse Practitioner* 3 (May/June 1978):6.

Tuma, J. L. B. v State of Idaho, Board of Nursing. Hearing, August 24, 1976.

Tuma, J. L. B. v Board of Nursing of the State of Idaho, Sup. Ct., No. 12587, 1977.

Tuma, J. L. B., Dist. Ct. Fifth Jud. Dist., State of Idaho, Brief No. 28732, 1977.

Tuma, J. L. B., Dist. Ct. Fifth Jud. Dist., State of Idaho, Reply Brief No. 28732, 1977.

Tuma, J. L. B., Dist. Ct. Fifth Jud. Dist., State of Idaho, Judgement No. 28732, 1977.

Tuma, J. L. B., Dist. Ct. Fifth Jud. Dist., State of Idaho, Brief (support of motion) No. 28732, 1977.

27.   Common Law as It Relates to Malpractice

Bonnie Bullough

Decision law, or common law as it is often called, is the older type of law. It originated with the English system or royal courts set up by Henry II in the twelfth century. It was called common law because all of the king's subjects fell under the decisions of the judges in the royal courts. The English system of looking to the precedents of decisions made in the past formed the basis for the decisions made by American judges in the colonial period. After the revolution the American body of decision law started developing as a separate entity, although the roots even today remain English.

American law, however, is unique because all laws, whether common or statutory, must conform to the Constitution of the United States. This is true not only of federal law but of state law since 1807, when the U.S. Supreme Court decided that state law in contravention of the Constitution was invalid even if it had been passed by the state legislature. Certain laws are more or less prohibited from being passed—namely, laws restricting freedom of religion, freedom of speech, and other freedoms mentioned in the Constitution and the Bill of Rights. The ultimate authority as to whether a given law contravenes these constitutional provisions is the U.S. Supreme Court.

In arriving at their decisions, judges rely on precedents, i.e., what has been decided before. The decision in one case will control the decision of like cases in the same court or in subordinate courts of the same jurisdiction. A lower court will not disregard a precedent by a higher court except in rare cases where the lower court concludes that the trend of other decisions by the higher court is such that it would overrule its own earlier decisions if again faced with the same legal problem. The Supreme Court does in fact sometimes change its opinion (Bullough, 1980).

Criminal and Civil Law

The two major divisions of law are criminal law and civil law. Criminal laws deal with crimes or offenses against the state; they are designed to protect all members of society from undesirable and detrimental forms of conduct. Murder, burglary, drug dealing, assault and battery, and other such actions are classified as crimes. Certainly, nurses can and do commit these crimes occasionally, even while on the job. Sometimes they do not even know they are committing a crime. This is particularly true of assault and battery. Assault is a threat to do bodily harm, while a battery is actual bodily harm. If a nurse threatened to carry out a procedure for which the patient did not give consent, it would be assault. If the procedure were actually carried out, it could be considered battery.

Most of the time, however, nurses are more concerned with civil law than criminal law. Civil law involves disputes between private persons, ranging from business contracts to divorce. An important concept in civil law is that known as torts. The term *tort* comes from the Latin word meaning twisted and involves a wrongful act resulting in an injury, loss, or damage, for which the injured party can bring civil action. The overriding objective of the tort law is to provide means for compensating those injured by the wrongful conduct of another. Its purpose is not so much to punish or penalize as to compensate the injured party. A nurse, for example, can be accused by a patient or the patient's heirs or family of negligence for failing to read the warning wrapper on a new drug or for wrongfully applying a restraining device. After a formal charge is made, the case goes to court, where a judge or jury renders a decision based on the evidence and awards appropriate damages. Since the assumption behind tort law is that someone is at fault, it is necessary to prove fault, although most of these cases involve negligence rather than an attempt to commit a deliberate wrong. Negligence in the medical and nursing field has been labeled malpractice, and so malpractice is one area of tort law (Bullough, 1980).

Proving Malpractice

In order to successfully prove malpractice the plaintiff who lodges the complaint must demonstrate that the following four conditions were present:

1. The defendant had a legal duty to the plaintiff.
2. That duty was breached, i.e., violated or not carried out.
3. Damage was caused by the defendant.
4. The plaintiff actually suffered damage (Viles, 1980; Hemelt and Mackert, 1978).

The standard for measuring the legal duty of the defendant is known as the "reasonable person" test. A nurse who is being sued is expected to function at the same level as a "reasonably prudent nurse" functions. If the nurse is an anesthetist or a clinical specialist, extra skills would be expected. Thus each level of professional is judged against peers. A reasonably prudent practical nurse is used as the standard for judging a practical nurse, a reasonably prudent registered nurse is used as the standard for a registered nurse, and a reasonably prudent nurse anesthetist is used as the standard for a nurse anesthetist. Usually expert witnesses are called to establish what is expected of a reasonably prudent nurse at the appropriate level. The expert witnesses are usually prestigious members of the profession who can describe the expectations for practice. This means that the standards change as the expectations for performance change and a prudent nurse in the 1980s may well be expected to know more than a nurse of the 1950s. Sometimes the testimony is buttressed by written standards of care including published documents such as the American Nurses' Association standards of care or the accreditation standards of the Joint Committee on the Accreditation of Hospitals. At other times less formal documents, such as a hospital job description, are used (Siedel, 1978; Holder, 1975).

Whether or not there was an actual breach of duty must be established by the plaintiff since the defendant is assumed innocent until it is demonstrated that he or she failed to carry out the assigned responsibilities. The hospital procedure manual and testimony of colleagues or expert witnesses can be used to establish this breach of duty.

Sometimes it is difficult to sort out who actually is liable for damage. Surgeons, for example, are ordinarily responsible for all operative negligence (Holder, pp. 207–210). If, however, a patient sues because a sponge allegedly was left in the operative wound, the court might well try to determine whether or not a sponge count was a common expectation in the hospital under question, whether sponge counts were common procedures in hospitals in the area, and whether or not a sponge count was carried out. If a sponge count had been done and the nursing staff had reported the missing sponge to the surgeon, they would not be negligent. If a sponge count was shown to be common practice and the nursing staff had failed to carry it out, they would be negligent. If the surgeon was the defendant, and nursing negligence could be shown, the surgeon might be able to use it as defense. Because the plaintiff seldom knows all of the details of the events which caused him or her harm before the suit is lodged, lawyers are now advising that all possible involved parties be named in the suit. This is one cause of the increased action against nurses.

Finally, the plaintiff must show actual harm. Errors in medication or other incidents which look negligent are not uncommon in health care settings, but if no harm follows, the incident is not a cause for legal action. The plaintiff must demonstrate that he has suffered harm in order to establish malpractice.

Who Is Legally Responsible for Nursing Negligence?

Since nurses are ordinarily employees rather than independent practitioners, the question arises as to who is legally responsible if the nurse is negligent. There is a legal doctrine called *respondeat superior* which means, "Let the master respond," or that the master is held accountable for actions of his servant. In more contemporary language this means that the employer is responsible for the actions of employees. This, however, is not always the case when nurses and hospitals are involved. Traditionally, for example, nonprofit hospitals could claim immunity from liability on the grounds that they were charitable institutions. It was assumed that they could not be expected to pay judgments for negligence because such payments would deplete their coffers, thereby threatening their continued existence. Not only was this principle well established in common law but many states had statutory laws spelling out charitable immunity.

A second defense used by hospitals was the doctrine of the borrowed servant. The first application of the borrowed servant concept to hospitals in the United States seems to have been the 1914 case of *Schloendorff v Society of New York Hospital.* In this case a distinction was made between the administrative tasks of hospital nurses and their delegated medical functions. This judgment made nurses responsible to the hospital for administrative tasks as servants of the hospital but considered them servants of the physician when they carried out medical tasks (*Schloendorff v. Society of New York Hospital,* 1914; Viles, 1980). Since the physician did not pay the hospital nursing staff, the nurses technically became borrowed servants. Sometimes this doctrine is termed the captain of the ship doctrine, a term which some nurses might prefer although it still makes the physician the captain. A 1950s example of the use of the doctrine occurred in a case involving a nurse who, in compliance with instructions from an obstetrician, applied pressure to the chest wall of a patient in the delivery room and cracked her ribs. The obstetrician was found, as captain of the ship, to be liable for the actions of the nurse. The hospital was not considered liable (*Minogue v Rutland Hospital,* 1956; Trandel-Korenchuk and Trandel-Korenchuk, 1982).

The effect of such a doctrine was to allow hospitals to conceptualize themselves as only offering hotel services for patients in order for physicians to carry out their work of healing. Obviously such an idea of hospitals had little correspondence with the reality of hospitalization. Moreover, while such a doctrine protected hospitals from liability, it downgraded the work of all nonphysician members of the health care team.

Several things happened to bring about change. One of the major reasons for change was the growth and extension of the insurance industry into various areas of liability. Thus all a charitable institution needed to do to protect itself was buy insurance, something that could be regarded as simply a cost of doing business. In addition, all kinds of charitable nonprofit groups sprang up to take advantage of the lack of legal liability. Consequently, legislatures repealed or altered state laws to allow limited liability for charitable institutions. Similarly, the federal government got into the act because traditionally federal and state hospitals were not liable for wrongs committed against their patients either. In 1945 the Federal Tort Claims Act was enacted allowing suits for negligence against such institutions (Creighton, 1980).

Courts do not operate in a vacuum, and as public perceptions changed, so did those of the court. The landmark case was *Bing v Thunig* in 1957, in which a hospital was held responsible for burns sustained by a patient as a result of a surgical prep performed by two hospital nurses (*Bing v Thunig,* 1957). In its ruling on this case the court explained that present day hospitals did more than furnish facilities for treatment, they also furnished treatment, a judgment which conformed more to the reality of what hospitals did than earlier ones.

In 1965 the Darling case went even further in establishing hospitals as liable for care given inside their walls. The plaintiff, who fractured his leg playing football, was taken to a local hospital where he was treated by a general practitioner with traction and a plaster cast. The cast was applied without stockinette or padding. It was also evidently too tight because the patient's toes became swollen, painful, and dark. When this was called to the physician's attention he ignored it for a time but eventually notched and split the cast. After this was done blood and foul-smelling drainage were noted by nursing staff. Eventually the patient was taken to another hospital where his leg was amputated. The hospital offered the traditional defenses—charitable immunity and borrowed servants—but these were rejected by the court. Written standards of care, including JCAH accreditation and state licensure standards, were used to establish the duty of the hospital and the hospital was cited for failing to meet these standards. It was considered negligent for not having required the attending general practitioner to consult with an orthopedic specialist.

The case also established a new duty for nurses, that of informing the hospital administration of any deviation from the norms of good physician care. The court held the hospital and its nurses negligent because there were not enough trained nurses capable of recognizing the gangrenous condition of the leg, the nurses did not test the circulation in the patient's foot frequently enough, they did not realize the developing symtoms were dangerous, and they did not call hospital authorities when the attending physician failed to act (*Darling v Charleston Community Hospital*, 1965; "The Darling Case," 1968; "The Darling Case Revisited," 1968; Murchinson and Nichols, 1970).

A more recent West Virginia case reiterated these findings. In this case the patient entered the hospital with a fractured wrist. During his hospital stay an infection developed; his arm became swollen, black, with a foul-smelling drainage. He became feverish, unable to retain oral antibiotics, and finally delirious. While he survived, his arm had to be amputated. The nursing staff reported these symptoms to the treating physician but he failed to act. The jury found, and the appellate court upheld the fact, that the hospital was negligent because the nurses did not report the failure of the attending physician to his department chairman.

The nursing procedure manual called for this further reporting, so that simply accepting the patient's deteriorating condition was considered negligent (*Utter v United Hospital Center*, 1977).

These cases expand the responsibilities of hospital staffs to include not only accountability for their own actions but also an added expectation that they will serve as patient advocates. Although this is still a beginning trend, it represents a radical change from past practices when physicians often carried the responsibility for their own actions plus those of hospital staffs.

The Malpractice Crisis

In spite of this trend, physicians still carry a heavier burden for malpractice claims than hospitals. The early 1970s were a time of a highly publicized malpractice crisis. The cost of physician malpractice insurance premiums escalated rapidly, and California doctors even went on strike to try to get the state government to come up with some solution to the problem. Some reforms were made to make insurance more available, and some hospitals started to take steps to improve patient care and hospital-patient relationships (American Hospital Association, 1980; Hogan, 1980). Yet when the closed-claims cases from 1975 to 1978 were reviewed by Curran he concluded that the problem was still significant. Dollar amounts awarded plaintiffs had continued to escalate; there were 23 awards of over one million dollars given in 1978. The majority of the claims were made by hospitalized patients, but attending physicians were still the primary defendants, paying indemnity in 71 percent of the claims, while hospitals paid in 25 percent of the cases and the nurses or other health professionals paid in 4 percent of the cases. Curran found, however, that juries continue to favor physician and hospital defendants in at least 80 percent of the cases. Curran argued that lay juries are not overly sympathetic to plaintiffs. Plaintiffs really have to prove malpractice to win judgments (Curran, 1981).

A study done by Campazzi focused on cases involving nurses. She examined all of the cases that had reached an appeal court during the decade from 1976 to 1977. Of the total 1,696 cases involving the health field, only 390 of the cases mentioned a nurse, nursing care, or nursing service. Emphasizing the time lag in legal actions, she noted that most cases had been filed 4 years before they reached the appeals level with a range between 1 and 25 years. The majority (88 percent) of the cases occurred in hospitals, 5 percent took place in nursing homes, 4 percent in psychiatric hospitals, and 3 percent in doctors' offices.

When she tabulated the defendants, she noted 390 first named defendants and 295 codefendants making a total of 685 defendants in 390 cases. Hospitals were defendants in 75 percent of the cases, physicians in 53 percent, insurance carriers in 11 percent, and nurses in 12 percent. Approximately half of the cases involving nurses were lost. In seven cases there was a judgment against a nurse ranging from $400 to $100,000.

In summarizing her findings, Campazzi noted a growing trend to name nurses in suits, although ordinarily hospitals or physicians were found liable for nursing negligence rather than nurses themselves. Problems in communication seemed to emerge as the basis for many suits, with patients and nurses not understanding each other or physicians and nurses failing to communicate. This was particularly true in emergency room cases when nurses would telephone physicians to report findings and physicians would give telephone orders. These situations not only led to litigation, they also resulted in fights in the courts between nurses and physicians about who said what. Surgical patients were often involved in suits because of infections, postoperative injuries, and foreign bodies left in operative wounds. Nurse anesthetists had a higher probability of suits than other nurses. Campazzi speculated that other specialists in the future may become the focus of suits like the anesthetists, although no case involving a nurse practitioner had reached the appellate level during the study period (Campazzi, 1980).

Since Campazzi's study there has been at least one major case involving a nurse practitioner (*Gugino v Harvard Community Health Plan et al.*, 1980). The patient had a Dalkon shield intrauterine device inserted in 1972. After reading an article about the dangers of these devices she called the health plan to which she belonged with concern. The physician indicated that he knew of no problems of infection involving the device. The patient did nothing until 1975 when she developed a foul vaginal odor. She called the health plan for an appointment but the nurse practitioner delayed seeing her and told her to douche with yogurt. A week later she developed intense pain and called again. The nurse practitioner told her she probably had a gastrointestinal flu and again failed to tell her to come in immediately. When the time of her appointment finally arrived she was found to have a severe infection with multiple abscesses and had to have a total hysterectomy. The plaintiff lost in the Medical Malpractice Tribunal but the case was overturned by the Supreme Judicial Court of Massachusetts and both the nurse practitioner and the physician were found to be negligent (Regan, 1980).

Avoiding Liability

What should nurses do to protect themselves and their employers from liability? The obvious major point to be made is that they should avoid negligence. The data show that juries are very prudent in their decisions; this is strong evidence that the major cause of negative outcomes of suits is negligence. This means that nurses must exercise caution in the care they give, checking medication labels carefully, calling for help when lifting heavy patients, and double-checking sponge counts. They should avoid working in an overtired condition or under the influence of drugs or alcohol.

A second point to be made is that nurses should take steps to keep their knowledge base up to date. They are judged on current standards of care, not the standard of care when they graduated, so course work and reading are needed to avoid negligence caused by ignorance.

A third observation is that careful charting or a system of incidence reports is clearly needed in situations where there is danger of a suit, including incidents when verbal orders are used, when there is conflict between the patient and nurse, or when there is a misunderstanding between other health professionals and the nurse. The lag time in law cases means that most participants in the events surrounding the case will have forgotten the details of what happened. An accurate written record is crucial.

Finally, nurses need to be more assertive when they see poor care being given. They need to complain about dangerous understaffing, or staffing with people who are poorly prepared. The precedent of the Darling case suggests that nurses should make sure that good care is given even if it involves conflict with a physician. Prudent hospital administrators will learn to appreciate this type of assertiveness on behalf of patients because it will save them money in malpractice suits and insurance premiums.

This raises one last question: Should nurses buy malpractice insurance? The answer is an equivocal one. Certainly nurse anesthetists should; perhaps other specialists should. Probably most other nurses started purchasing malpractice insurance several years too soon. The probability of a nurse being found liable is

still small considering the large number of working nurses. A nurse is much more likely to be sued for something involving an automobile than work. However, there is a small and growing danger of a judgment, and malpractice insurance for nurses is inexpensive. This small cost to insure peace of mind may not be unreasonable. Whether or not to buy malpractice insurance is a question that each nurse must consider. Hopefully the data presented here will be helpful in making that decision.

References

American Hospital Association, *Controlling Hospital Liability: A Systems Approach.* Chicago, 1980.

Bing v. Thunig, 143 N.E. 2d 3 (N.Y. 1957).

Bullough, V. "The Law: History and Basic Concepts." In *The Law and the Expanding Nursing Role,* edited by B. Bullough. New York: Appleton-Century-Crofts, 1980, pp. 3–19.

Campazzi, B. C. "Nurses, Nursing and Malpractice Litigation 1967–1977," *Nursing Administration Quarterly* 5 (Fall 1980):1–18.

Creighton, H. "Legal Aspects of Nosocomial Infection," *Nursing Clinics of North America* 15 (December 1980):789–801.

Curran, W. J. "Public Health and the Law: Closed-Claims Data for Malpractice Actions in the United States," *American Journal of Public Health* 71 (September 1981):1066–1067.

Darling v. Charleston Community Hospital, 200 N.E. 2d 145 (1964); 211 N.E. 2d 253 (Illinois, 1965).

"The Darling Case," *Journal of the American Medical Association* 206 (1968):1665.

"The Darling Case Revisited," *Journal of the American Medical Association* 206 (1968):1875.

Gugino v. Harvard Community Health Plan et al. 403 N.E. 2d 1166 (Mass., 1980).

Hemelt, M.D. and Mackert, M.E. *Dynamics of Law in Nursing and Health Care.* Reston, Va.: Reston, 1978.

Hogan, N.S. *Humanizing Health Care: Task of the Patient Representative.* Orodell, N.J.:Medical Economics Co., 1980.

Holder, A.R. *Medical Malpractice Law.* New York: John Wiley and Sons, 1975, pp. 40–43.

Minogue v. Rutland Hospital, 119 Vt. 336, 125 A 2d 796 (1956).

Murchison, I.A. and Nichols, T.S. *Legal Foundations of Nursing Practice.* New York: Macmillan, 1970.

Regan, W.A. "Nurse Practitioners and Professional Negligence," *Regan Report on Nursing Law* 21(3) (August 1980).

Schloendorff v. Society of New York Hospital, 105 N.E. 92 (N.Y. 1914).

Siedel, G.J., III. "Negligence." In *The Law of Hospital and Health Care*

Administration, edited by Arthur F. Southwick. Michigan: Health Administration Press, University of Michigan, 1978, pp. 114–128.

Trandel-Korenchuk, D. and Trandel-Korenchuk, K. "Borrowed Servant and Captain-of-the-Ship Doctrines," *Nurse Practitioner* 7 (February 1982):33–34.

Utter v. United Hospital Center, Incorporated, 236 S.E. 2d 213 (West Virginia, 1977).

Viles, S. M. "Liability for the Negligence of Hospital Nursing Personnel," *Nurse Administration Quarterly* 5 (Fall 1980):83–93.

28. A Nurse's Experience in Washington

Sister Rosemary Donley

In 1977–1978 Sister Rosemary Donley served as a Robert Wood Johnson Health Policy Fellow. She was the second nurse and the third woman to be chosen for this role. She spent the year learning about the legislative and administrative processes related to nursing and health care. The experience helped make her one of the outstanding authorities in the field of nursing legislation. Here she offers advice synthesized from her experience.

The Fellowship experience was rewarding. As time passed, I realized my opinions were respected and my political instincts were accurate. Was this to be explained by my Irish genes and childhood memories of the politics of Allegheny County? Did it have something to do with years in nursing?

The modern word *politics,* derived from an ancient Greek word for *city* or *state,* means the sharing of limited resources. Compromise and the sharing of resources are skills nurses use in practice. The political arena is an area where nurses will feel at home.

Donley, Sister Rosemary. "A Nurse's Experience in Washington." Reprinted with permission from *AORN Journal* 29 (June 1979):1279–1283. Copyrighted by the Association of Operating Room Nurses, Inc.

In asking you to locate your position in political action, my emphasis has been on movement from interest, to information, to involvement in the political process. Practice is a recognized way of developing and testing skill. Over the year, I thought about strategies, based on an insight into the democratic system. Simply, the good politician is always running for election. Name recognition and the development of constituencies around a variety of issues are important factors in winning an election. Using this principle, I suggest developing skills in the following areas.

1.   Become known by name to your representatives and senators. Develop personal and professional relationships with them and their staffs.

2.   Visit their district offices. If you are going to Washington, make plans to visit the office of your political association and the offices of your representatives and senators.

3.   Write brief notes to your congressmen. Someone, usually the staff person who has responsibility in the area, reads and answers the letters. Often the congressman is looking for a health issue. Your letter may focus his energy.

4.   Clarify your purpose and your communication. What do you want? (a) to acquaint the congressman with you and your interests? (b) to obtain information about or request a copy of a law, bill, or hearing report? (c) to express your concern and give a viewpoint about an issue that is being ignored or is before a committee of the House or Senate? (d) to ask your congressman to explore a question at a hearing? (e) to ask him to introduce an amendment or introduce a bill on a subject? (f) to ask for his vote on a particular issue? (g) to inform him of the impact that a bill or an issue would have on his constituents?

5.   In your communication, suggest positive approaches. Convey respect, information about the legislator's past record on the subject, and your sophistication about political realities.

6.   Identify yourself with the political action arm of your professional association. Invite the legislator or his representative to meetings where you can get publicity.

7.   Read the Washington commentaries from various points of view. Obtain the political commentary from your associations.

8.   Volunteer and help in election campaigns.

9.   Be patient. Politics, like love, takes time.

There is a classic stereotype of a politician. *He* smiles, kisses babies, smokes cigars, and shakes hands. Try to construct situations that are positive, and allow the legislator to do something for you. While in Washington, I learned something from the lobbyists. My favorite lobbyist would give us the position of his association; then he would smile and offer an option we would buy. By the time he had seen all the members and staffs of the Subcommittee on Health and the Environment, he had commitments for most of his package. The message is, play to win something.

A wise woman who represented a financially powerful lobby told me, "I never punish them when they vote against us. Anyone can make a mistake. Any bill is like a commuter train. There will be another one by in several hours." This good advice helped me gain perspective on how to deal with the congressmen and staffs.

I believe the key to effectiveness in the legislative process lies in the development of interpersonal relationships. In the Anglo-Saxon systems, laws develop out of experience, Cultivate a working and trusting relationship with your legislators and their staffs. Share your experience with them.

It is possible in Washington to have access to computerized information systems and to review abstracts of the literature. These are readily available to Congressmen and their staffs. Representatives need the local, human touch. Information about the impact of a program on a district or region, data to support the need for federal intervention, and facts that indicate government programs are being misused are politically vital. You can offer this.

I left Washington, DC, proud to be American. I respect the political process because, although it is somewhat chaotic, it is ultimately fair. I also realized the government needs me. I think it needs you, too.

Note

1. House Committee on Interstate and Foreign Commerce, *Compilation of Selected Acts within the Jurisdiction of the Committee on Interstate and Foreign Commerce* (Washington, DC: US Government Printing Office, Vol 1–4, 1977) 22.

29. Reimbursement for Nursing Services: Issues and Trends

Nancy Baker

Americans have long wanted a health care system that is accessible, comprehensive and affordable. Our failure to accomplish these goals has resulted in a resurgence of interest in national health insurance as a mechanism for increasing access, expanding the scope of services, and controlling costs.

Unfortunately, the health care industry (which is really a sick care industry) has fostered dependence on the two most expensive components of care: physician services and hospitalization. This situation has evolved from several historical themes, three of which threaten to perpetuate our inflationary system and prevent reimbursement for non-physicians:

1. failure to distinguish between medical care and health care
2. control of the industry by physicians and hospital administrators
3. lack of recognition for and undervaluing of the services of nurses

All of these factors have reduced the health options for consumers and have been demoralizing for nurses. This discussion will focus on various ways these issues impact upon the contributions nurses can make.

The first issue, **failure to distinguish between medical care and health care,** is a conceptual problem that has continually been reinforced by media, health service institutions and the existing benefit structure in the health care field. Medicine is one part of health care, but certainly not synonymous with it. The primary

Baker, N. "Reimbursement for Nursing Services: Issues and Trends." *Nursing Law and Ethics* 1 (April 1980):1, 2, 4. Reprinted with permission of the American Society of Law and Medicine, 765 Commonwealth Avenue, Boston, MA 02215.

focus of medical care is the diagnosis and treatment of disease entities. However, patients have other health needs that transcend medical diagnostic categories and fall within the nurse's scope of practice. A few examples of such areas are: patient teaching; psychosocial assessment, counseling and referral; health maintenance; illness prevention; and improvement of function in daily living. The nurse is the only health professional prepared to deliver this care in all types of settings.

Under most existing third party plans in the public and private sectors, nurses are not reimbursable care providers. Therefore, patients with nonmedical problems are financially limited in their access to other services because only physician care is covered by health insurance. In a system that overemphasizes medical problems, other health concerns of patients are often unidentified and untreated. For example, in my practice as a Family Nurse Practitioner in the nonacute Emergency Department of an urban hospital, I have become increasingly aware of patients' need for nursing care. Most of the clients that are triaged to the nonacute area do not need the services of a physician. Their problems usually involve the identification of a self-limiting illness, assessment of and referral for psychosocial concerns, need for health education and, sometimes, assistance in gaining entry into the health care system.

The second historical issue is **the power of physicians and hospital administrators to control access to and financing of health care services.**[1] This has increased the price of care by forcing the consumer to consult the most expensive health professional for all problems or be hospitalized in order to be reimbursed for some services. This control has even prompted the Federal Trade Commission to investigate the health insurance industry to determine if a conflict of interest exists.[2] (An amendment to the Federal Trade Commission Authorization Bill that would limit the Commission's authority to investigate the health care field was recently defeated in the United States Senate.)[3]

The limitation of reimbursement only to physicians results in an underutilization and inappropriate utilization of nurses. The physician "gatekeeper" role has been apparent in all practice arrangements. For example, nurses in "collaborative" practices must usually bill third party insurers for nursing services under the auspices of physicians. In other practice settings, such as the home, public health nursing services are reimbursable only if "ordered" by a doctor. This requirement increases the cost of care by assuming that patients are not capable of deciding for themselves when they need a nurse. Consulting the nurse directly would be much more economical and efficient.

The physician intermediary requirement and other obstacles caused by restrictive insurance and business corporation laws have generally limited nurses to employee status because they are unable to independently generate income. In states where the business corporation laws[4] exclude non-physicians from stock ownership in medical corporations these laws do more than hamper income. The exclusions have the additional effect of limiting nurses' power to control their own practices. This problem has been evident even in settings where the nursing components of care are particularly prominent such as Health Maintenance Organizations.

In addition to the negative effects of these requirements on consumers and nurses, the limitation of reimbursement to physicians is economically unsound. The enactment of any national health insurance plan will increase per capita patient visits. For example, the working poor are presently excluded from most private and public third party health insurance. Consequently, this group reports the lowest per capita number of visits to a health facility. One author has estimated that in New York City alone, health visits for the near-poor could be expected to increase by 2–3 million per year as a result of improved financial access to care under a comprehensive national health insurance program.[5] The system cannot afford to limit reimbursement to physicians for services that nurses can also perform, or to exclude nurses for their unique contributions.

Future cost containment through more prospective budgeting, particularly in hospital care, will be necessary to provide sufficient incentives for institutions to cut costs. In order to accomplish such a task, it will be necessary to provide improved financing mechanisms for home care and other nursing services such as preventive screening.

The third theme, **the undervaluing of nursing services,** relates to a broader problem in our society, that is, the socialization process that demeans the contributions of women. All women have had problems achieving status in our society, but "nursing is the most female sex stereotyped of all professions."[6]

The lack of recognition for the services rendered by nurses, coupled with the failure to achieve financial reimbursement under most health insurance plans, has greatly limited nurses' abilities to set up independent and collaborative practices and has also affected institutionally based nurses. Nurses in hospital practice have traditionally been undervalued and have suffered much economic discrimination. This situation has been well documented in a new book by Jo Ann Ashley entitled *Hospitals, Paternalism, and the Role of the Nurse.*[7]

The current practice of including the cost of nursing care under room rates has evolved from the nurse's historically low status in the hospital administrative and social hierarchy. This burying of the true monetary value and even identity of the nursing care rendered is not a sound fiscal practice. The lumping together of overhead costs, such as laundry service and nursing care, can provide the inefficient administrator with a mechanism for "covering costly and sometimes unjustifiable expenses."[8] This practice continues to limit nursing administrators' political clout by camouflaging the importance of their departments' services. One author, in pointing out the economic merits of prospective budgeting, states that all institutional rates must be determined by actual costs.[9] The itemization of care rendered to individuals in patient care hours should be the basis for the Nursing Department budget. This would promote the assignment of appropriate nurse-patient ratios in the hospital setting and would facilitate the appropriate recognition of the nursing components of care.

In addition, more complete identification and costing-out of nursing services could encourage more federal support for much-needed nursing research in such areas as the nurse's role in shortening hospitalization stays, in promoting improved self-care strategies, and in identifying methods to strengthen community nursing services.

Trends in Nursing Reimbursement Practices

Drastic changes in the financing of health care are needed to improve the quantity and quality of care and to broaden coverage to include more nursing services. This process has been accelerated by the emergence of better educated and politically assertive nurses. Moreover, the increased development of some areas in which nurses have always had great expertise, such as patient education, will no doubt be aided by the latest Surgeon General's Report, which has called for a "recasting" of the nation's health focus and more concentration on nursing areas.[10]

Federal Approaches

In 1972 the federal government amended the Social Security Act to allow for funding of several demonstration projects to study appropriate reimbursement mechanisms for nurse practitioners. Unfortunately, some of the resultant studies have primarily focused on methods to use nurses to expand physician practices and increase the delivery of "medical" services.

The practice of reimbursing nurses for "medical" services has created new problems for the profession. This approach not only continues to devalue the nursing role in primary care, but it inaccurately presents nurses as a type of physician extender. It places the nurse in the professionally unacceptable position of performing "medical" functions rather than "nursing" functions in order to be paid. These restrictions also require nurses to have "on site" physician consultation. This arrangement will never solve the current problems of geographic maldistribution of health care services.

Partially recognizing the limitations of this situation, Congress passed the Rural Health Clinics Act of 1977, which permits Medicare and Medicaid reimbursement for nurse practitioners for delivery of "medical" care but without "on site" physician consultation. However, there have been problems with implementation of this legislation due to restrictions in state nurse practice acts that forbid nurses to diagnose,[11] complex requirements for reporting, and resistance from local medical societies.

Another encouraging event has been the recent Congressional interest in extending health care benefits for Medicare recipients into some previously uncovered areas such as hospice care of the terminally ill. This type of care is primarily administered by nurses. Two amendments to the Medicare statutes that would extend these benefits are currently under review in the House of Representatives.[12]

Progress in institutional settings has been slow. However, Senator Edward Kennedy's (D. Mass) comprehensive health insurance proposal does recognize the need for change and calls for a delineation of nursing care costs in the hospital reimbursement formula.[13] This plan is a first step toward changing the professional and economic status of nurses in hospital practice.

State Approaches

A promising breakthrough has occurred in Maryland where the state legislature has recently passed two bills that mandate every health insurer to offer consumers the option of receiving care from a nurse practitioner or midwife.[14] These bills were sponsored by Marilyn Goldwater, a nurse, and widely supported by consumers and health professionals. The most significant aspect of this legislation is the fact that nurses are not required to practice "under the supervision" of physicians in order to be eligible for payment. The California Legislature has recently passed a bill that also demonstrates an increased recognition of the economic needs of professional nurses. It has amended the business corporation laws to allow nurses to hold up to 49 percent ownership in professional medical corporations.[15]

Conclusion

In the final analysis, legislation alone will not solve this country's health care problems. Everyone—patients *and* providers—must become more educated about the appropriate use of the system and wise utilization of different health care providers.

In the course of communicating about these issues with Congressional representatives, I have been dismayed by their continued view of nursing as a part of medicine and, also, by their lack of perspective about the underutilization of our skills. I believe that nurses have contributed to these impressions in our failure to standardize educational preparation at the baccalaureate level, our failure to develop sufficient peer review mechanisms for all types of practice, and in our reluctance to join collectively in addressing political issues that affect our profession.

It should be clear to nurses that for the profession to achieve more equitable status in the reimbursement system the present intermediaries' "gatekeeping" power must be challenged. To effect such a change, nurses must increase their political power. A group's influence can be enhanced by money, a high degree of internal unity, and individual members who are knowledgeable about issues and legislative process and can articulate their viewpoints to others. Obviously, the power of the American Nurses' Association would be increased if more nurses were members. It is also important that the state and national nurses' political action committees such as N-CAP (Nurses Coalition for Action in Politics) that can legally fund and endorse candidates be financially supported. In addition, more nurses must correspond with their legislators on the need for health care reimbursement reform. It is particularly imperative that nurses gain recognition as legitimate care providers before any national health insurance program is enacted. Otherwise, this country will never have a health care system that is affordable, comprehensive and universally accessible.

References

1. Welch, C. A., *Health Care Distribution and Third Party Payment for Nurses' Services.* American Journal of Nursing 75(10):1844 (October 1975).
2. *FTC Staff Recommends Termination of Physician Control over Blue Shield.* Behavior Today 10(20):1 (May 28, 1979).
3. McClure amendment to S. 1020, 96th Cong., 2nd Sess. (1980).
4. *See e.g.,* Article 15, New York State Business Corporation Law. (A unibill, sponsored by Senator Knorr is in Committee which would amend these regulations to allow nurses to own stock in medical corporations.)
5. Brecher, C., *et al., The Implications of National Health Insurance on Ambulatory Care Services in New York City,* Bulletin of the New York Academy of Medicine 53(2):193 (March 1977).
6. Cleland, V., *Sex Discrimination: Nursing's Most Pervasive Problem,* American Journal of Nursing 71(8):1542 (August 1971).
7. Ashley, J.A., Hospitals, Paternalism, and the Role of the Nurse. (Teachers College Press, New York) (1976).
8. Reimbursement for Nursing Services: A Position Statement of the Commission on Economic and General Welfare. (American Nurses' Association, Washington, D.C.) (1977) at 33.
9. Jennings, C.P. and T.F., *Containing Costs Through Prospective Reimbursement.* American Journal of Nursing 77(7):1159 (July 1977).
10. *Revolution in Health Care Urged in New Surgeon General's Report,* American Journal of Nursing 79(10):1671 (October 1979).
11. For example, the Attorney General of Missouri issued an opinion on January 2, 1980 that R.N.s cannot perform all of the duties outlined in the Rural Health Clinics Act, 42 U.S.C. § 1395, *as amended by* Rural Health Clinic Services Act, Pub. L. No. 95-210, 91 Stat 1485.
12. H.R. 3990, 96th Cong., 1st Sess. (1979) and H.R. 4000, 96th Cong., 1st Sess. (1979).
13. ANA Views the Current Proposals for National Health Insurance. (American Nurses' Association, Unpublished Report) (Revised October 1979).

14. *Maryland Assembly Approves Law for NP Reimbursement,* The American Nurse 11(5):3 (May 20, 1979).
15. *California Law Lets Nurses Share in Medical Corporations.* The American Nurse 11(8):1 (September 20, 1979).

30. Mandatory Continuing Education for Relicensure in Nursing: Issue of the Eighties?

Corinne T. Stuart

Should continuing education be mandated for relicensure? If it should be mandated, what factors should be considered when a compulsory continuing education law is passed? If mandatory continuing education is not the answer, how can the continued competence of nurses be assured?

Historical Perspective

Due to the growing public concern over professional obsolescence within the health professions, the National Advisory Commission on Health Manpower recommended in 1967 that professional associations and governmental regulatory agencies take immediate steps to establish systems 'designed to assist practitioners to maintain continuing competence (*Report of the National Advisory Commission,* 1967).

Again in 1971, the Department of Health, Education and Welfare's *Report on Licensure and Related Health Personnel Credentialing* cited professional obsolescence as a major basis for its recommendations that consideration be given to replacement of the present system of individual licensure with that of institutional licensure (U.S. Department of Health, Education and Welfare, 1971). Although the institutional licensure proposal never gained a significant following, it did serve as a stimulus to nurses to

search for alternative approaches to ensuring continued competence including, most notably, mandatory continuing education.

Existing Mandatory Continuing Education Laws

California in 1971 became the first state to pass a mandatory
continuing education law. Within the next 2 years Colorado, New
Mexico, New Hampshire, and South Dakota had followed suit
(Whitaker, 1974). A total of 18 states have now passed some sort
of continuing education statute although the focus in the states
varies. A summary of the existing laws is shown in Table 30–1. As
can be noted, 12 of the states have actually implemented requirements for registered nurses and 8 states have addressed additional requirements for nurse practitioners or other advanced clinicians including midwives. These additional requirements for
nurses in expanded roles are a more recent trend. Nebraska and
New Mexico have addressed the problem of inactive nurses returning to practice by writing mandatory educational requirements for them. Some states start out with just a small number of
hours and gradually increase the requirement, with 15 hours a
year being the eventual norm for registered nurses. The usual
attempt to provide quality assurance is to screen providers of the
programs.

Regulations in some states lessen the mandatory effect of the
statute. Exemptions have been promised for (1) persons living
outside the country for one year or longer, (2) absence from the
state due to military or missionary service for one year or longer,
and (3) unusual circumstances, poor health (require proof of
claim) (Waddle, 1980).

A Slowing Trend

In spite of the rapid spread of the idea of mandatory continuing
education during the decade of the 1970s there is definitely now a
hold on pushing the idea among the majority of state nurses'
associations. For example, in 1972 the New York State Nurses
Association established a Council on Continuing Education and
charged the group with responsibility for collection and dissemi-
nation of information concerning continuing education experiences and programs; the establishment of criteria for approving
continuing education experiences and programs; the review and
approval of continuing education experiences and programs; and

Table 30-1 State continuing education laws.

State	Starting Date	Providers Approved	Requirements for All RNs	Requirements for Certain Nurses
Alaska	1980	—	—	ARNP, 30 hr/2 yr or meet national certifying body's CE requirements
California	1978	Yes	30 hr/2 yr	—
Colorado	Not yet implemented	—	20 hr/2 yr	—
Florida	1981	Yes	30 hr/2 yr	ARNP, 15 hr/yr (can fill both requirements with same courses)
Idaho	1981	—	—	Nurse practitioners only, 60 hr/2 yr (includes midwives)
Iowa	1979	Yes	15 hr/yr	—
Kansas	1979	Yes	1979–80, 5 hr 1980–82, 15 hr 1982–on, 30 hr/2 yr	—
Kentucky	1981	Yes	1981, 5 hr 1983, 10 hr Each year after, 15 hr	—
Louisiana	Not yet implemented	—		—
Massachusetts	1982	Yes	1982, 5 hr/2 yr 1984, 10 hr/2 yr 1986, 15 hr/2 yr	—

State	Year		Proof of competency / CE one measure		
Michigan	1984	—	Proof of competency / CE one measure	—	
Minnesota	1980	—	1980, 15 hr/2 yr 1982, 30 hr/2 yr	—	
Mississippi					Nurse practitioners, 4 units/2 yr Midwives, hr not specified
Nebraska	1979	—	20 hr/5 yr		75 hr for nurses with less than 200 hr practice in last 5 yr
Nevada	1980	—	30 hr/2 yr		—
New Hampshire	1978	—	—		ARNP, hours not specified
New Mexico	1981	—	1981, 20 hr/2 yr 1983, 30 hr/2 yr		Refresher course for those not practicing for 5 yr
Oregon	1981	—	—		Nurse practitioners, 100 hr/2 yr Nurse practitioners, 100 hr/2 yr Nurse practitioners, 240 hr if inactive for 2 yr plus 25 hr pharmacology for nurse practitioners who prescribe
Washington	1981	—	Not yet implemented		Nurse practitioners who prescribe, 8 hr pharmacology

the collaboration with the State Education Department in developing and maintaining a system for validation of participation in continuing education experiences and programs (Driscoll, 1973).

A plan with specifications as to number of hours required every 2 years, appropriate fee schedules, approval control of programs, etc., was carefully designed. However, a decade later no law has been enacted and there are no serious efforts on the part of the association to sponsor one. This theme seems to be a recurrent one of late. State nurses' associations have either not introduced bills or when bills have been introduced state legislatures have turned them down. One of the reasons for such decisions has been the belief that increased health-care costs would result from the legislation of continuing education (Waddle, 1980).

Similarly, boards of nursing are questioning a mandatory continuing education requirement for relicensure. As can be noted in the table, the boards of nursing in Colorado, Louisiana, and Washington have delayed implementation of continuing education laws. The Colorado board was forced to take this action because the legislature did not approve implementation. In Florida a sunset review process failed to rescind the law but required that the rule-making process be carried out again. The California law has always been controversial. When it was first passed in 1971 it called for 30 contact hours a year. That law was repealed before it was implemented and the current substitute requirement for 30 hours every 2 years was passed. Again in 1981, members of the Board of Registered Nursing called for repeal, partly because they found the task of controlling the cost and quality of the offerings to be almost impossible. The law survived that call for repeal but it remains controversial.

The fact that the trend is slowing facilitates a careful reexamination of the arguments for and against mandatory continuing education.

Arguments in Support of Mandatory Continuing Education

As the health care delivery system becomes more complex the knowledge base needed to deliver good nursing care increases. The nurse who does not keep up with new equipment, new procedures, and new developments in nursing can be a danger to patients. Patient welfare, and sometimes even patient survival, are dependent on nurses' up-to-date knowledge. Consequently, continued competence is not just an individual professional concern; it is a public concern. For this reason various authorities had proposed reexamination for relicensure of key health professionals. This idea was, however, abandoned because of the expense and the fear on the part of professionals that they could not pass a general examination because they had concentrated their efforts to learn in specialized fields of practice. Because of these difficulties, documented continuing education was advocated as a substitute for retesting.

Although there has not been much empirical research about the actual outcomes of the continuing education movement, the studies that have been done are positive. Nurses who have worked in a state with mandatory continuing education tend to be supportive of the idea. In a dissertation finished in 1979, Pituch found that California nurses, who were forced to take courses for relicensure, were more supportive of such a practice than nurses in Michigan, who had a voluntary continuing education program at the time (Pituch, 1981).

Although the literature reveals little attention to monitoring postprogram outcomes in the clinical setting, an attempt to do just this was the purpose of an impact evaluation study done by the University of Iowa College of Nursing. The Iowa State Department of Health, Personal and Family Health Division was specifically concerned about the needs of registered nurses currently involved in county-community health providing maternal child health care. The nurses had been in maternal child health services for an extended period of time but had minimal opportunity for updating.

Impact evaluation as defined by Corbett is the evaluation of the impact of training on the problems and actual situations for which the training was prepared (Corbett, 1979). A course was designed to meet the identified learning needs of the practicing maternal child health nurses. It was conducted at four community sites covering each quadrant of the state of Iowa. Twelve 1-day sessions (meeting 1 day a week) were taught by faculty with expertise in the maternal child health area. Sixty-three nurses successfully completed the course. The funding covered a 15-month time frame.

A carefully devised interview survey was the evaluation tool. This same tool was used at the 2-month and 8-month evaluation following completion of the course. The nurse subjects as well as the nurse supervisors responded.

A comparison of nursing services before the maternal child health course and at 8 months following completion of the course depicted an improvement in practice with 50 percent or more of the enrollees in the following areas: prenatal classes, maternal child health counseling, hospital referrals, and conduct of Early Periodic Screening Diagnosis-Treatment. All subjects definitely showed an improvement in their level of self-confidence.

Other examples of achievement in this study are cited which indicate a high interest level in this specialty. One of the most positive indicators of success in the report of 70 percent of the supervisors was the observation of a more positive attitude toward maternal child health on the part of the program participants (Heick, 1981).

Arguments against Mandatory Continuing Education

Overlooking this study opponents of mandatory continuing education argue that there is as yet no definitive research findings that correlate continuing education with a change in nursing practice. They claim there are data to indicate that it increases the knowledge base of nurses, but there is no evidence to demonstrate that the practitioners change the way they practice nursing (Dodge, 1980). In other words, those nurses committed to currency in knowledge and updating of skills should not have a regulatory mandate imposed upon them just to force the few who do not respect this professional obligation (Dodge, 1980). If the nursing profession is theoretically committed to self-regulation, should the state then be asking for more rules to be imposed in a society already regulated to the point of intolerance?

Opposition to Mandatory Continuing Education

In 1972 mandatory continuing education was considered and rejected by the American Nurses House of Delegates. The ANA has subsequently supported voluntary, rather than mandatory, continuing education (Whitaker, 1974). However, the strongest note of concerned opposition is not from the ANA but from the American Hospital Association (AHA). They argue that there is little evidence to demonstrate that continuing education provides a safe practitioner. The AHA further believes it is the responsibility of a professional to keep his or her skills and knowledge current and that it is the health care institution's responsibility to evaluate and assure competence of its employees (AHA, 1979).

AHA Guidelines for Evaluating Proposals for Mandatory Continuing Education

In 1978, the AHA set forth guidelines to assist state legislators in evaluating proposals that mandate continuing education for licensed health care professionals. They define continuing education as "a planned series of activities that enables an individual to acquire skills, knowledge, and behavior needed to meet current job requirements or to remedy identified deficiencies" (AHA, 1979).

These guidelines cover three areas with specifics in each category. First, the AHA suggests that any proposal for mandatory continuing education legislation should include information on:

1. Current entry level practice standards as required by the licensure statute to indicate a minimal level of competency necessary to provide safe care.
2. Proposed plan and method of implementation.
3. Necessary resources for implementation of a mandatory continuing education system that is cost-effective as well as built-in evaluation measures specific to improved patient care and continued competence.
4. Plan to ensure the health care professional has met the mandatory continuing education requirements for renewal of license.

There should be a clear explanation of the problems and the specific nature of these problems that created the justification of mandatory continuing education. The AHA points out that job-specific problems related to changes in procedures, techniques, services, or assignments are responsibilities of the employer. Performance of patient care that is safe has been underscored by numerous court decisions that have held hospitals liable for negligence on the part of their employees that resulted in harm or injury to patients. The AHA argues that hospitals provide inservice education to maintain employee competence, and since a large percentage of health care professionals are employed by hospitals, it seems that mandatory continuing education would duplicate existing efforts and possibly dissipate limited resources.

The second list of questions addressed in the AHA guidelines concerns actual review of proposal content:

1. Are objectives clearly stated and specific to the identified problems?

2. Are data current on education and training needs, continuing education resources within the state, and geographic distribution of these resources?

3. What will be the cost to the state, the public, the professional, the employer, and the education system?

The third area deals with basic information on implementation of the structure and process. Therefore, the following questions should be addressed:

1. Is there opportunity for input at all stages by involved parties, including professionals, employers, professional associations, educational institutions, and regulatory agencies?

2. Who will be acting as the regulatory agency? If the state licensing board is to assume the task of mandatory continuing education, not only must added resources be allocated but the board should never appoint the concerned professional association (serving as a collective bargaining agent) as the approver of continuing education providers.

3. Is there flexibility to accommodate differences within the profession?

4. What are the requirements for the provider of the education? The AHA suggests the plan should include the provider's philosophy, descriptions of proposed offerings, objectives and anticipated outcomes, the intended audience, faculty credentials, sources of financial support, the record-keeping mechanism, and a valid method of evaluation (AHA, 1979).

5. What is the time cycle recommended for renewal of provider status?

6. Is there an appeals mechanism to ensure equity for both the professional and the provider of educational programs?

7. Is there an adequate phase-in period?

8. Is there a review process, and a termination or "sunset" date specified within the proposal?
9. Is there allowance for geographic mobility?

Professionals who apply for licensure by reciprocity or endorsement and individuals from foreign countries should be accommodated in this plan.

The intent of these guidelines by the AHA is to ensure a thorough examination of any proposal for mandatory continuing education. On completion of such a review, the substantive evidence should show whether the problem behind the statute request is a real one. It should ensure that the plan would be effective in the resolution of the problem and, lastly, it should identify the level of organizational and financial commitment necessary for successful implementation.

It is clear from these guidelines that the AHA considers mandatory continuing education to be a very complex issue. They hold that it is next to impossible to legislate learning and its subsequent application and argue that little evidence presently exists that continuing education in and of itself ensures continued competence. They continue to support and promote voluntary continuing education of health care professionals (AHA, 1979).

The AHA has considerable political "clout" and without a doubt has strongly influenced professional associations as well as the public and state legislative bodies to delay and actually oppose any measures supportive to mandatory continuing education for relicensure of nurses. This is not necessarily contrary to progress or efforts presently being made to ensure professional competence and safe practice in nursing.

Strategy for the Eighties

What, then, should the strategy be for mandatory continuing education in the 1980s? We cannot be oblivious to the economic climate and philosophical thinking of our present administration at the federal government level. The budget cuts and transfer of power to state governments may radically change our priorities. Nor can we ignore the present shortage of nurses as a critical concern of the health care delivery system.

One does not need a crystal ball to foresee the future of

mandatory continuing education for relicensure. I believe it will take a back seat! This will not necessarily be detrimental to maintaining professional competence. I am firmly convinced that continuing education for nurses on a voluntary basis is already a part of the philosophy and commitment of the truly professional nurse.

Strategies for success of voluntary participation in continuing education programs in nursing require:

1. Initiation of or continued effort in regional and/or state-wide planning
2. Efficient and effective use of higher educational resources to provide quality continuing education
3. Easy access to programs
4. Assessment of educational and practice needs of the nurse population
5. Establishment of data banks which would provide:
    a. Registration of statewide programs
    b. Dissemination of program information
    c. Library resource information:
        1. Computer retrieval system
            a. Need assessment-pretesting content areas
            b. Content learning units (audiovisual, programmed instruction, modular study)
            c. Posttesting evaluation
6. Use of telephone technology
    a. Establishment of or continued use of existing education telephone network systems (statewide)
    b. Dial access system (regional staff meeting, dissemination of emergency information) (Lutze, 1980)
7. Continuing education programs that allow for clinical practice and evaluation measures of performance
8. Research that will demonstrate the impact of continuing education on improvement of nursing care

Nursing fully recognizes that the nurse functioning within the confines of an institution or independently is liable for responsible, safe, and competent practice. Let us strive to provide continuing education programs that are of meaningful substantive content matched to the need of the practitioner. This commitment to excellence with some of the answers provided by research will enable the nursing profession to best serve the consumer of health care as well as maintain its own integrity.

References

American Hospital Association. "Landmark Statement: Consideration of Legislative Mandatory Continuing Education Proposals," *The Journal of Continuing Education in Nursing* (10)5 (1979):37–41.

Corbett, T. C. "Evaluations of Post-Implementation Strategies and Systems." In *The Evaluation of Continuing Education for Professionals: A Systems View*, edited by K. A. Murphy. Seattle: University of Washington, 1979, pp. 345–349.

Dodge, G. "Legislators Look Askance at Mandatory CE," *Association of Operating Room Nurses Journal* 31 (May 1980):1080–1091.

Driscoll, V. M. *Information and Guidelines for Approval of Continuing Education Programs and Experiences.* New York State Nurses Association Council on Continuing Education, 1973, pp. 1–2.

Heick, M. "Continuing Education Impact Evaluation," *Journal of Continuing Education in Nursing* 12(4) (1981):15–23.

Lutz, R. S. "The Telephone as a Teaching Medium," *Journal of Continuing Education in Nursing* 11(5) (1980):58–64.

Pituch, M. J. J. "Perceptions of Nurses Toward Mandatory Continuing Education" (Dissertation Abstract), *Journal of Continuing Education in Nursing* 12(2) (1981):15.

Report of the National Advisory Commission on Health Manpower, Vol. 1. Washington, D.C.: U.S. Government Printing Office, 1967.

U.S. Department of Health, Education and Welfare. *Report on Licensure and Related Health Personnel Credentialing.* Washington, D.C.: U.S. Government Printing Office, 1971, p. 60.

Waddle, F. I. "Trends in Mandatory Continuing Education," *Journal of Continuing Education in Nursing* 11(1) (1980):39–40.

Whitaker, J. G. "The Issue of Mandatory Continuing Education," *Nursing Clinics of North America* 9 (September 1974):475–483. Reprinted in *Expanding Horizons for Nurses*, edited by B. Bullough and V. Bullough. New York: Springer, 1977, pp. 178–187.

Index

Index

Accountability, 107, 171–172
  autonomy and, 115
  peer review, 115–127
Accreditation, *see* Certification of
  nurses
Acute care nurses, 134–135
  Adult education philosophy,
  236, 240–242
Advancement opportunity, 63
Advocacy, 107
Alcoholism among nurses, 93,
  289–290
Alverno College, 241
Ambulatory services, 171
American Academy of Nursing,
  173
American Association of Community and Junior Colleges, 213,
  225
American Association of Nurse
  Anesthetists (AANA), 160,
  162, 163–164, 165, 284
American College of Nurse Midwives, 284
American College of Surgeons, 162
American College Testing (ACT)
  Program, 244, 256–260
American Health Care Association, 213
American Hospital Association
  (AHA), 187, 215
  guidelines for evaluating proposals for mandatory continuing education, 318–319
American Medical Association
  (AMA), 162, 215, 279
American Nurses Association
  (ANA), 160, 161, 162, 199,
  280, 310–311, 318

accreditation system, 19–20, 284
  model definition of nursing, 281
  no-strike pledge, 8–9
  professional versus technical
    nursing, *see* ANA 1978 Resolutions; ANA 1985 Proposals
    representation in, 206
ANA Code for Nurses (1976)
  statement 1 of, 90–92
  statement 3 of, 92–94
  text of, 89–90
ANA 1965 position paper, 226–
  227, 256, 258, 285
ANA 1978 Resolutions, 184–188,
  197, 225
  Buckeye State Nurses Association position on, 197–203
ANA 1985 Proposals, 184–188,
  195–196, 205–215, 225
American Nursing Home Association, 213
American Society of Anesthesiologists (ASA), 163–164
American Vocational Association,
  214
ANA, *see* American Nurses Association (ANA)
Anesthesia, 156–164
Anesthesiologists versus nurse
  anesthetists, 156, 158–164
Articulation, 260–262. *See also* Career ladder
Assault, 293
Assessment programs, 236–238,
  240–244. *See also* Regents External Degree Nursing Programs (REDNP)
Assistant technical nurse, *see* Technical nursing

327

Certification of nurses, 171, 282,
285, 286–287. *See also* Licens-
ing of nurses; Nursing prac-
tice law
Civil law and nursing, 293
Clinical Anesthesia, 163
Clinical nurse specialists, 133–134,
136
certification of, 286–287
Code for nurses, *see* ANA Code
for Nurses
Collective bargaining, 8–9, 19, 20,
34
work satisfaction and, 67–68
College Level Examination Pro-
gram (CLEP) tests, 258–260
College Proficiency Examination
(CPE), 258–260, 263
College training for nurses, *see*
Associate degree programs;
Baccalaureate programs;
Education
Commission on Nontraditional
Study, 238
Common law
history of, 292
malpractice and, 292–301
Communication
definition of, 106
between nurses and physicians,
6–7
Community colleges, 183. *See also*
Associate degree programs
Competency-based education, 236,
240–242. *See also* Regents External Degree Nursing Programs (REDNP)
Competition in health care, role of
nursing in, 169–174
Consumer perception of nursing,
108–112
changing, 112–114
consumer, definition of,
105–106
nurses' perception of their services, 107–108

nurses' responsibilities to consumers, 107
Continuing education, mandatory,
312–323
AHA guidelines for evaluating
proposals for, 319–321
arguments against, 318
arguments in support of,
316–318
opposition to, 318–319
state laws, 313, 314–315 (tab.),
316
strategy for the eighties,
321–323
Conway, Shirl, 73
Costs of health care
and costs of nursing education,
207–208
nursing contribution to control
of, 24–25, 135, 169–174
Costs of nursing service, *see* Reimbursement of nursing care
Council of Baccalaureate and
Higher Degrees of the Na-
tional League for Nursing, 20,
184, 186, 225, 256–257
Council on Postsecondary Accreditation (COPA), 250
Crile, George, 159
Criminal law and nursing, 293
Curriculum, *see* Education

Darling versus *Charleston Community
Hospital,* 297
Defamation, 102–104
Definition of Nursing Practice
(1972), 191–192, 195
Delegated tasks, GMENAC Report
on, 145–147, 149–150, 152,
154
Demand for nurses, 15–16. *See
also* Shortage of nurses; Sur-
plus of nurses
Demography of nursing profes-
sion, 7–9
IOM 1981 Report, 14–15

Ned Lowry (character), 75
Negligence, ANA Code for Nurses
on, 92–94. *See also*
Malpractice
Nelson, Dagmar, 161
New Jersey Supreme Court, 91
New York Performance Assess-
ment Centers, 244, 246
New York Postgraduate Hospital,
New York City, 157
New York Regents External De-
gree Program (NYREDP),
183, 235, 238–239, 244, 246,
247, 251, 259, 263–264
New York State Nurses Associa-
tion, 184, 186, 187, 225, 313
New York State study on turnover
in nursing, 60–69
Nightingale, Florence, 3–5, 38, 181
Noonan, Barbara R., 135
No-strike pledge, 8–9
Nurse, 71, 83–84
Nurse administrators, 19
Nurse aided family care, 172
Nurse anesthetists, 132, 169
versus anesthesiologists, 156,
158–164
certification of, 286–287
development of specialty,
156–164
Nurse midwives, 132–133, 169
certification of, 286–287
GMENAC recommendations on,
145–147, 149–152
laws and regulations affecting,
146–147, 150
reimbursement of, 147, 151
substitution, 145–147, 149–150,
152
supply of, 145–146, 153
Nurse-patient relationship
consumer perception of,
108–112
ethics of, 95–101
See also Ethical relationship
models

Nurse practitioners, 134, 135–136,
138–139, 169, 228–231
certification of, 282–283, 284–
285, 286–287
GMENAC recommendations on,
145–147, 149–152
laws and regulations affecting,
146–147, 150, 152
reimbursement of, 147, 151
substitution, 145–147, 149–150,
152
supply of, 145–146, 153
The Nurses, 71–72
compared to analogous hospital
dramas, 76–77
impact on patient welfare,
78
inventory of nursing activities,
78–81
main characters, 72–74
personal attributes of nurse
characters, 81–83
supporting cast, 74–75
thematic orientation, 75–76
Nurses' aides, 28, 32
Nurses' Associated Alumnae of
United States and Canada,
280
Nurses' Association of the American College of Obstetricians
and Gynecologists (NAA-
COG), 284
Nurses Coalition for Action in Politics (N-CAP), 311
Nurse Training Act, 12
Nursing diagnosis versus medical
diagnosis, 283–284
Nursing education, *see* Education
Nursing practice law
civil law suits, 289
disciplinary actions by boards of
nursing, 285, 288–289
malpractice, 293–301
state nurse practice laws,
279–282
See also Licensing of nurses

SOUTHERN MISSIONARY COLLEGE
Division of Nursing Library
711 Lake Estelle Drive
Orlando, Florida 32803